SFIMMS SERIES IN NEUROMUSCULOSKELETAL MEDICINE

OSTEOPATHIC MANIPULATIVE MEDICINE APPROACHES TO THE PRIMARY RESPIRATORY MECHANISM

Harry D. Friedman, D.O.
Wolfgang G. Gilliar, D.O.
Jerel H. Glassman, D.O.

Published by SFIMMS Press

San Francisco International Manual Medicine Society

email: admin@sfimms.com
www.sfimms.com.

First Edition
Library of congress card catalog number 00-133447
ISBN 0-9701841-2-3

San Francisco International Manual Medicine Society

The San Francisco International Manual Medicine Society (SFIMMS) is an association of physicians and health professionals founded in 1995 to establish high educational standards and practice in the field of manual medicine.

The Society's courses are designed to provide health professionals with a strong foundation in manual medicine. The courses are offered at basic, intermediate and advanced levels with appropriate textbooks and course manuals provided. The educational format utilizes a variety of approaches including: Didactic Teaching, Step-By-Step Presentation, Hands-on Laboratory Sessions and Clinical Problem Solving.

These high quality educational programs facilitate the acquisition of palpatory skills and clinical problem solving approaches using a low student-teacher ratio in a direct, hands-on format.

Founding Members

Wolfgang G. Gilliar, DO (right)

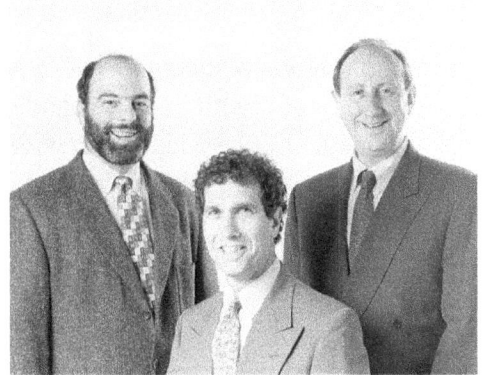

Dr. Gilliar is in private practice in San Mateo, CA. He is board certified in Physical Medicine and Rehabilitation, and Osteopathic Manipulative Medicine. He is an assistant clinical professor at Michigan State University College of Osteopathic Medicine. He is also the editor and co-author of many Manual Medicine texts and scientific papers. Dr. Gilliar lectures and teaches extensively at national and international meetings. His specific research interests include neurophysiologic processes in their application to manual medicine and exercise principles, as well as practice parameter development.

Harry D. Friedman, DO (left)

Dr Friedman is in private practice in Corte Madera, CA. He is board certified in Family Practice and Osteopathic Manipulative Medicine. He is an assistant clinical professor at Michigan State University College of Osteopathic Medicine and Touro University College of Osteopathic Medicine.

Dr. Friedman has participated in various research studies concerning uniform osteopathic documentation. He is the author of a chapter for the Foundations of Osteopathic Medicine textbook and has co-authored the text Functional Methods. Dr. Friedman lectures and teaches extensively in the US and abroad, and is one of the faculty developing manual medicine programs for the American Academy of Family Physicians.

Jerel H. Glassman, MPH, DO (middle)

Dr. Glassman is a staff physician at St. Mary's Spine Center in San Francisco, CA. He is board certified in Physical Medicine and Rehabilitation, and Osteopathic Manipulative Medicine, and is an assistant clinical professor at Michigan State University College of Osteopathic Medicine and Touro University College of Osteopathic Medicine. He is also a clinical instructor at Stanford University Medical School.

Dr. Glassman lectures frequently at many national meetings, including the American Academy of Physical Medicine and Rehabilitation, the American Back Society, the California Medical Association and American Osteopathic Association among others. Through his clinical and teaching activities he has pursued the integration of manual medicine into the multi-disciplinary rehabilitation model.

Foreward

The inspiration for this and the other books in the SFIMMS series in Neuromusculoskeletal Medicine came from our students and their desire for educational excellence. Quality instruction requires a level of clarity and correctness that reflects the subject's complexity but also allows for its comprehension on many different levels; conceptual, perceptual, and practical.

This material and the format in which it is presented have been developed to facilitate an understanding of Osteopathic Manipulative Medicine that encompasses its philosophy, science, and its practical clinical application. It is not the author's intention in writing this book to impart an Osteopathic education. Rather, we realize that such learning requires extensive study, supervision and clinical experience and cannot be acquired by simply reading this, or any other, book. We caution against the non-professional use of this book as it is intended as a textbook for Neuromusculoskeletal instruction in conjunction with a scientific education in the healing arts. Independent self-study of these approaches without the proper background and supervision is expressly against the authors' recommendation and wishes.

It is impossible to recognize every person who shared their knowledge and inspired our efforts. The community of practitioners expanding the limits of the cranial concept first articulated by W. G. Sutherland, D.O., are many. As with A.T. Still before him, Dr. Sutherland inspired a generation to seek and define the fundamental healing qualities of the life force itself. In our generation, we were inspired by, and are grateful to many, including: V. Frymann, D.O., F. Mitchell, Jr., D.O., R. Fulford, D.O., A. Becker, D.O., R. Becker, D.O., A. Chila, D.O., J. Upledger, D.O., H. Miller, D.O., J. Jealous, D.O., J. Barral, D.O. (UK), B. Briner, D.O., and P. Greeman D.O.

We want to especially thank Hollis King, D.O., and the Cranial Academy, for making the Academy bibliography available to be included in the text.

Finally, we wish to thank our wives, Denise, Barbara, and Beth for all their support, and Eric Shilland, for his computer and graphic assistance.

Contents

Level I: The Basics

Course Objectives	2
Osteopathic Philosophy and History of the Cranial Concept	3
Scientific Understanding of the Primary Respiratory Mechanism	4
Components of the Primary Respiratory Mechanism	10
Osteology of the Skull	11
Cranial Articulations	16
Meninges	17
Cranial Dura	18
Cerebrospinal Fluid Fluctuation	19
Inherent Motility of the CNS	20
Flexion and Extension of the Sphenoid and Occiput	21
Flexion and Extension of the Sacrum	23
Lumbosacral Decompression- Table Session	25
Intraosseous Sacral Lesions- Table Session	26
Individual Bones- Anatomy and Physiological Motion	27
Occiput	27
Sphenoid	28
Temporal	31
Parietal	35
Frontal	35
Ethmoid	36
Vomer	36
Frontal Lift- Table Session	38
Parietal Lift- Table Session	39
Temporal Bone Motion Testing and Decompression- Table Session	40
Direct Membranous Release- Table Session	42
Pelvis	42
Occipital Condyles	45
Home Occiput Release	47
Sphenobasilar Strain Patterns	48
Torsion Strains	49
Sidebending- Rotation Strains	50
Lateral Strains	52
Vertical Strains	53
Compression Strains	55
Treatment With Balanced Membranous Tension- Table Session	56
Fluid Wave	57
V-Spread and Fluid Wave Technique- Table Session	58
Temporal Bone Checkup- Table Session	59
Temporal Bone Balancing- Table Session	61
Treatment of Transverse Diaphragms: Body Molding and Balancing- Table Session	62
Pelvic Diaphragm	62
Thoracic Diaphragm	62
Thoracic Outlet	62
Transverse Cranial Diaphragm	62
Compression of the Fourth Ventricle- Table Session	64

Sequence of Treatment 66
Goals and Principles of Treatment 68
Psychological Aspects of Treatment 69
Cranial Exam Record 70
Finding the Area of Primary Restriction Using the CRI- Table Session 71
Two-Operator Technique- Table Session 74
Level I Course Schedule 76

Level II: Embryology, Newborns, Trauma, and the Rest of the Body

Course Objectives 82
Basic Course Review- Table Session 83
Osteopathic Approach to Infants 85
     Embryology 85
     Birth Mechanics 87
     Infant Anatomy 88
     Infant Evaluation 90
     Principles of Newborn Treatment 92
     Craniofascial Exam Record 93
Effects of Trauma on Breathing and Diaphragm Function 94
Breathing and Diaphragm Function- Table Session 95
     Shock Release Technique 95
     Rib Cage Release 96
     Anterior Diaphragm Release 97
     Sternum 99
     Clavicle 100
     Shoulder 101
Daily Supplemental Exercises 102
Technique to Bring the Three Diaphragms Into Phase- Table Session 105
Diagonal Vector Release- Table Session 107
Facial Trauma 108
Intraoral Techniques- Table Session 109
     Cruciate Suture 109
     Maxilla 110
     Palatine 112
     Zygoma 113
     Vomer 114
     Ethmoid (Fronto-maxillary) 115
     Sphenopalatine Ganglion 116
     Frontosphenoid Articulation 117
     Sphenosquamous Pivot 118
Orbital Techniques- Table Session 119
     Compression of the Fronto-nasal Articulation 120
     Compression of the Naso-maxillary Articulation 121
     The Orbit 122
     The Eyeball 123
Temporomandibular Joint Dysfunctions- Table Session 125
     Sphenomandibular Ligament 125
     Stylomandibular Ligament 126

Capsular Elements 127
Hyoid 127
Geometric Axes in the Cranium 128
Orbital/Auditory Axis Release of Tentorium Cerebelli- Table Session 129
Facial Bones- Sequence of Treatment 130
Venous Sinus Drainage Technique- Table Session 131
Two-Operator Technique- Table Session 136
Face Lift 136
Dural Stretch: Sacro-occipital Release 137
Level II Course Schedule 139

Level III: Harnessing the Fulcrum, Unleashing the Tide

Course Objectives 146
Fluid Matrix and Midline Function 147
Biodynamic vs. Biomechanical Approach 150
Palpating the Fluid Membrane Matrix and the Breath of Life- Table Session 151
Occipital Approach 151
Temporal Approach 152
Tidal Potency and Respiratory Function 153
Structural and Functional Midline 154
Intraosseous Motion and Membranous Function 155
Treatment Sequence for Harnessing the Fulcrum, Unleashing the Tide 156
Sacral Evaluation and Treatment- Table Session 157
Sacral Apex 157
Intraosseous Sacral Dysfunction 158
Thoracolumbar Junction 159
Sacrosternal Axis 160
Occipital Evaluation and Treatment- Table Session 161
Occipitocervical/Thoracic Junctions 161
Occipitoatlantal Junction 162
Occipitosternal Axis 163
Cranial Vault Evaluation and Treatment- Table Session 164
Inion/SBS 164
Bregma/Frontoparietal 165
AP Axis Evaluation and Treatment- Table Session 166
Bregma-Inion Axis 166
Nasion-Inion Axis 167
Four Quadrant Diagnosis and Treatment- Table Session 168
Venous Sinus Dural Technique- Table Session 170
Transverse venous sinus 170
Occipital Sinus 171
Straight Sinus 172
Superior Sagittal Sinus 173
Dural Ring Balancing- Table Session 174
Mandibular Rami 175
Maxillary Arches 176
Tentorium Cerebelli 177
Sphenoid 178

Two-Operator Technique- Table Session 179

    Dural Tube Release 179

    Occipital-Sternal-Sacral Release 180

Level III Course Schedule 181

Level IV: Osteopathic Approach to Infants and Children

Course Objectives 186

Embryonic Intelligence: Its Design and Function 187

Clinical Implications of Embryonic Intelligence 188

Maternal and Fetal Relationships 189

Osteopathic Manipulative Treatment of the Pregnant Mother- Table Session 190

    Fetal Release 190

    Thoracolumbar/Lumbosacral Junction Release 191

    Seated Hip Release 192

Osteopathic Manipulative Treatment of the Postpartum Mother- Table Session 193

Perinatal Health Promotion 194

Brain Growth Time Chart 195

Infant Brain Function 196

Functional Brain Stages 198

Developmental Checklist 199

Development of Neurological Organization 200

Neurological Organization and Patterning 201

Interventions to Enhance Sensory and Motor Integration

   in Relation to Movement Patterning- Table Session 203

Evaluation and Treatment of Compressed Sutures:

  Articular and Membranous Approaches- Table Session 204

    Pterion 205

    Asterion 205

    Coronal Suture 205

Osteopathic View of Health and Illness 206

Related Health Topics 207

    Nightime Parenting 207

    Upper Respiratory Congestion 207

    Asthma 207

    Learning and Emotional Disabilities 207

    Cerebral Palsy 208

    Downs Syndrome 208

    Visual Disturbances 209

    Upper Respiratory Tract and Ear Infections 209

Pediatric Ecology 210

Developmental Interfaces in Pediatric Ecology 212

Family Systems Assessment from an Osteopathic Perspective 213

Level IV Course Schedule 216

Osteopathic Clinical Problem Solving 219

Examination of the Adult Patient 220

Bibliography of Research Related to Cranial Osteopathy and

  Fetal and Infant Development 221

List of Figures

Figure 1: Connective Tissue Histology of Cranial Sutures 16

Figure 2: Intracranial Dural Membranes 17

Figure 3: Flexion/Extension Axes of Sphenoid and Occiput 19

Figure 4: The Skull in Extension 20

Figure 5: The Skull in Flexion 20

Figure 6: The Sacral Mechanism in Flexion 21

Figure 7: Extension of SBS and Sacrum 22

Figure 8: Flexion of SBS and Sacrum 22

Figure 9: Interrelated Motions of the Cranial Base Bones During Flexion 35

Figure 10: Torsion Right 47

Figure 11: Sidebending-Rotation Right 48

Figure 12: Lateral Strain Right 50

Figure 13: Vertical Strain Superior 51

Figure 14: Vertical Strain Inferior 51

Figure 15: SBS Stacking 54

Figure 16: Symmetric Orbital Axes 126

Figure 17: Distortion of Orbital Axes in Right Lateral Sphenobasilar Strain 126

Figure 18: Symmetric Petrous Axes 126

Figure 19: Distortion of Petrous Axes in Right Lateral Sphenobasilar Strain 126

Figure 20: Dural Venous Sinuses- Lateral View 130

Figure 21: Dural Venous Sinuses- Posterior View 130

Figure 22: The Motility of the Neural Tube 147

Figure 23: Directional Potency 151

Figure 24: Soft Potency 151

Figure 25: Depictions of Dural Ring Imbalances 172

Figure 26: Crawling Patterns 200

Figure 27: Creeping Patterns 200

Figure 28: Pediatric Ecology 209

List of Tables

Table 1: Foramina and Canals of the Cranium 13

Table 2: Jugular Foramen Contents 14

Table 3: Development of the Cranial Bones 15

Table 4: Overview of CNS Embryology: Theory and Function 86

Table 5: Birth History 91

Table 6: Developmental History 91

Table 7: Facial Bones Sequence of Treatment 131

Table 8: Difference Between Biodynamic and Traditional Biomechanical Approach 150

Table 9: Brain Growth Time Chart 195

Table 10: Infant Brain Function 196

Table 11: Functional Brain Stages 198

Table 12: Developmental Checklist (Modified Denver) 199

Table 13: Development of Neurological Organization (Brain Function)
in Children Without Significant Brain Injuries 200

Table 14: Examination of the Adult Patient 220

OSTEOPATHIC MANIPULATIVE MEDICINE APPROACHES TO THE PRIMARY RESPIRATORY MECHANISM

Level I
The Basics

OMM Approaches to the Primary Respiratory Mechanism

Level I
Course Objectives

Aquire an understanding of the five
components of the Primary Respiratory
Mechanism (*i.e.*, the cranial concept)
and their anatomic and physiologic basis

Demonstrate manual skills and
understanding of the principles of
craniosacral diagnosis

Demonstrate manual skills and understanding of
the principles of craniosacral treatment

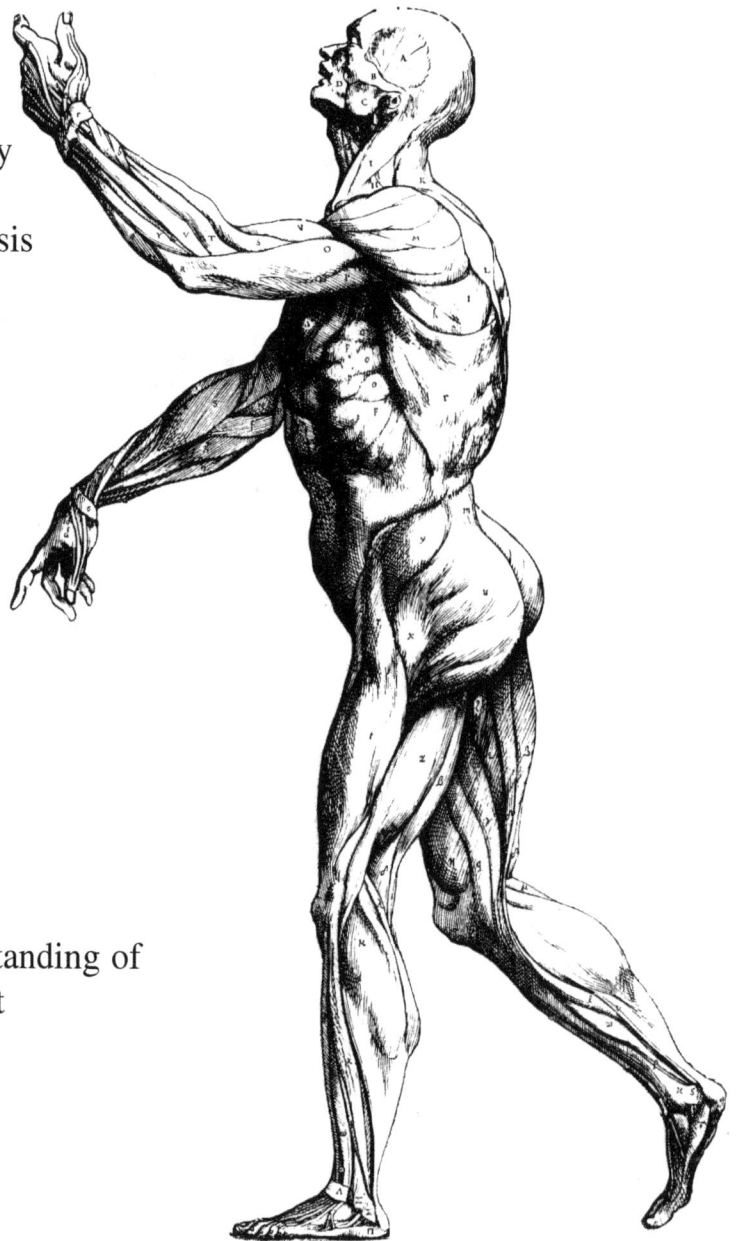

Osteopathic Philosophy and History of the Cranial Concept

The philosophical foundations of an osteopathic approach to patient care should be clearly understood before introducing the cranial concept. Osteopathic philosophy has always emphasized the somatic component in both health and illness. The efficiency and/or inefficiency of the living body, especially the musculoskeletal system and its integrating functions, are at the foundation of this philosophical framework.

Current medical thinking appears to be dominated by two common theories: one is the disease theory, the other is the external intervention theory. The prevailing standards of allopathic medicine are based on "disease" entities which can be described, named and classified into diagnostic categories and associated therapeutic measures. Within the context of this disease theory, current treatment of disease processes all share one basic assumption: externally controlled therapy is necessary for treatment of the pathology whether structural or functional.

Within the Western medical world there does exist a system of medicine that approaches pathology from a different perspective. Osteopathic medicine, while utilizing diagnostic labels and tests, as well as external agents for therapy, does not limit itself to the "disease" or "external intervention" theories in philosophy or in therapeutic technique. Dr. Andrew Taylor Still, the founder of osteopathy in post Civil War America, formulated three general principles that are fundamental to the osteopathic concept:

1. The inter-relationships between structure and function are reciprocal. Improved structure maximizes function, while increasing function improves structure.

2. The inherent healing capacity of the body cures all ailments. Dr. Still recognized that the human body manufactures all necessary substances for the maintenance and repairs of life, including responding correctly to external interventions. Osteopathic medicine aims to enhance the body's healing potential by optimizing the structure and function of its integrating functions.

3. The rule of the artery is supreme. In order to function efficiently, any body part must have a continuous arterial blood supply and proper venous and lymphatic drainage of waste products. To the degree that this blood supply or drainage mechanism is compromised dysfunction, pathology and disease are likely to begin.

Osteopathic treatment methods aim specifically to restore autonomic balance; increase arterial, venous, and lymphatic function; and relieve biomechanical stress patterns from myofascial and membranous tissues to optimize their mobile function.

The question that Dr. Still posed was relatively simple; "How does a physician stimulate this natural capacity of the body?" The answer to this question gave birth to osteopathic medicine whereby therapeutic alteration of the structural relationships in the musculoskeletal system might influence the internal workings of various body functions. "The job of the physician is to find health and give it motion, anyone can find disease." (A.T. Still.)

The Cranial Concept

The cranial concept was first conceived by a medical student at the American School of Osteopathy in Kirksville, Missouri. In 1899, William Garner Sutherland was observing a disarticulated human skull when an idea came to him that he was unable to dismiss in spite of his standard anatomical training. He thought to himself that the beveled articular surfaces of the sphenosquamous area were "beveled like the gills of a fish indicating articular mobility for a respiratory mechanism." Finding it impossible to prove that the bones of the cranium did not move, Sutherland discovered that all the articular surfaces of the cranial bones were designed for movement; furthermore, that the articular configurations within the sutures were similar in every living human.

Dr. Sutherland hypothesized a "primary respiratory mechanism" consisting of the central and peripheral nervous system, the cerebrospinal fluid fluctuation, the intracranial and intraspinal membranes, the articular mobility of the cranial bones, and the involuntary mobility of the sacrum between the ilia. He stressed that the functional interdependence of these components of the primary respiratory mechanism determines the efficiency of the whole system.

This mobility between the cranial bones and between the sacrum and the ilia is not muscular in origin, but rather an involuntary movement that functions in concert with the mobility of the intracranial and intraspinal membranes. When this primary respiratory system is altered, homeostasis is disrupted and susceptibility to illness is increased. These alterations are manifested in the musculoskeletal system as a loss of motion; motion that is based in the osseous, fluid and soft tissues of the craniosacral mechanism.

Sutherland introduced craniosacral manipulation to the osteopathic profession in the 1930's and began teaching the principles by the 1940's. His courses typically extended for two weeks, the first week being all anatomy, and the second week mostly lectures about the cranial concept as Sutherland came to know it. Few techniques were taught during this "introductory" course.

Cranial manipulation adds significantly to the portion of the nervous system that can be influenced through manual medicine. Spinal manipulation addresses one-third of the central nervous system in the spinal cord, two-thirds of the autonomic nervous system in the sympathetic nerves, and two-thirds of the peripheral nervous system via the spinal nerves. Cranial manipulation adds two-thirds of the central nervous system in the brain, one-third of the autonomic nervous system through the parasympathetics, (in both the cranium and sacral regions), one-third of the peripheral nervous system in the cranial nerves and the nerves of special senses, additionally, it influences the neurochemical and neuro-endocrine processes occurring in the central nervous system.

Scientific Understanding of the Primary Respiratory Mechanism (PRM)

Current scientific understanding of the cranial mechanism has proposed a pressure-stat model that offers an explanation of cranial motility. In this model, the cerebrospinal fluid production by the choroid plexus is more rapid than the resorption of the cerebrospinal fluid by the arachnoid bodies. When an upper threshold of pressure is attained, a homeostatic mechanism stops production of the cerebrospinal fluid. When the intercranial pressure causes the suture to open to a specific dimension, a stretch reflex is activated that signals the ventricle system to stop production of cerebrospinal fluid. When the suture begins to compress, the intracranial cerebrospinal fluid pressure is reduced, and the brain is signaled to produce more cerebrospinal fluid. This relay system has been histologically confirmed by Dr. Ernest Retzlaff at Michigan State University. Dr. Retzlaff has traced single nerve axons extending from the sagittal suture through meningeal membranes to the wall of the third ventricle. A pulse waveform of cerebral spinal fluid has been shown intracranially and intraspinally. This has been observed repeatedly during the performance of a spinal tap with the subsequent observation of a pulsatile fluctuation of the cerebral spinal fluid in the manometer. Studies of the choroid plexuses show the transference of arterial pulsation to the cerebral spinal fluid (Bering, 1955). Blockage of the choroid may increase intracranial pressure. MR image studies show the mobility of the brain related to the arterial pulse wave, and this mobility influences the fluctuation of cerebral spinal fluid (Feinbegr, 1987). Additional research points to a rhythmic contraction of the oligodendroglial cells of the neuroglia as a possible cause of motility and/or fluctuation in the cerebral spinal fluid system.

Mobility Studies

Rhythmic motions of the human cranium have been detected by both physicians trained in osteopathic cranial manipulation, as well as scientists in other disciplines, who have described similar phenomena. Ruch and Fulton observed inherent automaticity in the neuronal activity of the vasomotor center; waves of changing pressure, slower and longer than those associated with respiration were observed, as were rhythms associated directly with both cardiac and respiratory rates. These changing pressure waves are termed Traube Herring phenomenon. Sears also postulated these longer waves originating in the respiratory center of the medulla through spinal respiratory motor neurons. Isolated central respiratory drive potentials (CRDP'S) were observed in his study. Among cranial osteopathic researchers, Dr. Frymann notes the similarities of these potentials to some of the cranial recordings in her studies. Dr. Frymann conducted a series of experiments in 1971 and 1978 designed to investigate the motion of the living cranium. An apparatus was constructed with the help of an electrical engineer to measure this motion and it is described in her 1971 article, "A Study of the Rhythmic Motions of the Living Cranium." Dr. Frymann's device measured signals from thoracic respiration, cardio-vascular pulse, and voluntary muscular activities, as well as the oscillatory motion of the cranial bones. Her experiments were done using force transducers attached to the suture and demonstrated cyclical wave formations on polygraphs independent of pulse and respiratory measurements in multiple subjects, both human and animal.

Motility studies on squirrel monkeys using two different measurements of transparietal motion also showed a cyclic cranial bone movement ranging from 5 to 7 cycles per minute and differing from cardiac and respiratory rates (Michael, 1975; St. Pierre, 1976). More recent studies of sagittal suture motion in cats showed rotary and translatory movement (Adams, 1992). The motion of bone was altered by externally applied force and by changes in intracranial pressure, which was manipulated by induced hypercapnia, intravenous norepinephrine, and injection of artificial cerebral spinal fluid into the lateral ventricle.

Although the amount of mobility in each of these studies has been small across a single suture, it appears that when aggregated with all the sutures in the skull, there is sufficient motion for the human hand to palpate. The palpable capability of the human hand was studied by using a clamshell device to simulate motion of the parietal bones computer-driven for rate and amplitude (Mitchell, 1978; Roppel, 1978). Skilled clinicians and untrained observers were asked to palpate the simulated internal and external rotational movement of the parietal bones and to report expansion, contraction, or nonmovement. Verbal reports of the blinded evaluators were compared with the computer program. These studies showed that accuracy of palpation related directly to the rate of motion and that decisional delay was related inversely. The perception threshold was found to be 0.5 to 0.25 mm per second. Trained and untrained evaluators showed similar performance.

Anatomic Studies

The sutures in animals and humans have been studied extensively (Magoun, 1966). Sutures in primates showed no sutural obliteration at any age (Kovich, 1976; Retzlaff, 1978,1979). Animal sutures showed ligaments with a consistent fiber organization and many free nerve endings. The waviness of Sharpey's fibers within the sutures appears to result from stretch applied during movement of the cranial bone (Retzlaff,1976).

Histologic Studies

Histological research has also been conducted on the structure of the cranial bone suture. In 1956, Pritchard investigated the development and structure of sutures in various animal models and in man. They found five intervening layers of cells and fibers between cranial articulations and two uniting layers of fibrous strata joining the inner and outer boundaries of the suture. This study inferred that sutures allow for expansion during bone growth and form a strong bond between articular surfaces that allows for slight movement. Retzlaff, in '76, confirmed these five layers of cells in the adult squirrel monkey and showed that there are three types of connective tissue found in the suture: collagenous, reticular and elastic. Collagen fibers are the most abundant connective tissue present in the suture. Bundles of collagen fiber, also known as Sharpey's fibers, penetrate the cranial bone and extend across sutures connecting one bone to the opposite bone. An arteriole and one or more non-myelinated nerve fibers accompany each Sharpey's fiber upon penetration of the cranial bone. The nerve fiber and arteriole enter the Haversian canal system and extend into the myeloid spaces. Sharpey's fibers are most numerous in areas where bones are subjected to the greatest separation forces. Thus, Sharpey's fiber bundles serve functionally as anchors for cranial bones, allowing firm, but moveable attachments between bones. A reticular type of connective tissue is seen in conjunction with the collagen bundles, they also penetrate the cranial bone and may serve as anchors for the Sharpey's fiber bundles of the bone. Elastic tissue is observed to criss-cross the collagen bundles, perhaps serving as a contractile mechanism. This sutural matrix is highly vascularized and possesses nerve fibers. Retzlaff hypothesizes that an autonomic nervous system reflex is mediated by these nerve fibers. This reflex is, in part, vasomotor and part sensory in function. Nonmyelinated autonomic fibers, innervating the arterioles in the dura and sutures, are thought to be neurosecretory in function and to control vascular constriction. Free-ending fiber types are found in all of the major vessels in the dura, in the suture, and in the walls of the third ventricle of the brain. Dr. Retzlaff and others suggest that these free-endings represent the origin of the dendrites, which are involved in sensation from the sutures, dura and in the walls of the third ventricle. Compression of the sutures may result in tissue ischemia and, in turn, ischemic conditions may lead to localized, as well as referred pain and alterations in the neurochemistry of the brain. (i.e. endorphins.) Alterations of brain chemistry have been shown to modulate pain perception, as well.

Interexaminer Reliability Studies

The earliest interrater reliability study was performed by Upledger in 1977. The principal investigator and one of three other cranial evaluators examined the same patient. They evaluated 24 characteristics of cranial motion, and a three-point scale was used for assessment of each motion. Normal and symptomatic patients were included. The interrater reliability averaged 0.87.

One of the authors of this text (Friedman) conducted two studies of multiple operators performing examinations of the cranial sacral system. The first study involved 24 subjects evaluated by six examiners using four different screening tests. A total of 96 comparisons were made, one for each test, on each patient (24 subjects x 4 tests = 96 comparisons). Results were tabulated based on the presence or absence of asymmetry (+ or - test) and the side of the restricted motion (L or R). For + or - test asymmetry, 87 of 96 test comparisons showed clear agreement between the six examiners (maximum one examiner disagreeing with the rest). 60 of 96 showed all examiners in agreement. 9 of 96 demonstrated lack of agreement between examiners. With respect to the side of restriction for each test, 63 of 96 comparisons showed a majority of examiners in agreement (four of six examiners).

In the second study, three patients were examined by nine operators using a single test for asymmetry. All three comparisons demonstrated complete agreement between the nine examiners for the presence of asymmetry, but examiners were split on the side of restriction. A clear majority of these test comparisons (25 of 27) agreed on improvement of the asymmetry after treatment was applied.

Clinical and Efficacy Studies

A study of 1250 infants with symptoms of vomiting, hyperactive peristalsis, tremor, hypertonicity, and hyperirritability were assessed for disturbances of the craniosacral mechanism (Frymann, 1966). With increased restriction of craniosacral strain patterns, there was increased prevalence of symptoms in this infant population.

In another study, 200 grade-school children were studied by craniosacral examination and a blinded psychological and educational test to examine the relationship of craniosacral dysfunctional findings in problems in childhood development (Upledger, 1978). The results showed a positive correlation of cranial motion restriction in the children who displayed multiple psychosocial and educational problems.

A study was made of the prevalence of cranial dysfunction in children with a history of otitis media (Degenhardt, 1992). As the number of cranial strain patterns increased, there was an increased incidence of otitis media in this population.

A 3-year study of children from 18 months to 12 years old with and without recognized neurologic deficits was made assessing their response to craniosacral manipulative treatment. Houle's profile of development was used to compare neurologic and chronologic age and rate of development, and scores were adjusted for age (Frymann, 1992). A comparison was made with children whose treatment was initiated promptly versus those whose treatment was delayed. The data supported the statistic significance of the use of craniosacral manipulative treatment in significantly improving the sensory performance of children with neurologic deficits.

This is only a brief overview of some of the research studies into the field of craniosacral manipulation. Much work needs to be performed, particularly efficacy studies and controlled clinical trials in patients with a variety of clinical presentations.

Clinical Applications

Dysfunction of the craniosacral mechanism can have a variety of symptoms. Dysfunction of the cranial base can have significant influence on the function of the 12 cranial nerves. They are all at risk for potential entrapment neuropathy. The major areas of potential problems include the area of the sphenoid and the apex of the temporal bone influencing the trigeminal ganglion and the cavernous sinus and its relationship to cranial nerves three, four, and six. Dysfunction in the region of the greater and lesser wings of the sphenoid and the apex of the temporal bone can profoundly influence orbital function and facial pain. A second area of major clinical significance involves dysfunction of the posterior quadrant articulations of the occiput and the temporal bone. The jugular foramen is found within a suture between these two bones. Through it run the ninth, tenth, and eleventh cranial nerves and the dural venous sinuses drain to the internal jugular vein. Restricted motion at this region can result in passive congestion within the skull and entrapment neuropathy of the associated ninth, tenth, and eleventh cranial nerves. Involvement of the vagus nerve can manifest in a myriad of internal organ symptoms of the viscera from the root of the neck to the midportion of the descending colon. The third major area of symptom production involves dysfunction of the temporal bone. It can influence the jugular foramen but also includes the auditory and vestibular portions of the eighth cranial nerve. Asymmetric imbalance of temporal bones is a frequent finding in patients with symptoms of dizziness and vertigo. The facial nerve traverses the temporal bone from the internal acoustic meatus to the facial canal, and temporal dysfunction is a common finding in the presentation of Bell's palsy. A dysfunctional temporal bone has been categorized as a major troublemaker (Magoun, 1974).

Because of the intimate relationship with all the cranial nerves, particularly the vagus, it is common for patients with significant craniosacral dysfunction to present with a myriad of multisystem symptoms. These patients frequently undergo extensive evaluation of the cardiovascular, pulmonary, gastrointestinal, and genitourinary systems to no avail. Unexplained respiratory problems, cardiac arrhythmias, indigestion, irritable bowel syndrome, urgency, and frequency are all common presenting complaints of patients with significant craniosacral problems.

Headache is another common presentation in this patient population. Headaches may manifest as classic occipital tension-type headache, to significant vascular components similar to classic migraine. Trigeminal neuralgia symptoms are common in patients with dysfunction of the front quadrants of the skull.

Temporomandibular joint syndromes commonly are associated with imbalance of the temporal bones and restriction of mobility of the face. Some have described the opposing surfaces of the upper and lower teeth as being one of the largest sutures found within the cranial system. Abnormal bite and poor dental care contribute to dysfunction of the face and temporomandibular joint with frequent alteration in muscular balance at the craniocervical junction. In addition to appropriate dental care, a patient with temporomandibular joint syndrome frequently will benefit from concurrent craniosacral treatment to balance the temporal side of the temporomandibular joint.

Individuals with traumatic brain injury (TBI) can present months after their trauma with a broad spectrum of continued complaints and findings. These include cognitive and perceptual deficits, impaired balance, dizziness and vertigo, motor weakness, coordination problems, and symptoms of autonomic dysfunction (Binder, 1986). Recently, a high incidence of somatic complaints also has been noted. Fifty-six percent of all patients with TBI and 89% of those with mild TBIs reported continued pain issues 6 or more months postinjury (Esselman, 1991). Headaches were the most frequent complaint followed by neck and shoulder pain. It is now recognized that many individuals with brain injury enter the medical system as patients with chronic pain (Anderson, 1990). Both these groups can manifest behaviors of impaired concentration, easy fatigability, depression, anxiety, and psychosocial adjustment issues.

Cranial findings in 55 patients with TBI revealed all had reduction in amplitude or rate of CRI. 95% of patients had sutural and bony restrictions of the cranial vault. 95% also had mobile strain patterns of the sphenobasilar synchondrosis (Greenman, 1996).

Contraindications and Complications

As subtle as this form of manual medicine may appear, it apparently is not innocuous. Three of the 55 patients (5%) treated in the Michigan State University TBI program experienced some form of iatrogenic reaction to the treatment (Greenman, 1995). These reactions included worsening of vertiginous symptoms with onset of cardiac, respiratory, and gastrointestinal visceral symptoms after treatment, increase in psychiatric symptoms involving anger with outbursts, paranoia and other ideations requiring hospitalization, and onset of significant opisthotonos or spasm of much of the body. This population is one that would be perceived as being at greatest risk for potential complications. Although this rate is low, it should alert all practitioners of craniosacral manipulation to be cautious. In a majority of the cases, the potential benefit exceeds any concern for potential complications.

Contraindications to craniosacral treatment include patients who present with acute, unstable neurologic signs, increased intracranial pressure, intracranial bleeding, and nonhealed fractures of the vault, cranial base, and upper cervical spine, particularly depressed fractures. Caution also must be used in patients with a history of seizure. Although not an absolute contraindication, seizure states should be managed with extreme caution.

Because of the intricate relationship of the craniosacral system with CNS function, it is common to have a patient experience some exacerbation of symptoms during the process of treatment. Each patient responds uniquely to craniosacral intervention, and unlike other forms of manual medicine treatment, it is more difficult to predict the patient's response to treatment intervention. A high degree of experience and clinical judgment are essential for the successful craniosacral practitioner.

Components of the Primary Respiratory Mechanism

1.   **The osseous articular mechanism** - anatomic design of the cranial bones by and for motion.

2.   **The reciprocal tension membrane**- the intracranial and intraspinous dural membranes.

3.   **The fluctuation of the cerebrospinal fluid** - NOTE: fluctuating rather than circulating.

4.   **The inherent motility of the central nervous system.**

5.   **The articular mobility of the sacrum between the ilia** - An involuntary motion around the transverse axis of the sacrum (located at the level of the second sacral segment).

Osteology of the Skull

There are twenty-nine bones in the adult skull:

A.   Eight in the cranial group, the occiput. sphenoid, ethmoid, and frontal, as well as the paired temporals and parietals.

B.   Fourteen in the facial group, the vomer and mandible, as well as the paired maxillae, palatines, zygomatics, lacrimals, nasals and inferior conchae.

C.   Seven in the miscellaneous group, the six ossicles of the internal ears, as well as the hyoid. These are only indirectly concerned in the cranial concept.

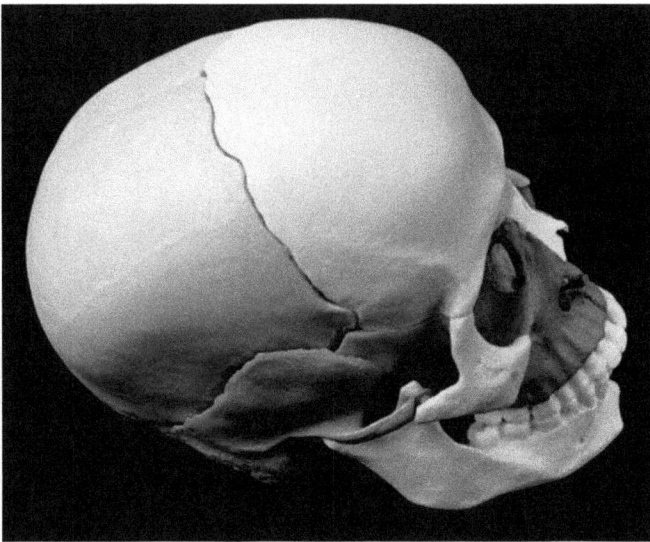

Superolateral View of Skull

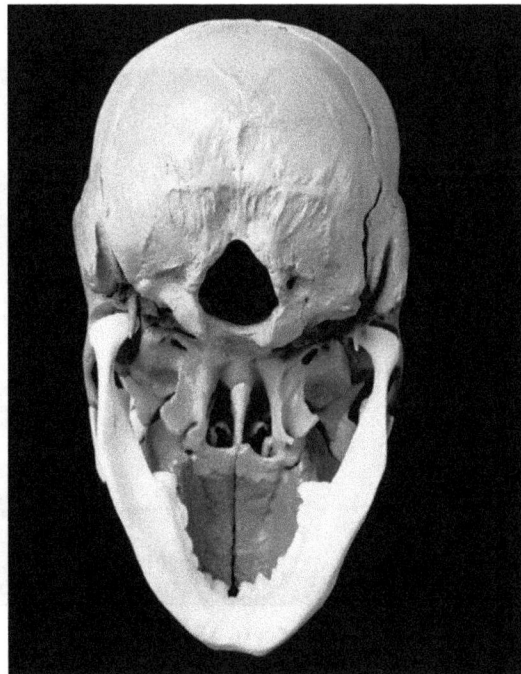

Inferior View of Skull

Most sutures are named for the two bones which approximate each other (e.g., temporoparietal, zygomaticomaxillary, etc.). One should <u>know</u> which bones articulate with each other. There are exceptions to the above named sutures. They are:

1. Metopic (Frontal-Frontal) present in 10% of adult skulls

2. Coronal (Frontal-Parietal)

3. Sagittal (Parietal-Parietal)

4. Squamosal (Parietal-Squamous Temporal)

5. Lambdoidal (Parietal-Occiput)

In addition there exist several important junctional areas within the skull. These are:

6. Bregma - Junction of coronal & sagittal sutures
   (area of Anterior Fontanel - closes at 18 mos.)

7. Lambda - Junction of sagittal & lambdoidal sutures
   (area of Posterior Fontanel - closes at 2 mos.)

8. Pterion - Junction of frontal, parietal, sphenoid & temporal bones.
   These four bones overlap each other- in alphabetical order from within outward.
   (area of anterior-lateral Fontanel - closes at 2 mos.)

9. Asterion - Junction of temporal, parietal & occipital bones
   (area of posterior-lateral Fontanel - closes at 2 mos.)

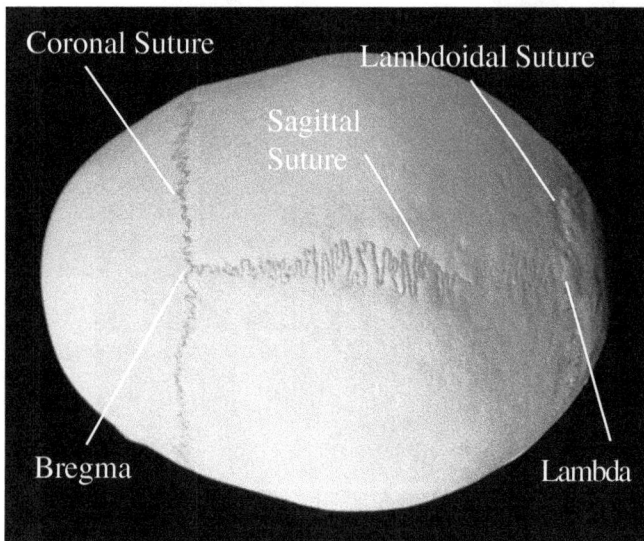

Superior View of Cranial Sutures

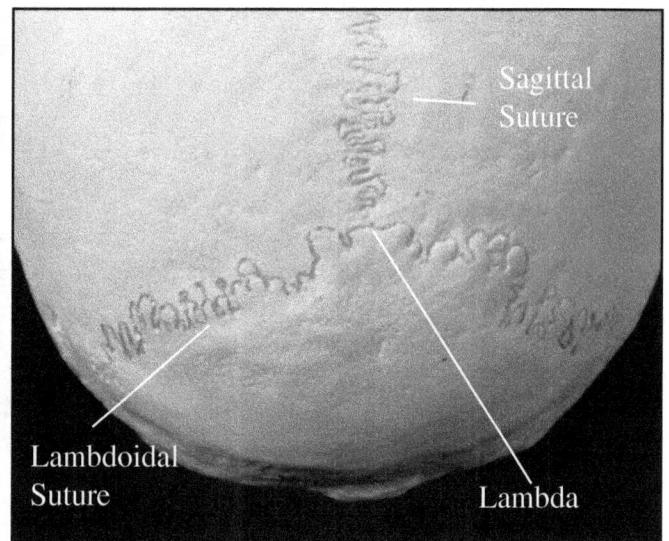

Superoposterior View of Cranial Sutures

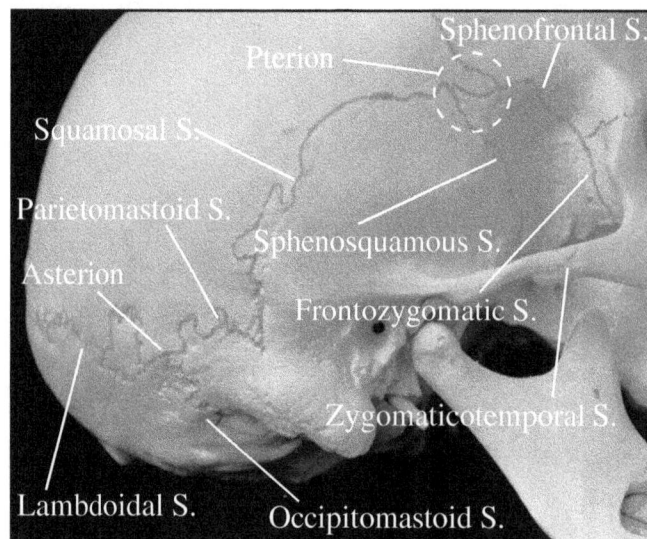

Lateral View of Cranial Sutures

Table 1: Foramina and Canals of the Cranium

Name	Contents	Description and Course
Olfactory foramina	Olfactory nerve filaments	Nasal fossa via the cribriform plate to the nasal bulb in the anterior cranial fossa.
Optic foramen	Optic nerve and ophthalmic artery	Apex of the orbit between the roots of the lesser wing to the anterior cranial fossa under the posterior angle of the lesser wing.
Superior orbital fissure	CN III, IV, and VI; first division of CN V; ophthalmic vein	From middle cranial fossa to orbit passing between the greater and lesser wings of the sphenoid
Interior orbital fissure	Second division of CN V and intraorbital vessels	From the pterygopalatine and infratemporal fossae to the orbit, between the maxillary tuberosity and the greater wing of the sphenoid
Foramen ovale	Third division of CN V; meningeal artery and emissary vein	From the middle cranial fossa through the greater wing of the sphenoid to the infratemporal fossa near the lateral pterygoid plate.
Greater and lesser palatine foramena	Palatine nerves from spheno-palatine ganglion and vessels	The opening of the pterygopalatine canal at the posteriolateral corner of the hard palate.
Pterygoid canal	Vidian nerve (greater and deep petrosal)	Near the border of the foramen lacerum this canal runs forward through the medial pterygoid plate to the pterygopalatine fossa.
Pterygopalatine canal	Vessels and descending branches of sphenopalatine ganglion	Between the tuberosity of the maxilla and the perpendicular plate of the palatine, this canal runs from the interior apex of the pterygopalatine fossa to the posterolateral surface of the hard palate.
Foramen rotundum	Second division of CN V to pterygopalatine fossa	Through the anterior of the greater wing between the middle cranial fossa and the the pterygopalatine fossa.
Sphenopalatine foramen	Ascending nasal nerve from the sphenopalatine ganglion and vessels	Through the notch at the upper end of the perpendicular plate of the palatine, made into a foramen by the sphenoid body. Pterygo-palatine fossa to nasal fossa
Foramen spinosum	Recurrent branches of third division of CN V and middle meningeal artery.	Through the angular spine of the sphenoid from the infratemporal fossa to the middle cranial fossa.
Stylomastoid foramen	CN VII and stylomastoid artery	External opening of facial canal posterior to the base of the styloid process.
Supraorbital notch	Supraorbital nerve and vessels	Inferomedial aspect of superior orbital rim.
Zygomaticofacial foramen	Zygomaticofacial nerve from second division of CN V	Orbital to malar surface of zygoma.
Foramen magnum	Medulla and meninges, vertebral arteries, spinal roots of CN XI, dural veins, anterior and posterior spinal arteries.	Through base of occiput.
Hypoglossal canal	CN XII	superolateral to foramen magnum.
Carotid canal	Internal carotid artery and carotid sympathetic plexus	Passes through the petrous temporal to open anterior to the jugular foramen and superior to foramen lacerum.
Internal auditory meatus	CN VIII and labyrinthine artery	Starts superolateral to the jugular foramen in the petrous ridge of the temporal bone passing into the inner ear.

Table 2: Jugular Foramen Contents

Cranial Nerve IX (Glossopharyngeal)	*Motor*: Stylopharyngeus *Sensory*: Pharyngeal constrictors, carotid body and sinus *Gen. & Spec. Sense*: post. 1/3 tongue *PNS*: Parotid gland (via otic ganglion & Lesser petrosal nerve from Inf. Salivatory Nucl.)
Cranial Nerve X (Vagus)	*Motor*: Pharyngeal constrictors, larynx, palatoglossus, muscles of palate (except tensor veli palatini) *Sensory*: base of tongue, larynx, inf. constrictor. *Sensory & PNS*: gut, heart, trachea, bronchi, lungs *Spec. sense*: taste - epiglottis & palate
Cranial Nerve XI (Accessory)	*Motor*: Sternocleidomastoid (also C-3) trapezius (also C3 4)
Internal Jugular Vein	begins here
Inferior Petrosal & Sigmoid Sinuses	end here

Table 3: Development of the Cranial Bones

Bones	Birth	One Year	Three Years	Six years	7 to 9 Years	10 to 25 Years
	At birth all cranial bones are single layer bones joined by cartilage. Six fontanelles are present, one at each corner of the two parietals.	Skull has doubled in size, bones are still only a single layer. Serrations beginning to form, all fontanelles are closed except the anterior, which may persist until 18 months.	All sutures are closed and serrations developing, but little interlocking present.			
Occiput	In four parts: Two condylar parts, a basilar part and a squamous portion divided by fissures at the lateral angles.	Still in four parts; squamosal features have disappeared.	Condylosquamal junction closing.	Condylosquamal junction completely fused.	Basio-occiput fuses with condylar parts.	Sphenobasilar synchondrosis fused by 20 to 25 years.
Sphenoid	In three parts; Basiosphenoid with lingula and two alisphenoids.	Fused into one piece.				
Temporal	In three parts: Petrosal, Squama, and Tympanic ring.	Fused into one bone; mastoid process forming.		Petrous full size.		
Frontal	In two parts: right and left portions separated by metopic suture.	Metopic suture persists.	Metopic suture starting to close.	Metopic suture closed.		
Parietal	Large- offers protection to all lobes of the brain.	Sagittal suture presists; serrations begin to form.	Serrations developing.			
Ethmoid	Two lateral masses separated by ethmovomerine plate.					Completely ossified by 18 years of age.
Maxilla	Incisive suture separates premaxilla and maxilla.	Getting taller as face lengthens.	Getting taller.			Incisive suture may persist to mid-life.
Mandible	Two parts joined by fibrous symphysis.	Two parts have fused.				
Atlas	Three parts: anterior and two lateral arches joined by cartilage.	In three parts.	Posterior arch fusing.	Atlas completely fused.		
Vertebra	Three pieces: body and two halves of the vertebral arch.	Halves of arch unite behind, moving lumbar to cervical.	Cervical bodies join to arches. Moves cephalad.	Union of arch to body in lower lumbars complete.		Body height, transverse process grows.
Sacrum	At birth the sacrum is made up of five developing vertebrae. The bodies of the sacral vertebrae are separated in early life by intervertebral cartilages. Each vertebra develops from at least seven ossification centers.	By the 18th year the two lowest segments become united by bone and the process of bony union gradually extends upward so that the five sacral vertebrae are united into one bone by the 30th year.				

Cranial Articulations

Synchrondrosis: a cartilaginous union such as the sphenobasilar synchondrosis

Suture: "A form of articulation characterized by the presence of a thin layer of fibrous tissue uniting the margins of the contiguous bones; found only in the skull."

The histology of this thin layer of fibrous tissue has been studied in man and animals, and suggests that it is the "site of active bone growth, and that it is at the same time a firm bond of union between the neighboring bones, which nevertheless allows a little movement."

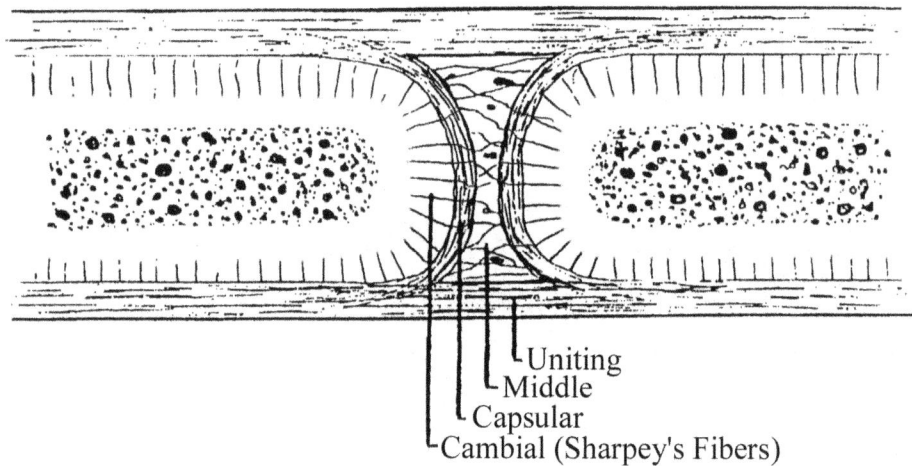

Uniting
Middle
Capsular
Cambial (Sharpey's Fibers)

<u>Fig. 1</u>: Connective Tissue Histology of Cranial Sutures

Meninges

The meninges enveloping the Central Nervous System are separated into three layers: the pia, arachnoid and dura. The cranial portion of the dura has two layers, the external layer being continuous with the periosteum and the internal layer which has several folds that separate the parts of the brain and enclose the venous sinuses. The falx cerebri is a sickle-shaped fold separating the cerebral hemispheres. It attaches to the crista galli of the ethmoid, to the frontal, parietal and occipital bones. The tentorium cerebelli is a sickle-shaped fold between the cerebrum and cerebellum. It attaches to the occipital, parietal and temporal bones. The free border of the tent attaches to the anterior clinoid processes and the attached border to the posterior clinoid processes. It attaches to the falx cerebri where it encloses the straight sinus. These two membranes, the falx and the tent, are referred to as the reciprocal tension membranes because they operate as a shifting suspension fulcrum. This fulcrum is located along the straight sinus where the falx cerebri and tentorium cerebelli meet and is called the Sutherland fulcrum. The dura continues down the spine, attaching to C2 and C3 and finally to the second sacral segment. This is the spinal reciprocal tension membrane, uniting and coordinating the involuntary movement of the sacrum with the cranial bones. Other dural folds to review are the falx cerebelli and the diaphragm sellae. The filum terminale is a continuation of the pia mater which blends with the dura within the sacral canal and attaches to the coccyx.

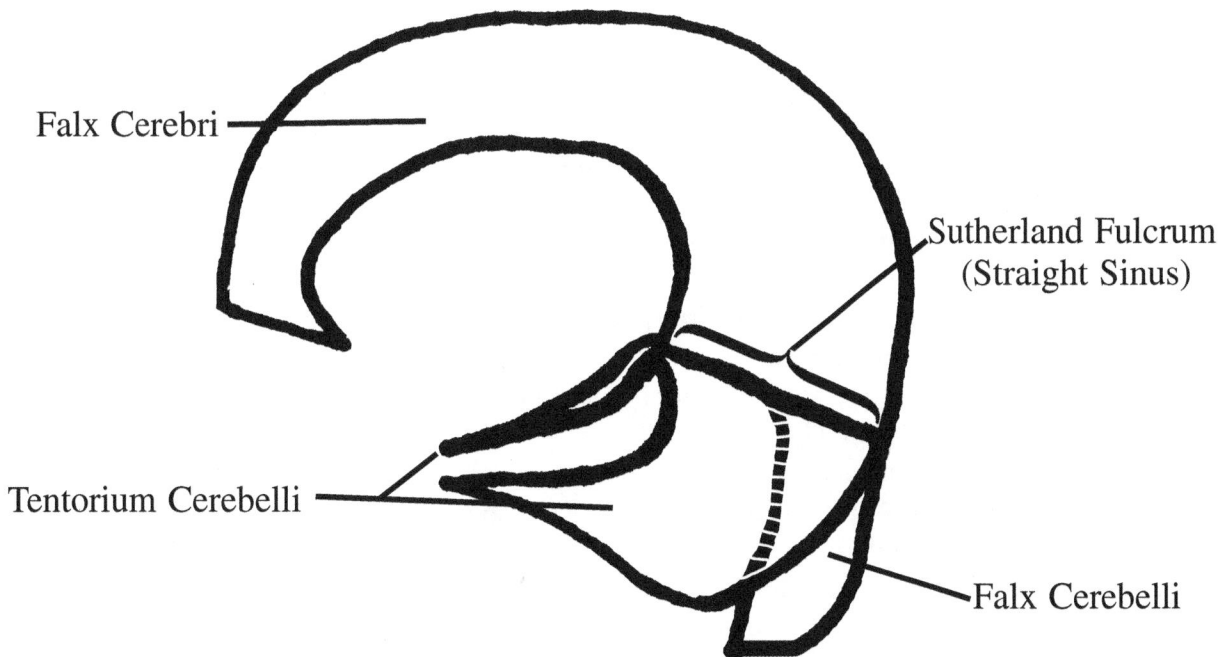

Fig. 2: Intracranial Dural Membranes

Cranial Dura

Periosteal Layer (↔periosteum of spinal canal)
Meningeal Layer (↔spinal dura)
        thrown into folds: Falx Cerebri
                                Tentorium Cerebelli
                                Falx Cerebelli
                                Diaphragma Selli

Cranial sinuses are formed within the meningeal layer

A. FALX CEREBRI
    1. Origin: Straight Sinus
    2. Attachments:
        a. Internal Occipital Protuberance
        b. Sagittal Ridge of Occiput
        c. Interparietal Suture
        d. Metopic Suture
        e. Crista Galli of Ethmoid (Anterior superior pole of attachment)

B. TENTORIUM CEREBELLI
    1. Origin: Straight Sinus
    2. Attachments:
        a. Posterior border attachments
            i. Internal Protuberance of Occiput
            ii. Along Transverse Ridges
            iii. This is posterior pole of attachment.
        b. Mastoid angles of parietals
        c. Ridge at top of Petrous Portion of Temporal Bone
            i. Divided insertion for superior Petrosal Sinus
            ii. Lateral poles of attachment
        d. Petrosphenoid ligament
        e. Anterior termination of outer border to POSTERIOR CLINOID PROCESS of
           body of Sphenoid
        f. Internal (medial) border of Tentorium cross over the petrosphenoid ligament and
           inserts on ANTERIOR CLINOID PROCESSES.
        g. Anterior inferior poles of attachment
            i. Anterior Clinoid Processes
            ii. Posterior Clinoid Processes

Cerebrospinal Fluid Fluctuation

Fluid within the ventricular system has an important role from its beginning in the embryonic growth and development of the Central Nervous System to its ongoing role in neurochemical and humoral regulation of the CNS.

The system consists of two lateral and two central ventricles. The two central ones include the 3rd ventricle, situated just superior to the brainstem and pituitary gland, posterior to lamina terminalis and anterior to the pineal gland. The 4th ventricle is inferior to the 3rd and rests posterior to the brainstem, and anterior to the cerebellum. All four ventricles communicate with each other, the lateral two with the 3rd and the 3rd with the 4th. From the 4th ventricle, CSF passes into the subarachnoid space within the dura that surrounds the brain and spinal cord. CSF fluctuation occurs within the subarachnoid space, emptying out into the venous dural sinuses through arachnoid granulations. Fluid also passes out the dural sheaths surrounding nerve roots as they leave the CNS. CSF within these sheaths become part of the peripheral circulation where it is believed to impart nutritive factors.

CSF fluid production by choroid plexuses within each ventricle controls the fluctuation of CSF and is thought to occur in association with the flexion and extension movements of the CRI. Flexion is associated with expansion of fluid volume in the ventricular system, and extension with contraction of the ventricular fluid volume.

Inherent Motility of the Central Nervous System

Originating from the embryologic development of the CNS, this inherent motility is inseparable from the fluid and membranous elements of the Primary Respiratory Mechanism. Together, they function to produce the CRI, elaborating an involuntary, rhythmic coiling and uncoiling of the CNS. Rhythmic coiling and uncoiling of the CNS is associated with expansion and contraction phases of the CRI. (see Osteopathic Embryology, pg. 87)

Specific properties of the cellular components of the CNS also exhibit inherent motility. This includes contractility of the neuroglial cells as well as the automaticity of electrical potentials firing in the brain. Rhythmic variations in neurochemical and neurohumoral activities may also be associated with variations of the inherent motility of the CNS. Motile functions of the CNS relating to fluid fluctuation and membranous tension are readily palpated by the trained examiner.

Flexion/Extension of Sphenoid and Occiput

Axes: Two transverse axes

Through sphenosquamous pivots of the sphenoid
Just above jugular processes of occiput

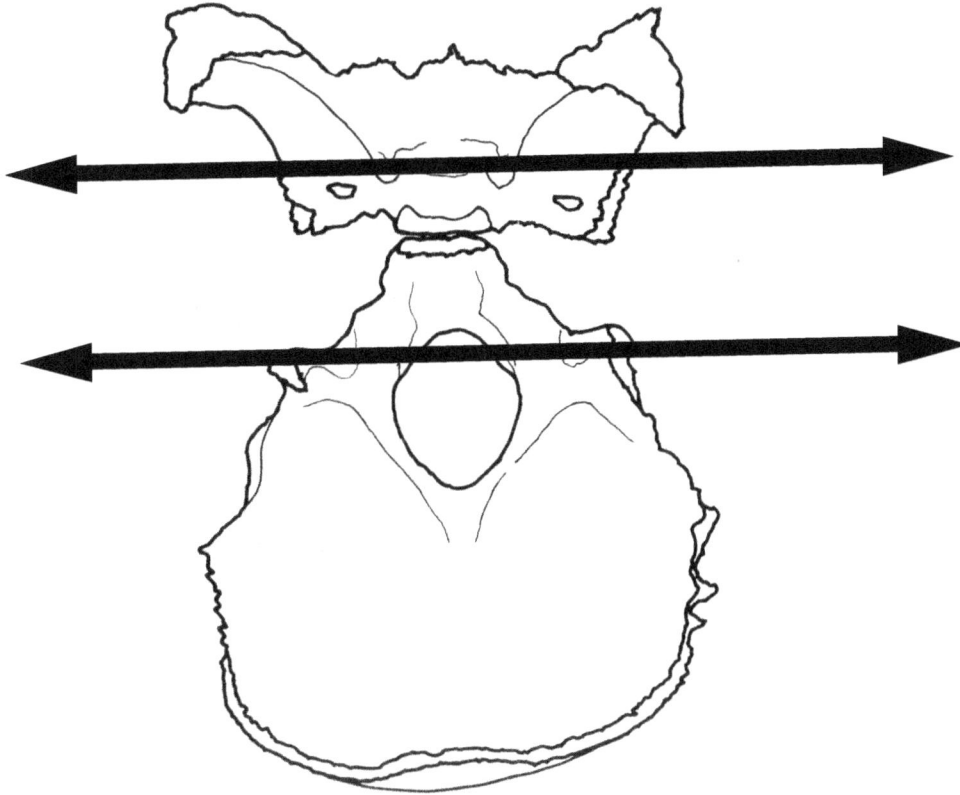

Fig. 3: Flexion/ Extension Axes of Sphenoid and Occiput

Naming of Motion: Sphenoid and occiput move in opposite directions. Bases of both bones rise in flexion. Bases of both bones descend in extension. Note that the occipital lateral angles and greater wings of the sphenoid (your palpatory landmarks) move opposite to the bases forming the sphenobasilar synchondrosis, as they are on opposite sides of the "gears."

Palpatory experience: Take the vault hold, with forefingers on the greater wings of the sphenoid, and the little fingers on the lateral angles of the occiput. In flexion all four landmarks will move away from you inferiorly as the sphenobasilar synchondrosis rises between your hands. As the SBS descends in extension your hands will move toward you (superiorly, away from the patient's feet).

Palpatory experience: As both hands move towards the patient's feet in flexion the sides of the head will widen slightly, separating the hands from each other through the mechanism of the widening, externally rotating the temporals. Conversely, In extension your hands move toward you and the head narrows slightly from side to side as the temporals internally rotate.

The skull widens laterally with external rotation of the temporals and shortens slightly front to back. It is as if the head has filled with air during inspiration. Conversely, the lateral narrowing of internal rotation (during extension) is accompanied by slight anteroposterior elongation of the cranium and the sides pull as if they are deflating during exhalation.

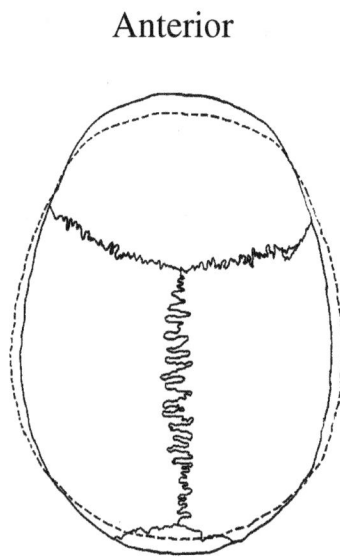

Anterior   Anterior

Fig. 4: The Skull in Extension   Fig. 5: The Skull in Flexion

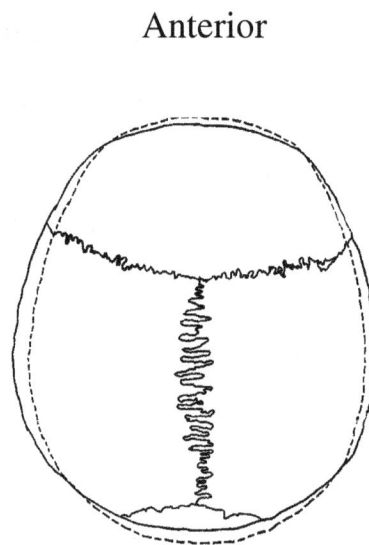

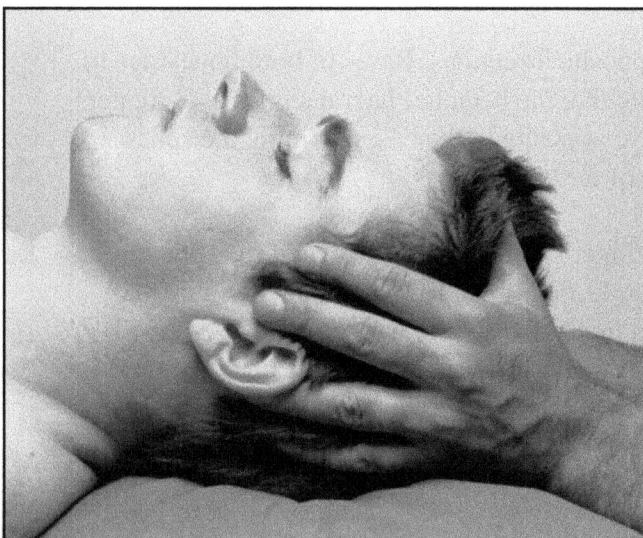

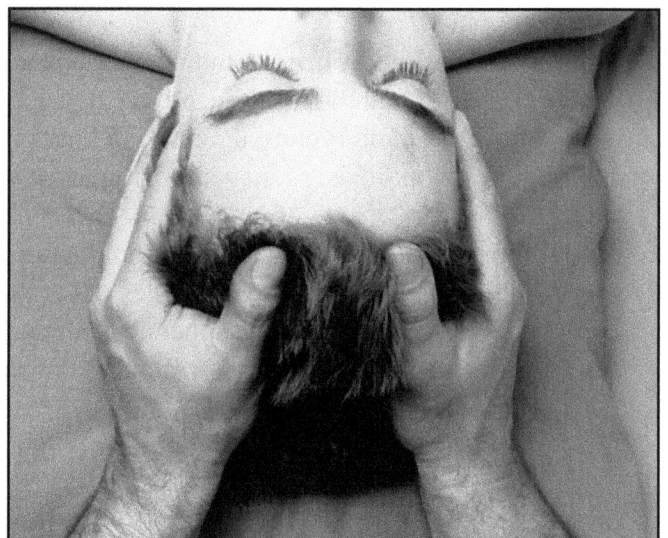

Vault Hold

Flexion/Extension of the Sacrum

Axis: Transverse, through S2

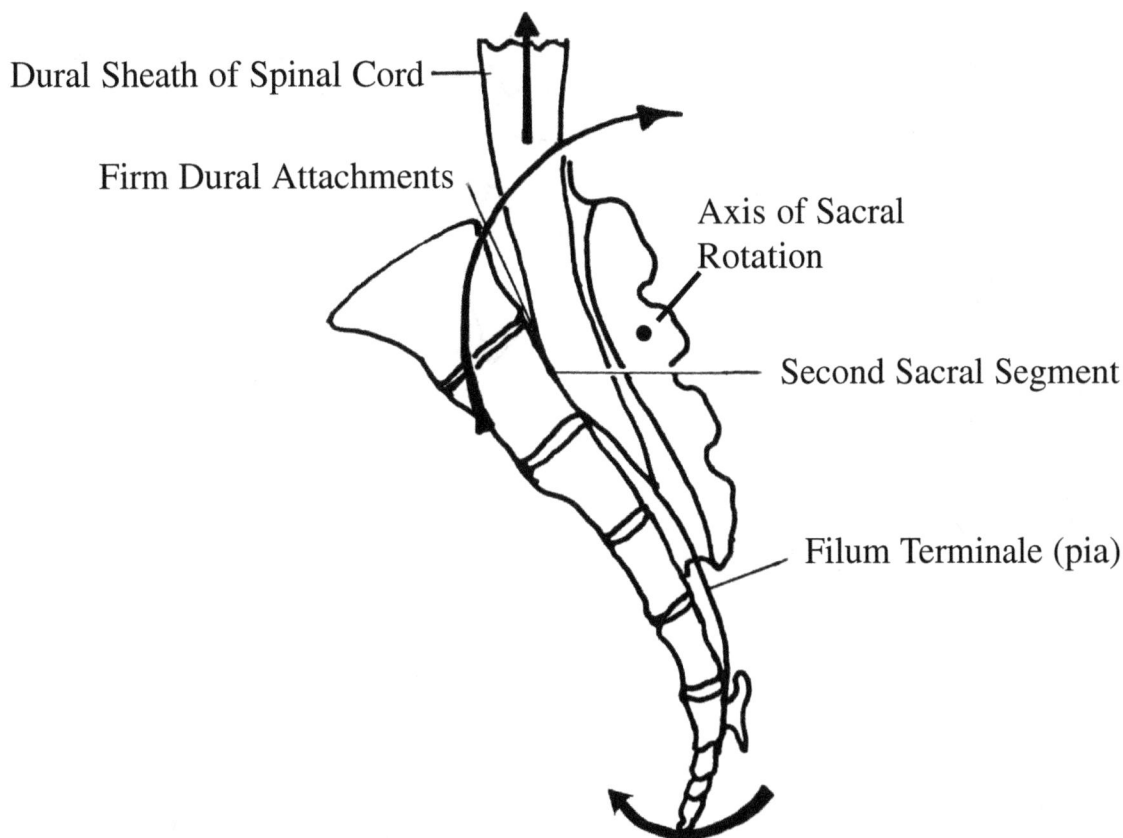

Dural Sheath of Spinal Cord

Firm Dural Attachments

Axis of Sacral Rotation

Second Sacral Segment

Filum Terminale (pia)

Fig. 6: The Sacral Mechanism in Flexion.

Motion: In the flexion phase the sacral base tips posteriorly, coccyx moves anteriorly and the whole sacrum is pulled somewhat superiorly by the upward 'tug' of the dura. In extension, the base tips anteriorly, and the coccyx moves posteriorly, and the sacrum moves slightly inferiorly.

Palpatory experience:
Sacrum of supine patient is held in the palm of the hand with the base of the sacrum at the fingertips and the coccyx near the wrist.

In flexion the base moves posteriorly to 'push' against the fingertips and the whole hand moves slightly superiorly.

In extension the base moves anteriorly and pressure against the fingertips is lessened as the sacral base moves anteriorly and upward. Dural tension is lessened, allowing the whole sacrum to move toward the patient's feet.

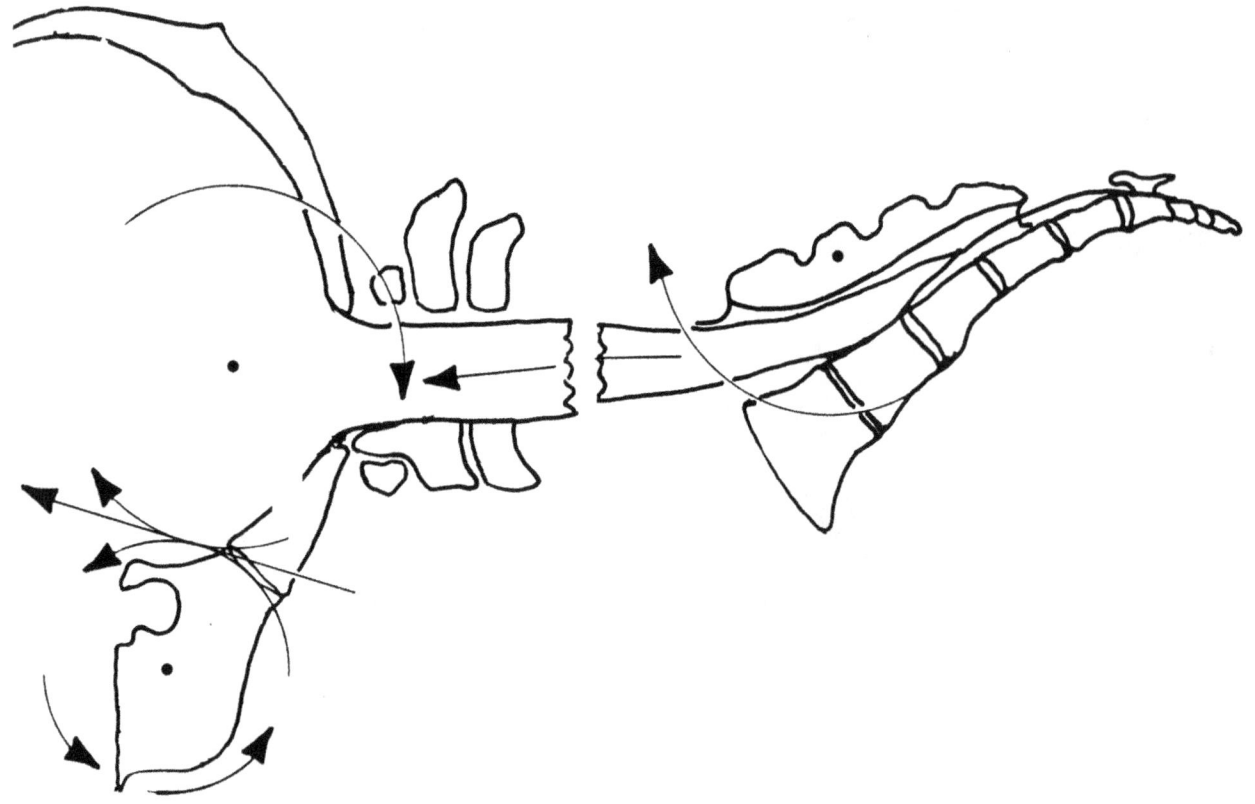

Fig. 8: Flexion of SBS and Sacrum

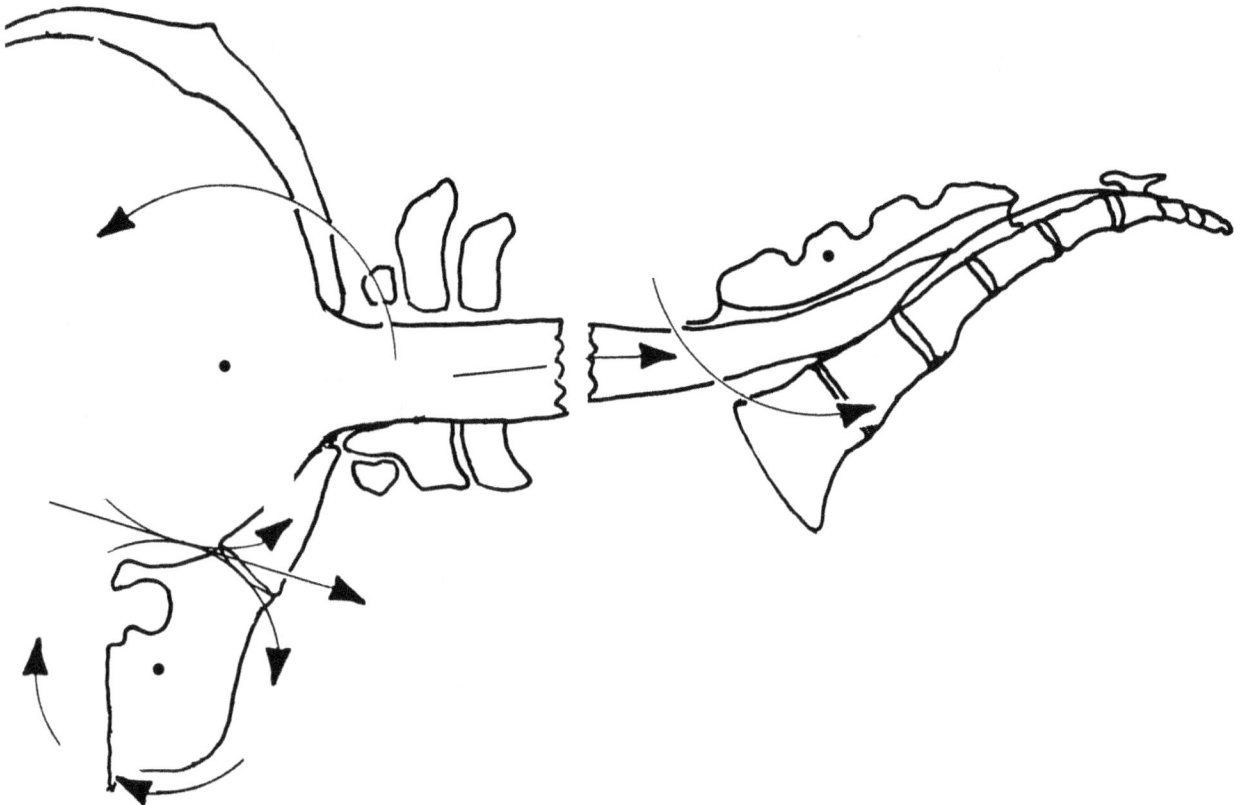

Fig. 7: Extension of SBS and Sacrum

24

Lumbosacral Decompression

Patient supine. Physician sits beside the patient's pelvis, facing the patient's head. If the physician is right-handed, sit on the right side of the patient (if you are left-handed please reverse the following instructions and read left for right and vice versa). Place the right hand between the patient's legs and under the sacrum so that the sacral base rests on the pads of the terminal phalanges. (In the infant two fingers will encompass the whole sacrum.) The inherent respiratory motion of flexion and extension around the transverse axis is evaluated.

Motion around any other axes of motion is noted if it occurs consistently or intermittently (i.e., sidebending or rotation). <u>There is no need for passive motion testing</u>. However, resilience or joint play at the lumbosacral junction can be tested by drawing the sacrum down toward the feet. Wait a few moments to feel the membranous response of the sacrum. This is a passive test of motion performed by the physician. If this is absent or difficult on one or both sides, lumbosacral compression is present.

The texture, solidity or "heaviness" of the sacrum is noted. The compressed sacrum has a distinctive absence of resilience and flexibility, a solid heavy feel. To treat this condition the operator maintains contact with the sacrum with finger tips at the first sacral segment. The other hand contacts the fifth lumbar at the transverse processes, a thumb and finger may be the most comfortable. Gently compress the two hands together until a sense of "swelling" and separation develops between them. Note the freedom of motion now occurring between them.

For intraosseous sacral lesions repeat the same technique between S1 - S2 and after release here, repeat at S2 - S3. It is wise to check all the sacral segments, but by the time S2 - S3 is decompressed the remainder are usually moving freely.

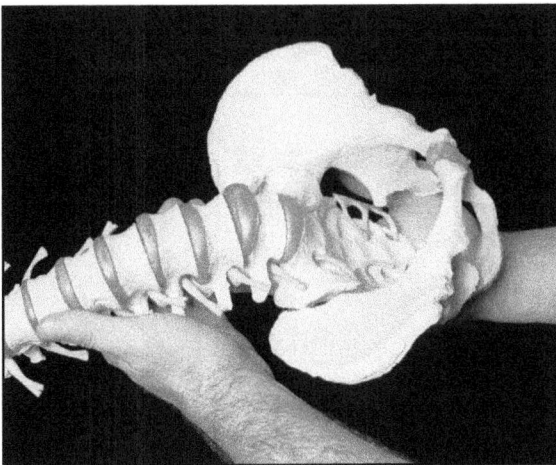

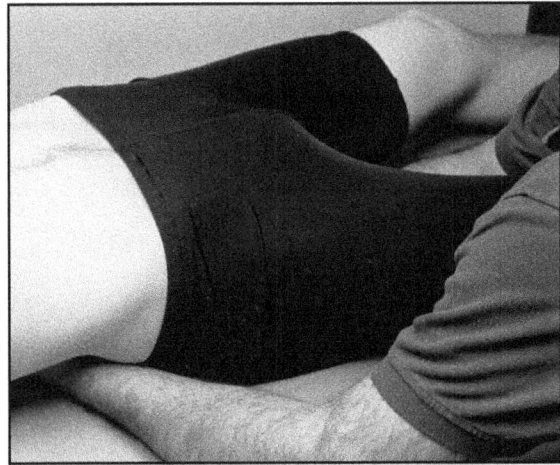

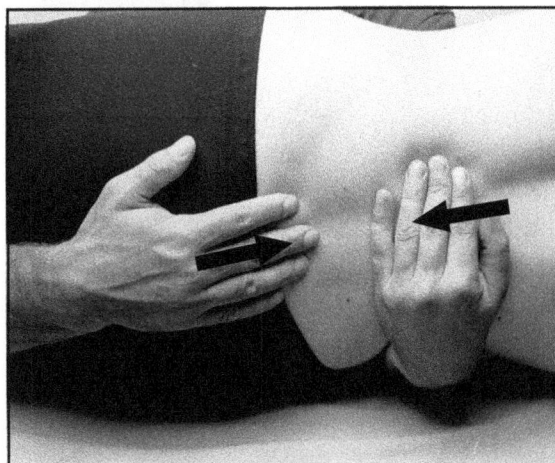

Lumbosacral Decompression

Intraosseous Lesions

During sacral and cranial bone development, strains may develop within the growth plates as well as later at the time of fusion. which then become part of the intraosseous bone structure. These strains may be the result of labor and delivery, during which time the head and rump must withstand pressure of up to 200 pounds per square inch. They may also be due to impact from falls, particularly to the head and tailbone, and altered weight bearing/postural mechanics due to abnormal musculoskeletal development.

Membranous elements which surround the bone reflect intraosseous strain patterns, disturbing interosseous relationships and the functional characteristsics of the dural tube and reciprocal tension membrane. Intraosseous dysfunction exhibits an unusual rigidity and heaviness which seems unresponsive to treatment. Locating the focus of membranous pull within the bone, e.g the sacrum, allows activation of the fluid mechanism of the CRI. Bone remodelling and growth are sensitive to external forces (e.g. gravity) and may be influenced by cranial rhytmic impulse approaches (see Level III, page 155).

Individual Bones - Anatomy and Physiological Motion

A. Occiput

1. Structure - Function

   a. The occiput is formed from four parts during infancy

      1) Squama
      2) Two condylar parts
      3) Basilar process

   b. The occipital condyle is made up of 1/4 basilar portion and 3/4 condylar portion.

   c. Osseous union of condylar parts with squama not complete until the fifth year, not complete with basilar part until the seventh year.

   d. The articulations of the occiput

      1) Parietals
      2) Temporals
      3) Sphenoid
      4) Atlas

   e. Review structures related to the occipital region, e.g. hypoglossal canal, falx cerebri and cerebelli, tentorium cerebelli, jugular notch and fossa.

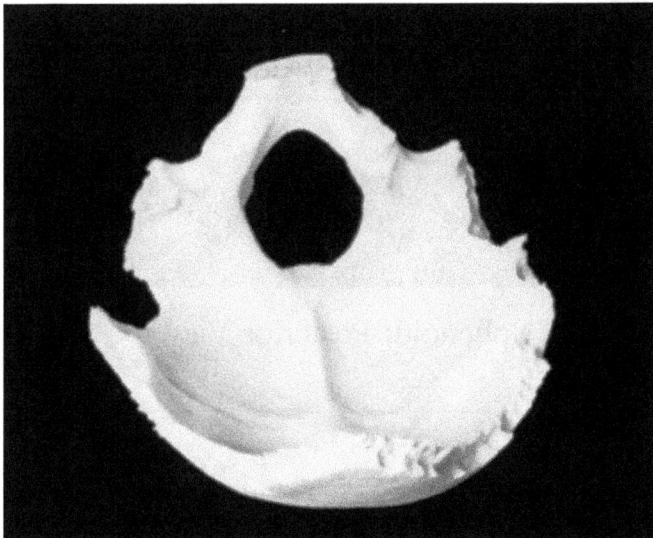

Occiput: Superior View   Occiput: Inferior View

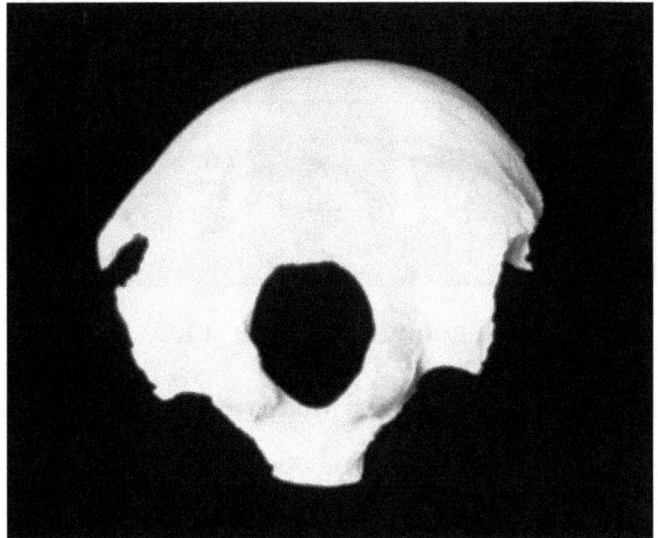

2. Physiological Motion - The axis of motion for flexion and extension is a transverse axis directly above the foramen magnum at the level of the confluence of sinuses.

3. Intraosseous Lesions

These occur easily between the unossified parts of the occiput during the stresses of labor and delivery. They can have significant impact on the development of the child and should be treated early. Compression of the condylar parts is especially common.

B.   Sphenoid

1. Structure - Function

    a. At birth, the sphenoid consists of three osseous parts: body and lesser wings, and two greater wings. These osseous parts are separated by cartilaginous tissue

    b. The articulations of the sphenoid (12)

        1) Paired bones

            (a) parietals

            (b) temporals

            (c) palatine

            (d) zygoma

        2) Unpaired bones

            (a) frontal

            (b) ethmoid

            (c) vomer

            (d) occiput

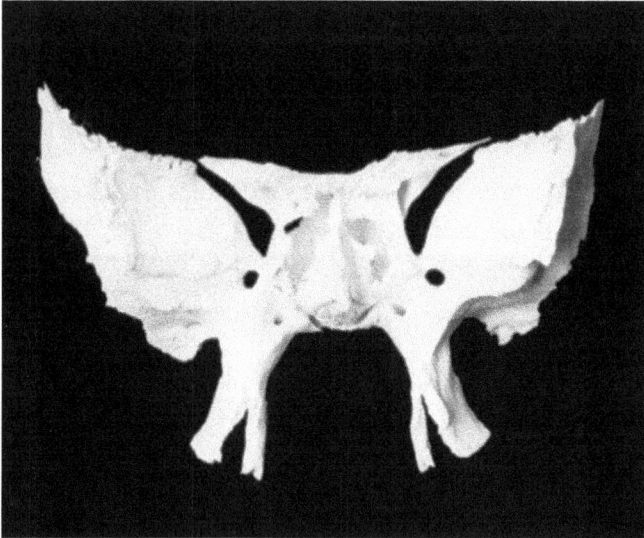

Sphenoid: Anterior View   Sphenoid: Posterior View

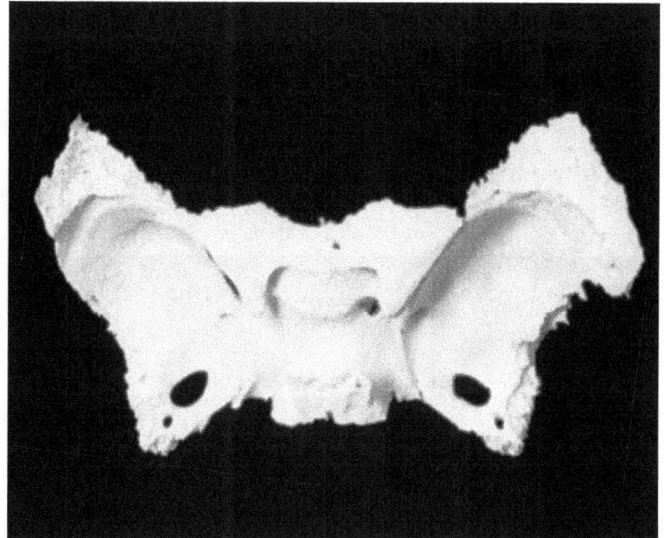

2. Physiological Motion

    a. The sphenoid moves around a transverse axis through the center of its body

    b. In flexion, the greater wing moves forward, laterally and inferiorly. The pterygoid processes move posteriorly and slightly laterally while the body expands slightly.

3. Intraosseous lesions - The parts of the sphenoid are separated by cartilage at birth and are thus vulnerable to warping during the stresses of labor and delivery.

4. Palpation of Occiput and Sphenoid

    a. **Vault hold**. Thumbs parallel or interlocked over the vault. Fingers are spread with the index fingers over the lateral surface of the greater wings of the sphenoid; the middle fingers just in front of the ears; the ring fingers posterior to the ears; the little fingers on the occipital squama. Use palmar surface of fingers, not the tips.

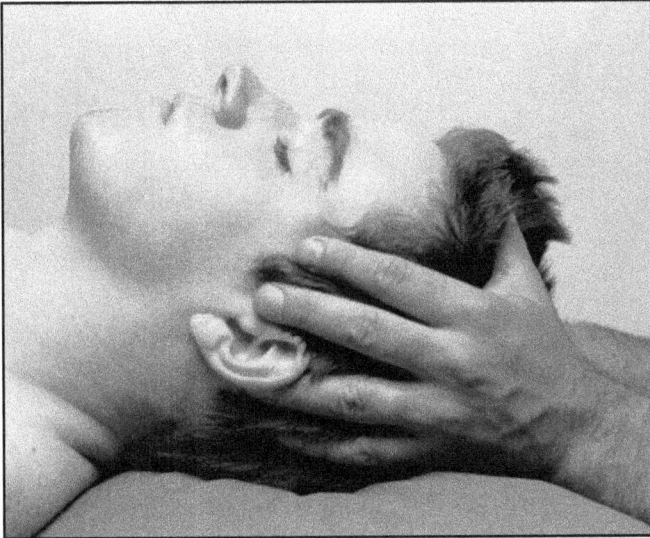

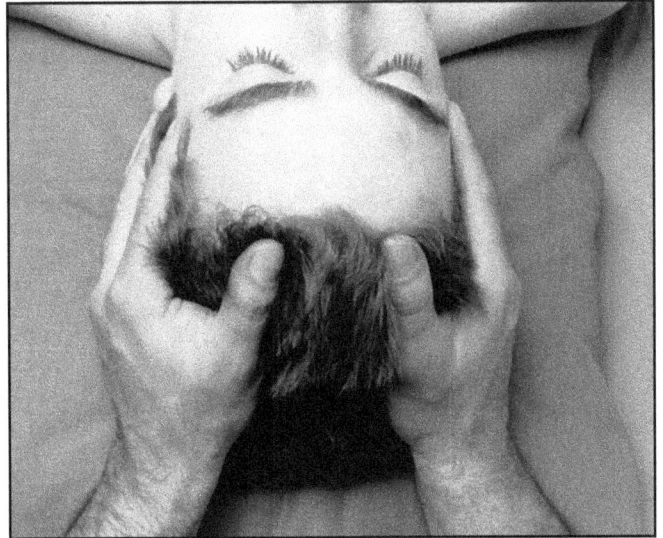

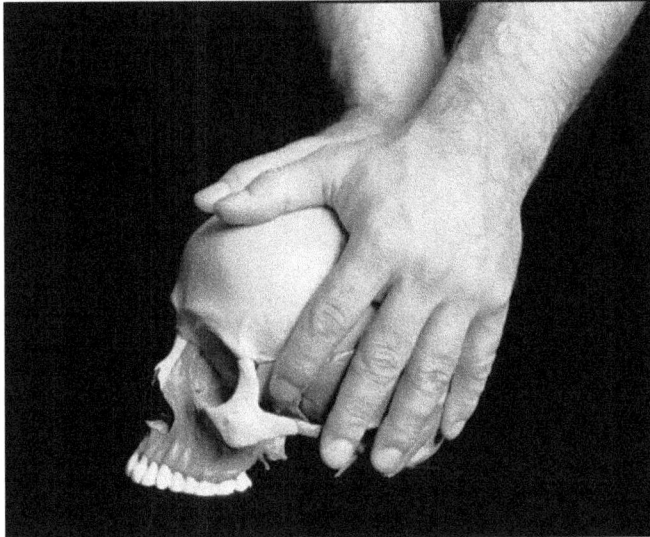

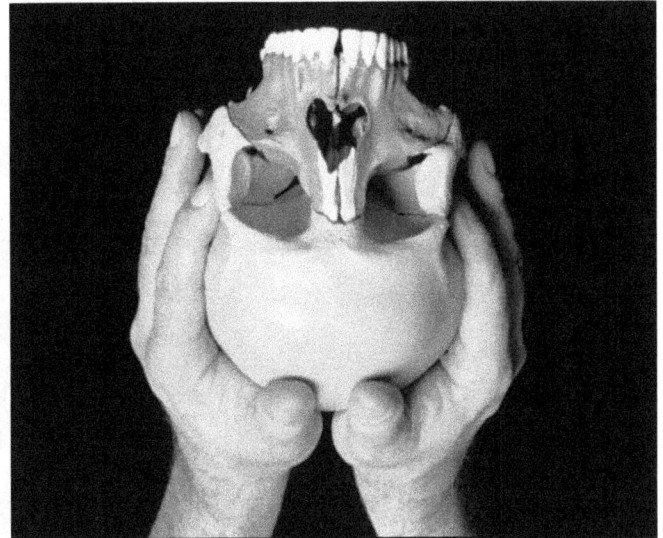

Vault Hold

b. **<u>Fronto-occipital vault hold</u>**. One hand is cupped under the occipital squama, medial to the lateral angles. The other hand is held with the palm approximating the frontal squama, the middle finger on one greater wing, the thumb on the other. Keep touch light.

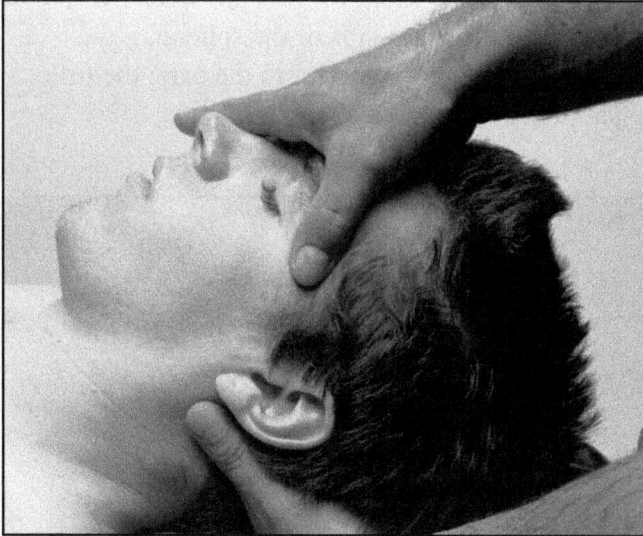

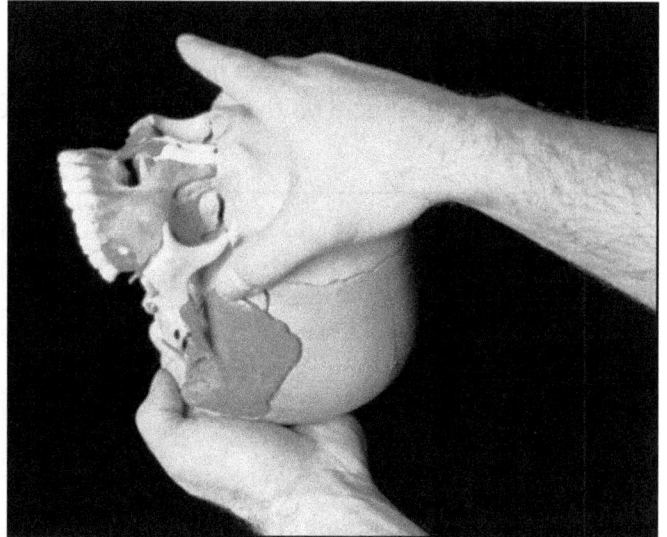

Fronto-Occipital Vault Hold

c. **<u>Occipital vault hold</u>**. Both hands cup underneath the occiput, fingers contacting the inferior lateral squama, thumbs contacting the greater wings of the sphenoid.

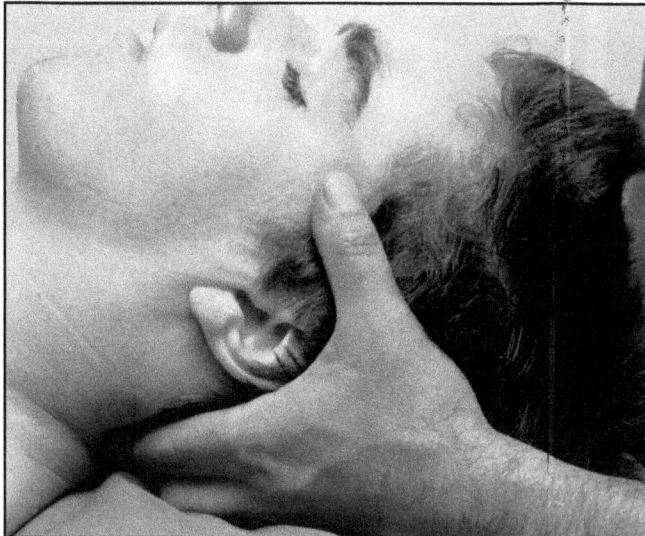

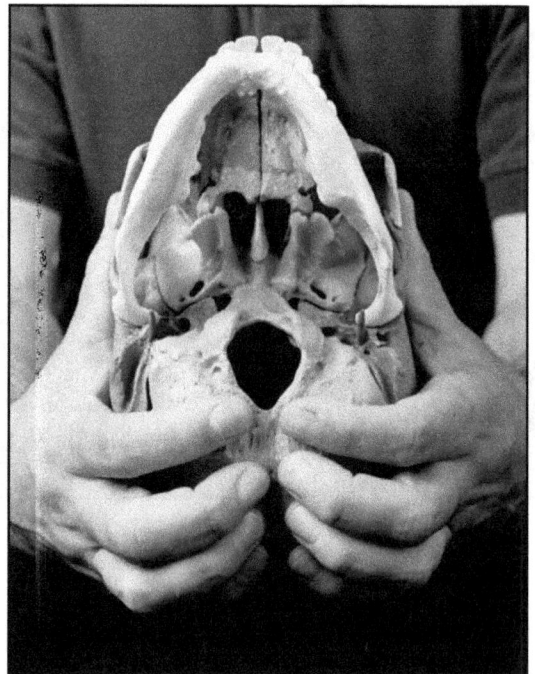

Occipital Vault Hold

These holds are used to palpate inherent motion of vault, sphenoid and occiput in diagnosis and later for treatment.

C.   Temporal Bone

1. Structure - Function

a. There are four parts of the temporal bone

1) squama
2) styloid process
3) mastoid portion
4) petrous portion

b. The articulations of the temporal bone include

1) mandible
2) parietal
3) sphenoid
4) zygoma
5) occiput

c. Review the anatomy of the temporal bone and the structures that pass through and
around it.

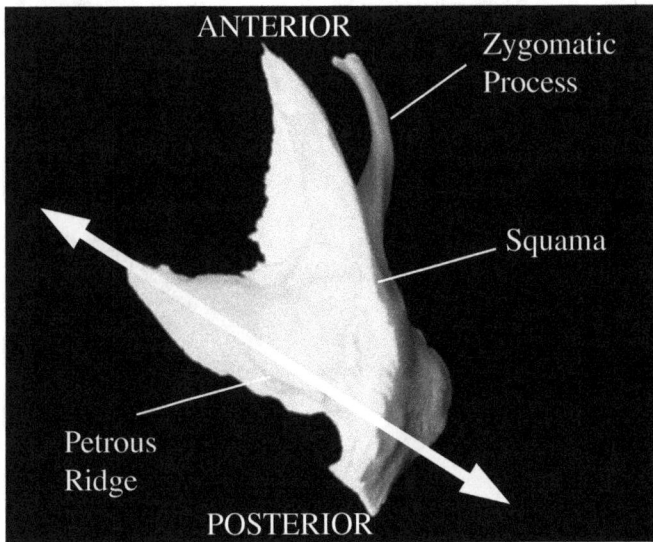

Superior View of Temporal Bone With
Axis of Rotation

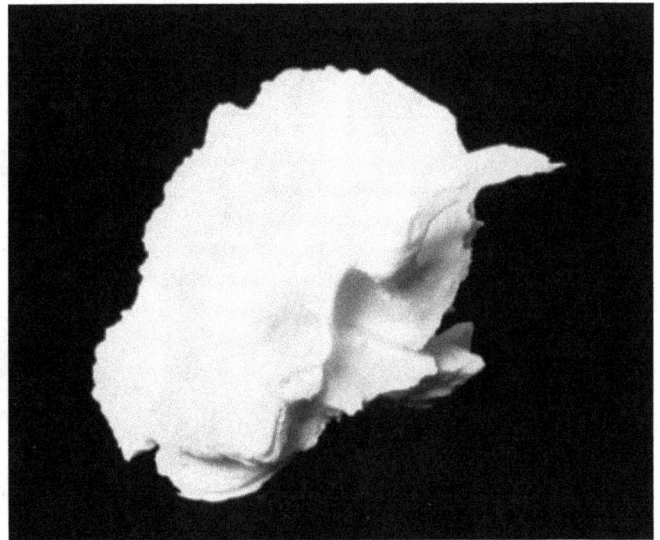

Lateral View of Temporal Bone

2. Physiological Motion

    a. Physiological motion of the temporal is guided and influenced by the occiput

    b. As the occiput moves into flexion, the temporals externally rotate. With extension of the occiput, the temporals internally rotate.

    c. The axis of rotation upon which the temporal moves runs approximately from the jugular surface to the petrous apex of the temporal bone. During external rotation the squama moves anterolaterally, the mastoid process moves medialward and slightly posterior.

Internal/external rotation of the temporals

Axis: Along the petrous ridge; the axis of the two temporals converge anteriorly.

Motion and how named: In external rotation (during flexion of the SBS) the temporals rotate anteriorly, the squama widen from each other, the mastoid process move posteromedially. The opposite occurs in internal rotation (during SBS extension).

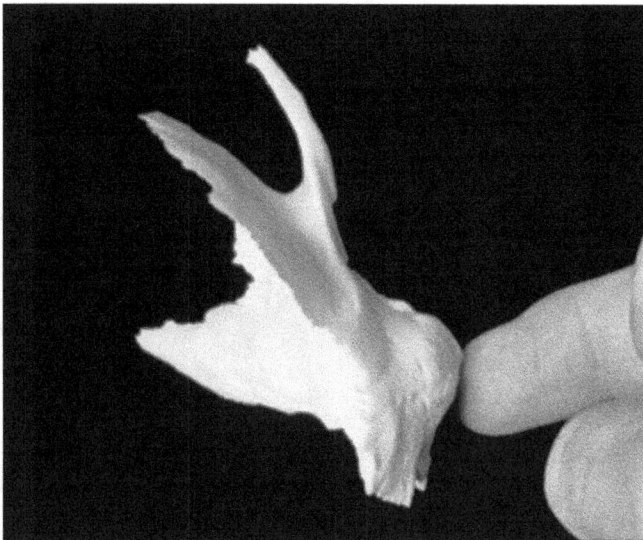

Temporal Bone in Internal Rotation

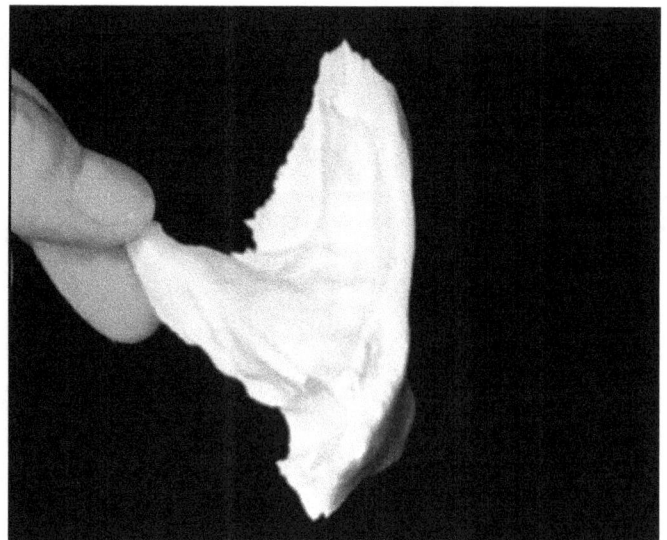

Temporal Bone in External Rotation

3. Palpation of Temporals

a. **<u>Temporal hold with thumbs</u>** - place thumbs behind the ears overlying the mastoid portion of each temporal bone. Place each thumb so that the metacarpal-phalangeal joint is directly posterior to the external auditory meatus.

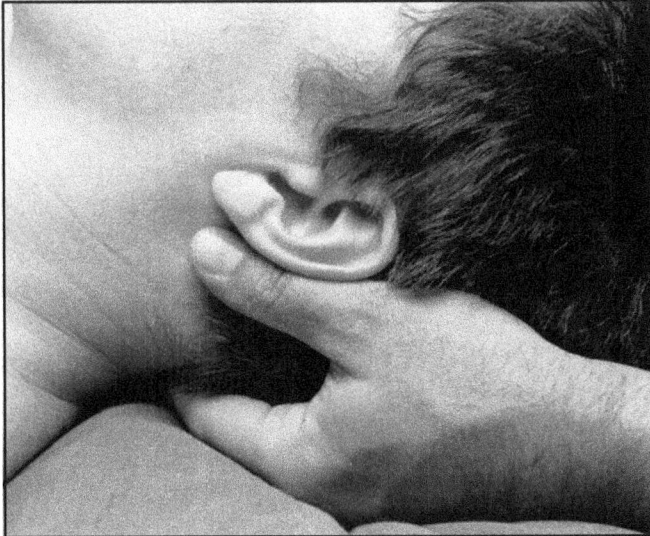

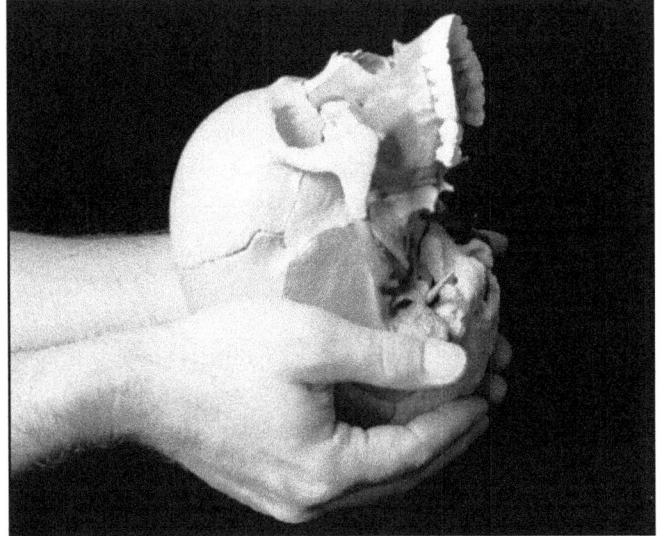

Temporal Hold With Thumbs

b. **<u>Temporal hold with fingers</u>**
   1) place third digit into external auditory meatus
   2) place thumb and index finger on the zygomatic process of the temporal bone
   3) Place fourth finger on mastoid process and fifth finger superior to fourth on squamous portion of the temporal bone
   4) Observe motion present. Slight influence with thumb and fourth finger increases external rotation. Slight influence with index and fifth finger increases internal rotation.

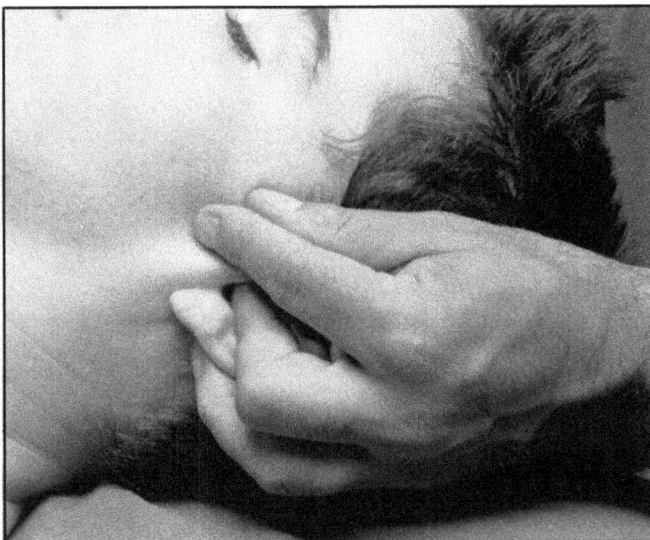

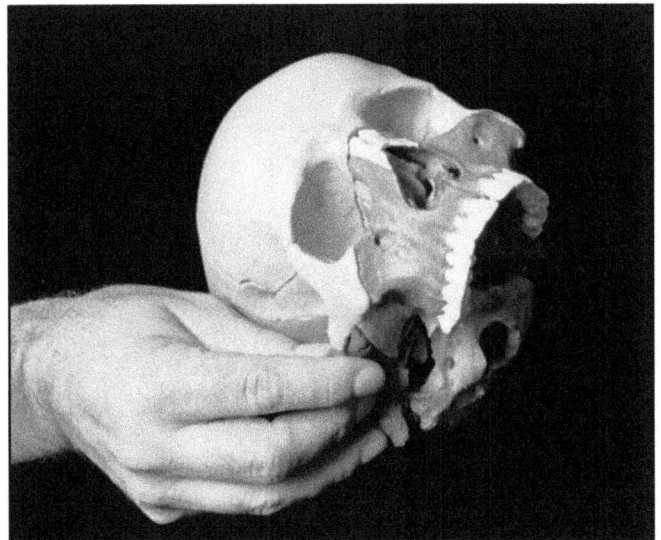

Temporal Hold With Fingers

These holds are used to diagnose and treat imbalance and somatic dysfunction of the temporal bones.

D. Parietal Bones

1. Structure - Function

    a. Articulations of the parietal

        1) sphenoid
        2) occiput
        3) temporal
        4) frontal
        5) opposite parietal

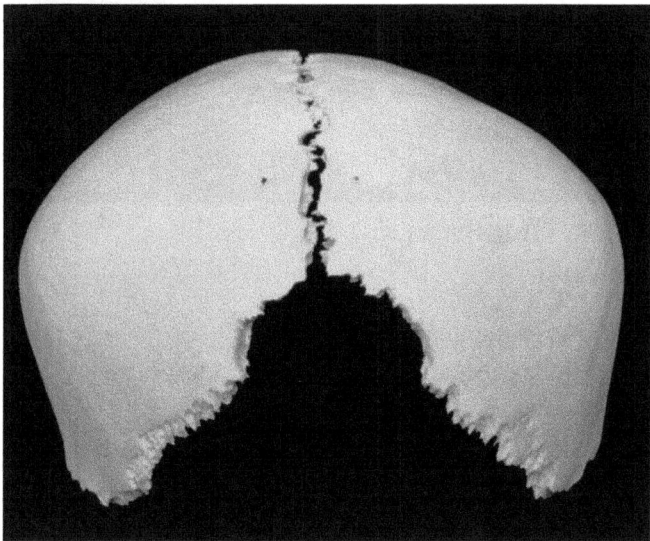

Posterior View of Parietal Bones

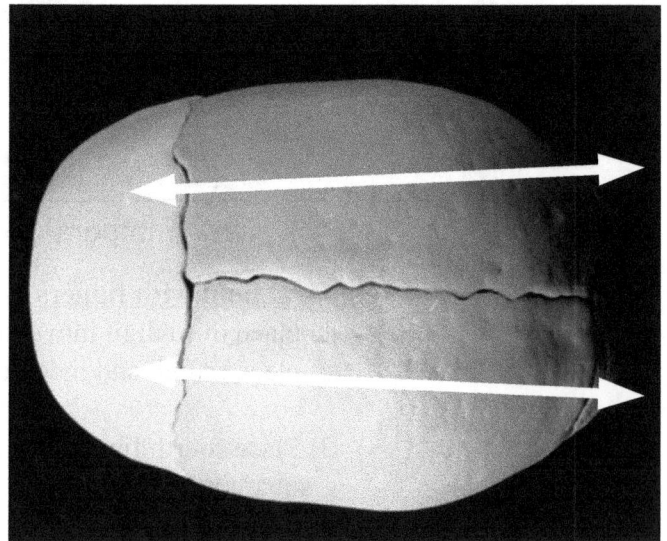

Superior View of Parietal Bones with Axes of Rotation

2. Physiological Motion

    a. External rotation occurs with flexion of the spheno-basilar synchondrosis. The inferior borders move laterally with external rotation and medially with internal rotation. The widening of the parietals is greater at the posterior aspect of the bones

    b. The axis of rotation occurs at the change of bevel through the anterior and posterior borders of each parietal bone.

E. Frontal Bone

1. Structure - Function

   a. Frontal bone articulates with

      1) nasal bones   5) sphenoid
      2) maxillae   6) ethmoid
      3) zygomae   7) lacrimals
      4) parietals

   b. The mechanical importance in the articulation between the frontal and parietal bones is that there is a change in the bevel. The coronal suture can be divided into thirds with the middle third beveled at the expense of the inner table and the lateral 2/3rds at the expense of the outer table. Thus, the frontal overlaps the parietal bones in the middle third and the opposite is true for the lateral two thirds.

2. Physiological Motion

   a. Axis of rotation of each frontal passes from the change of bevel at the coronal border, downward and forward through the center of the orbital plate.

   b. Embryogically the frontal bone is formed in two parts. They remain as paired bones in 10% of the population. Thus, functionally it is considered a paired structure having the motions of external and internal rotation.

   c. The inferior lateral angles of the frontal bone move laterally, inferiorly, and slightly forward in external rotation. The opposite is true for internal rotation.

   d. The glabella may recede slightly in external rotation due to the pull of the falx cerebri.

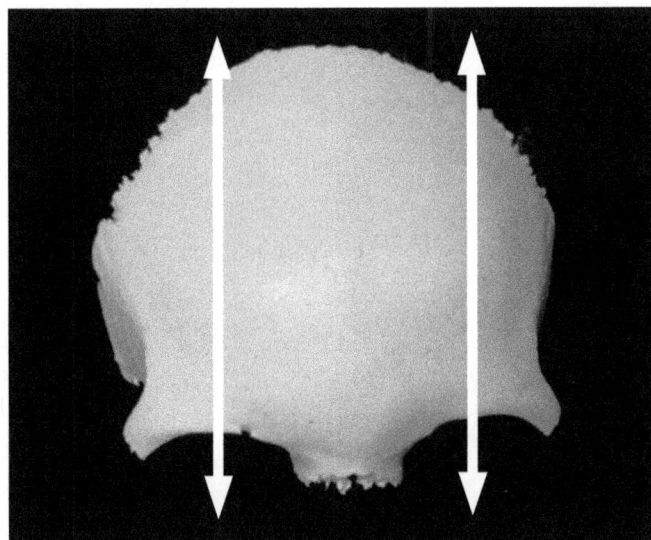

Frontal Bone with Axes of Rotation

F. Ethmoid

    1. Structure - Function

        a. Articulations of the ethmoid

1) frontal	6) palatines
2) sphenoid	7) inferior conchae
3) nasals	8) vomer
4) maxillae	9) septal cartilage
5) lacrimals	10) sphenoid conchae

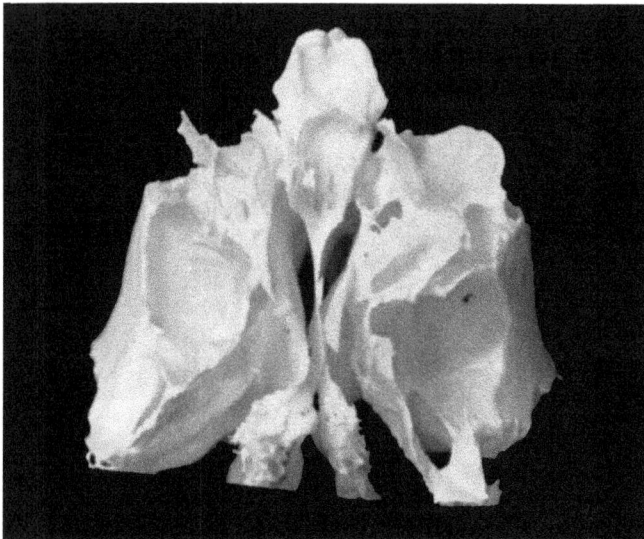

Posterior View of Ethmoid Bone   Anterior View of Ethmoid Bone

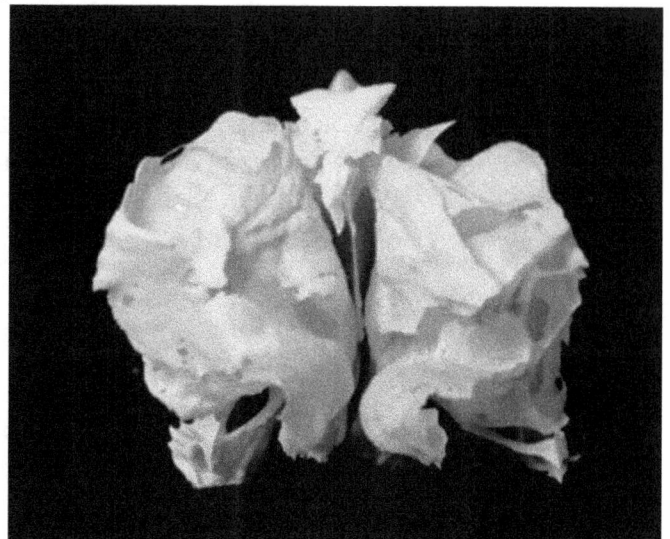

    2. Physiological Motion
        a. The axis of physiological movement is a transverse axis through the middle of the ethmoid.
        b. The ethmoid is considered a midline bone with movements of flexion and extension. It moves around its axis in the same direction as the occiput.
        c. The lateral masses (labyrinths), of the ethmoid move as paired bones; internal and external rotation, being influenced by the maxillae.

G. Vomer

    1. Structure - Function
        a. Articulations of the vomer

           1) sphenoid
           2) ethmoid
           3) palatines
           4) maxillae
           5) septal cartilage

    2. Physiological Motion
        a. The axis of rotation is slightly inferior in the middle of the vomer. This is a transverse axis.
        b. Vomer functions as a midline bone, moving into flexion and extension.

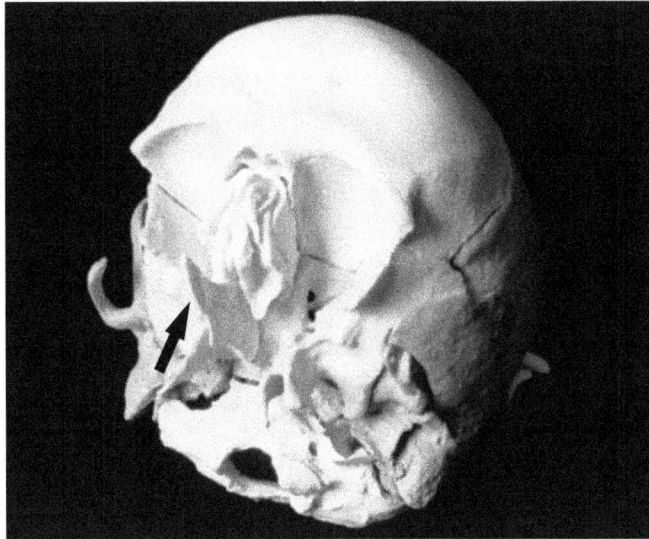

Partial Skull Revealing Vomer

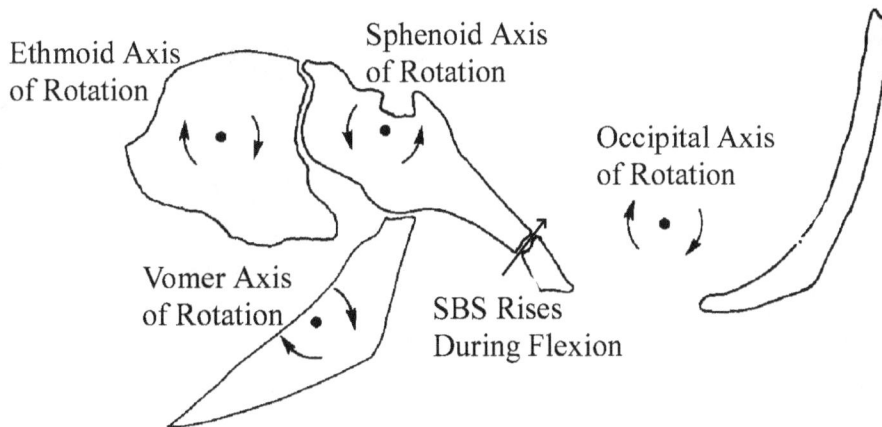

Ethmoid Axis of Rotation

Sphenoid Axis of Rotation

Occipital Axis of Rotation

Vomer Axis of Rotation

SBS Rises During Flexion

Fig. 9: Interrelated Motions of the Cranial Base Bones During Flexion

Frontal Lift

The effective performance of this technique rests on an understanding of the anatomic relationships of the frontal bone to the parietal bone, the greater wing of the sphenoid bone and the temporal bone at pterion. Review the bony structure. The frontal bone is the deepest and most medial of all the bones. The principle of the technique is 1) to internally rotate the frontals to disengage them from their related bones, 2) to lift them anterior and 3) permit them to externally rotate and widen the ethmoid notch.

The Treatment:

Patient is supine, operator sits at the head at the table. Rest your elbows on the table. Place your hypothenar eminences on the lateral angles of the frontal and interlace the fingers over, but not in contact with, the forehead. Attempt to draw the fingers of one hand from the fingers of the other while resisting this motion by adducting the fingers (action of the lumbrical muscles.) In this way the hypothenar eminences exert an influence of internal rotation on the lateral angles of the frontal bone. Coordinate this action with a lifting of the frontal anteriorly (toward the ceiling) until you feel the lateral angles moving into external rotation. Gently release your hands. An alternate treatment method is to use the fingertips to guide the lift.

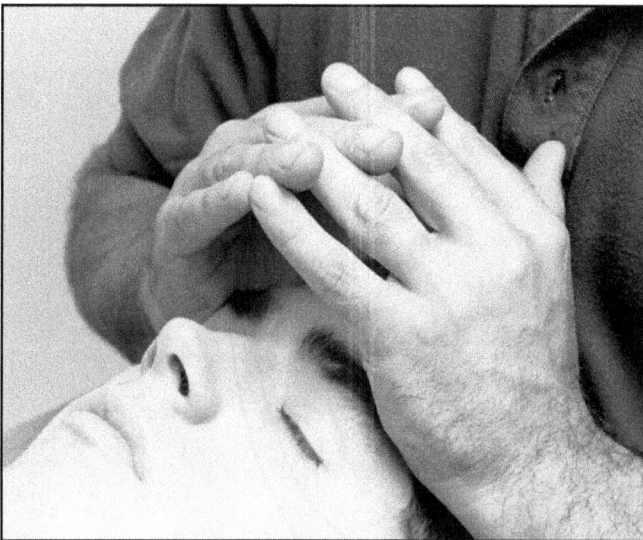

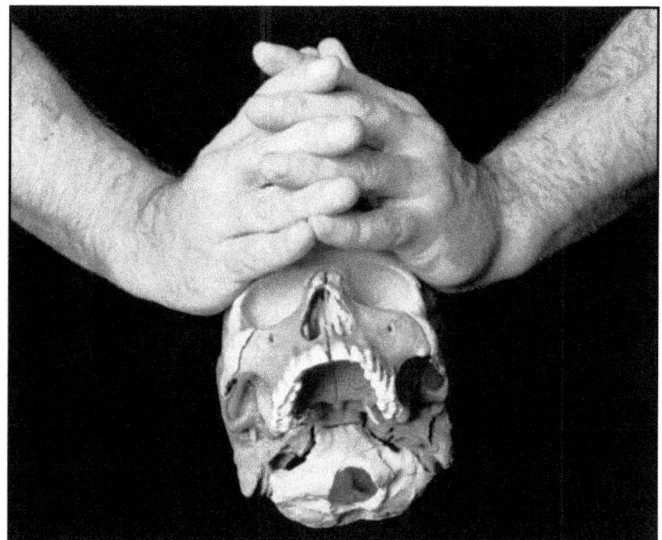

Frontal Lift (above), Alternate Method Frontal Lift (below)

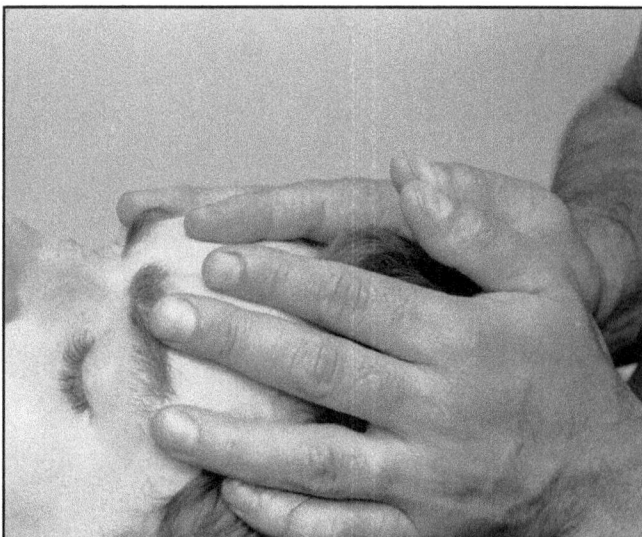

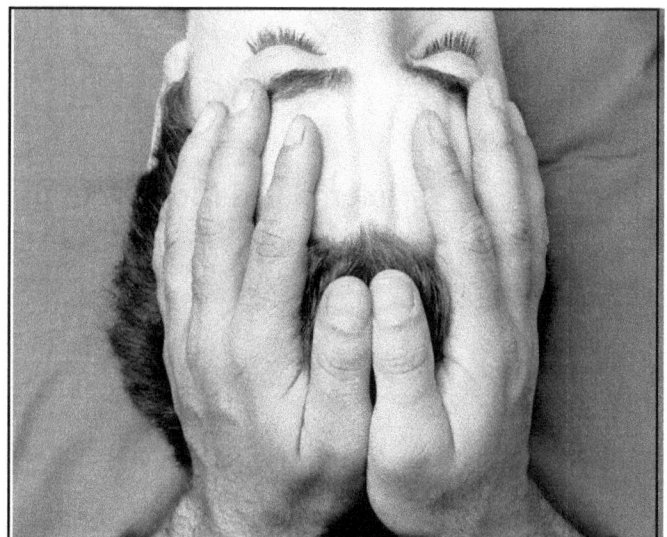

Parietal Lift

Note the anatomic position of the parietal bone. Its anterior border is at the coronal suture which Is approximately at the junction of the anterior and middle thirds of the vault. Study the relationship of the parietal as it glides deep to the squamous temporal. In internal rotation the parietal bone approximates the squamous portion of the temporal bone and in external rotation they separate.

The Treatment:

Patient supine, operator sits at the head of the table. Rest your forearms on the table. Place your finger tips on the inferior border of each of the two parietals just above the squamous temporal. Cross the thumbs above but not In contact with the sagittal suture. Firmly press one thumb against another, i.e., one thumb presses upward as the other resists this motion by pressing downward. Thus the fingers will approximate and induce internal rotation of the inferior border of the parietal bones. At the some time lift both hands in a cephalad direction (towards the operator) until the parietal bones move into external rotation. Release the head gently.

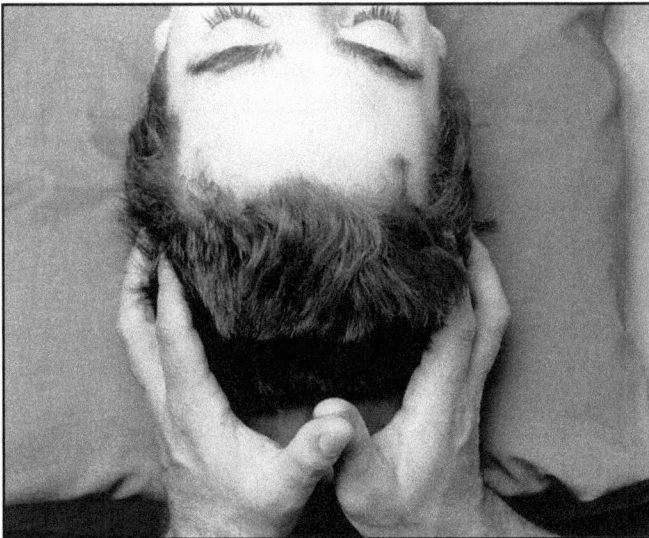

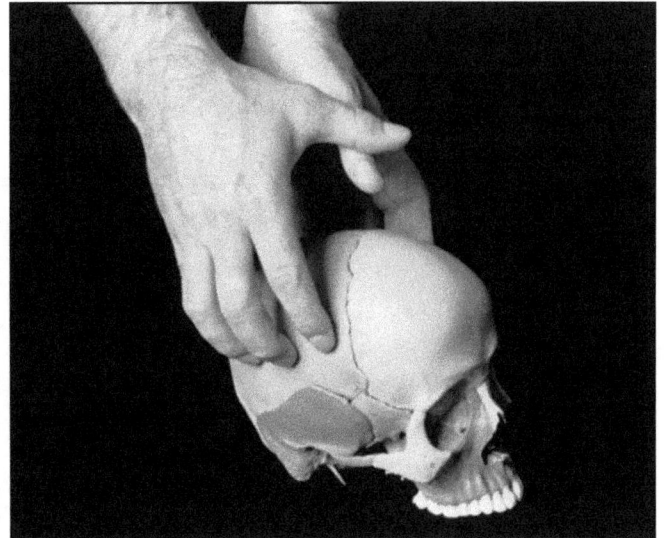

Parietal Lift

Temporal Bone Motion Testing and Decompression Technique

1. **Draw test.**   The operator sits at the head of the table and contacts the inferior portion of the mastoid with his index finger, gently drawing the temporal bones cephalward, either simultaneously or one at a time. Restriction of motion indicates a positive draw test.

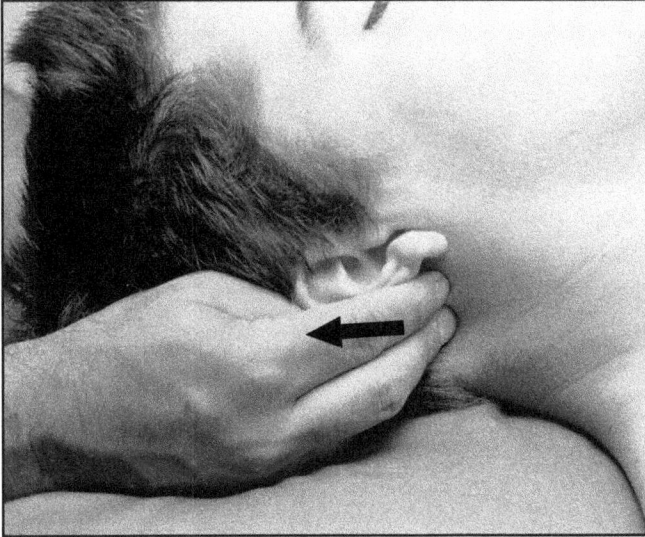

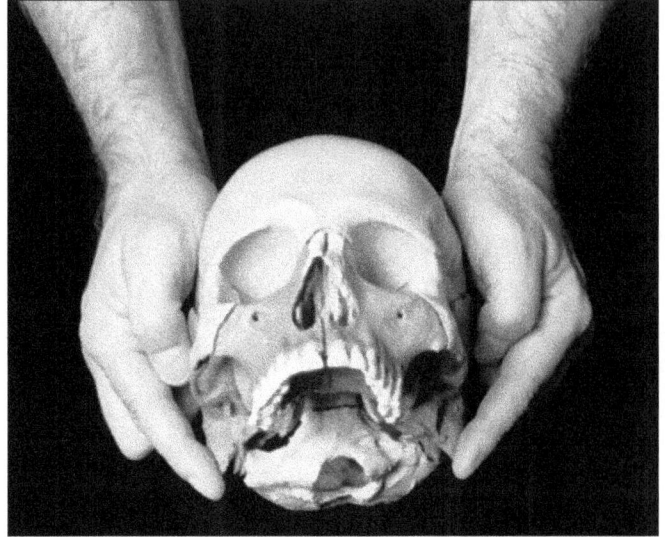

Temporal Bone Draw Test

2. **Bilateral temporal bone hold** with active and passive testing to determine internal and external rotation restriction of movement.

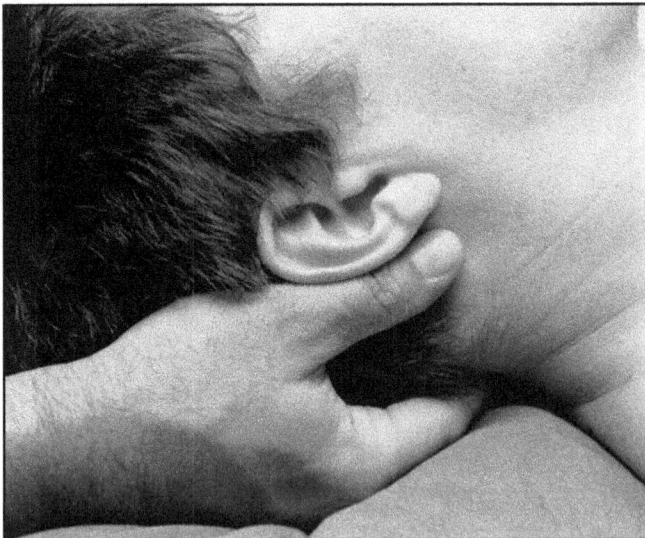

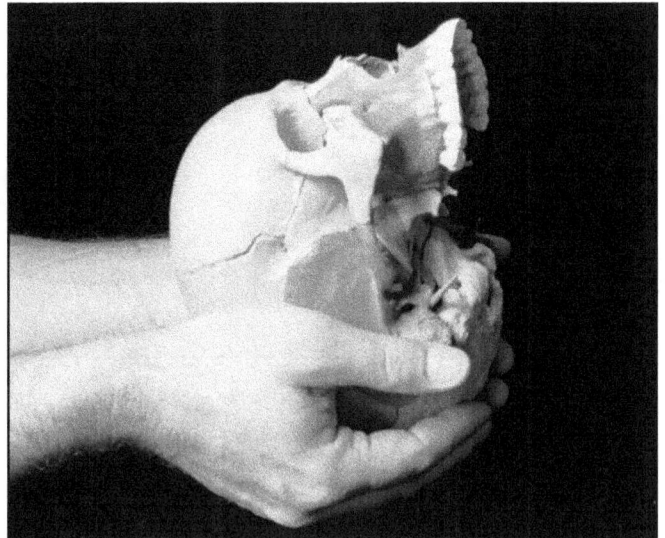

Bilateral Temporal Hold with Thumbs

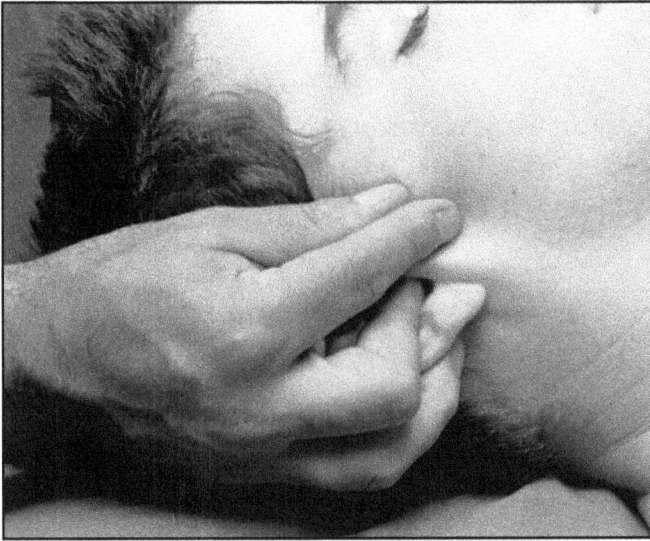

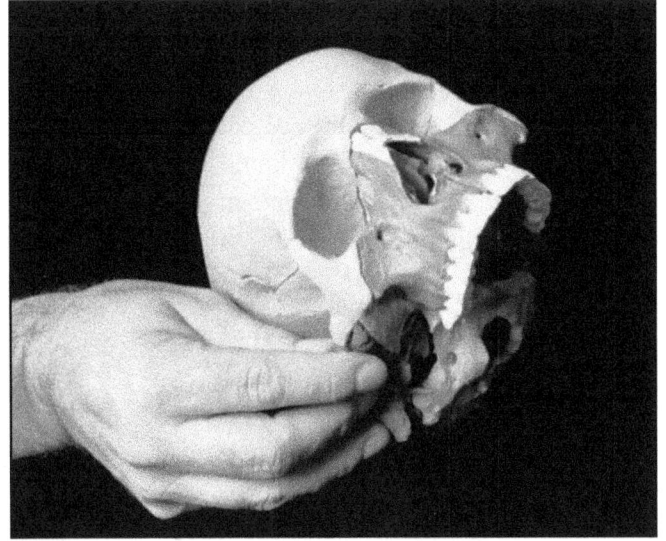

Bilateral Temporal Hold with Fingers

3. **Temporal bone decompression**. The patient is supine, operator sitting at the head of the table, holding the pinna of each ear in his fingers, apply a gentle traction in a posterolateral direction. Resistance to gentle traction indicates that compression is present, and the gentle traction should be maintained with equal pressure bilaterally until a release of tension is appreciated. Retest 1 and 2 above; if restriction is still present, then additional temporal bone dysfunctions must be diagnosed and treated.

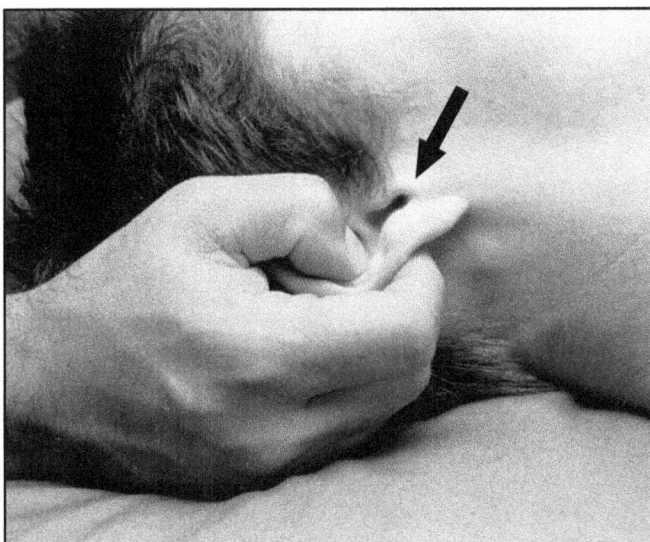

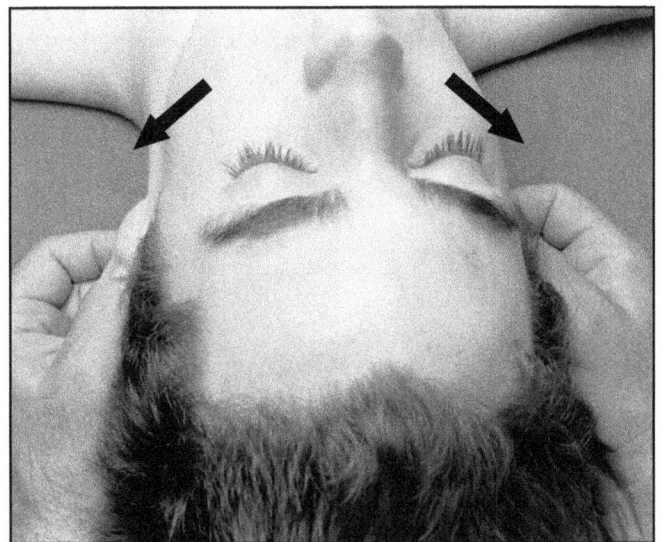

Temporal Bone Decompression

Direct Membranous Release

Pelvis

1. **Rock test**. Evaluation of pelvic motion is accomplished with the patient supine, the operator standing at the patient's side, contacting the patient's ASIS bilaterally. Gentle posterior force is applied one side at a time, assessing the compliance of the pelvic motion at the beginning and mid range of motion. End range of motion is not as important in determining a positive rock test.

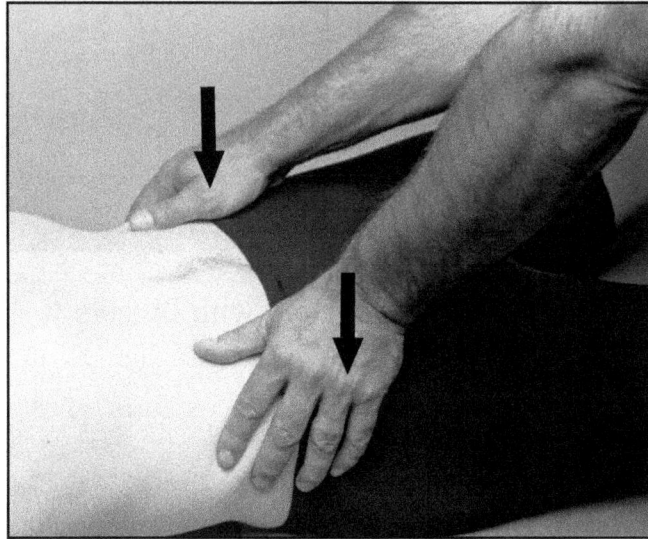

Pelvic Rock Test

2. **Traction test**. To confirm which side of the pelvis is restricted and to better assess changes after treatment, the operator may stand at the foot of the table, hold onto the heels of the feet bilaterally, and apply a gentle traction force through each leg individually, again assessing for the compliance of motion at the beginning and mid ranges of motion.

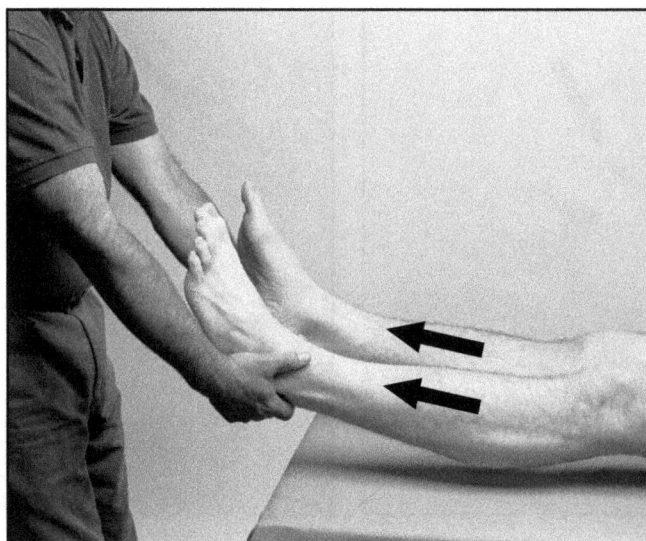

Pelvic Traction Test

3. **Unilateral treatment** with patient supine, operator sitting on the side of the patient where the dysfunction has been identified. The operator places one hand under the sacrum as in the lumbosacral decompression technique. The other hand contacts the sacral sulcus just medial to the PSIS, applying lateral traction through the PSIS while the other hand applies gentle sacral traction. This position is held until a tissue relaxation is felt between the two hands.

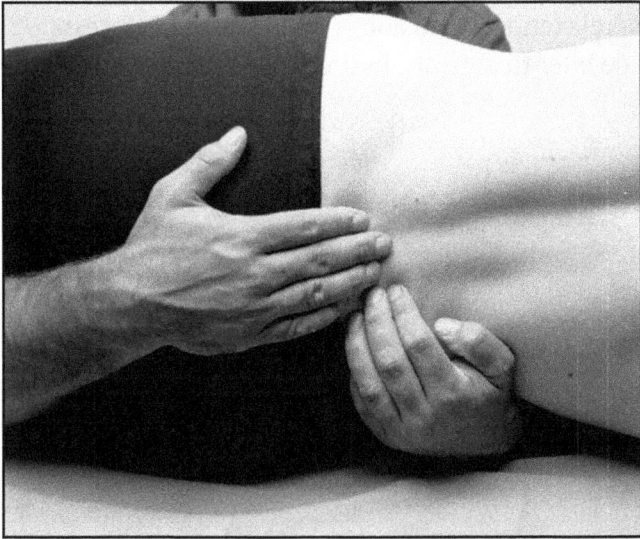

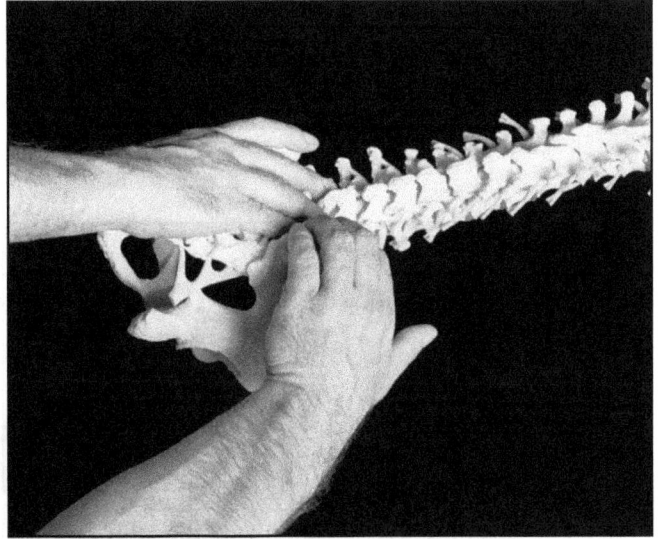

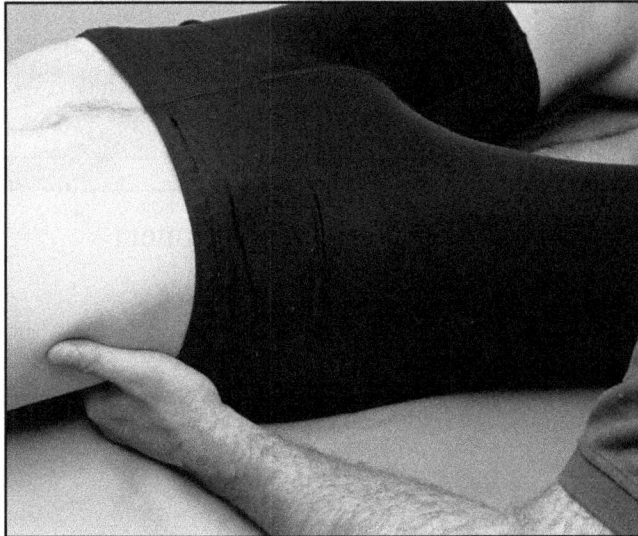

Unilateral Pelvic Treatment

4. **Bilateral treatment** with patient supine, operator sitting on the side of the dysfunction, with one hand on the sacrum and the other arm contacting the bilateral ASIS with the hand and forearm. Using this ASIS contact, the pelvis is translated left-right, sidebent, and rotated into the direction of mobile restrictions. The sacral contact is directed also in the direction that increases tissue tension in the pelvis. This position is held until a relaxation of tension is appreciated. Reassessment of the rock and traction tests should be made after treatment. Indirect positioning can also be used.

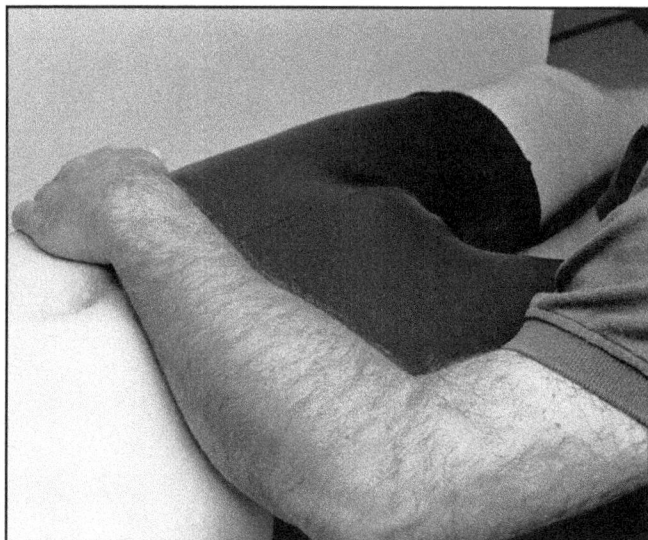

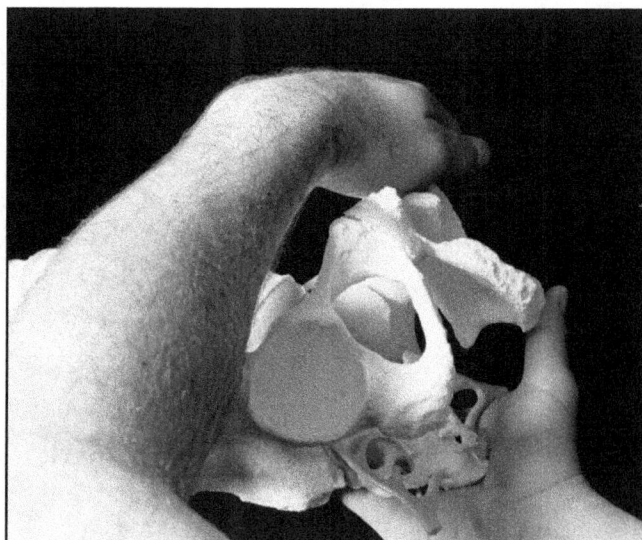

Bilateral Pelvic Treatment

Direct Membranous Release

<u>Occipital Condyle</u>

1. **Assessment** of occipital condylar compression is made with the operator sitting at the head of the table, contacting the inferior aspect of the occiput bilaterally. Gentle occipital traction is induced unilaterally, bringing the occiput into flexion, and any resistance to this motion is consistent with condylar compression on the same side. The occiput is positioned anteromedially on the side of condylar compression and won't move posterolaterally. Condylar compression may also present with hard, rigid and sensitive suboccipital tissues and may make the patient feel slightly nauseous.

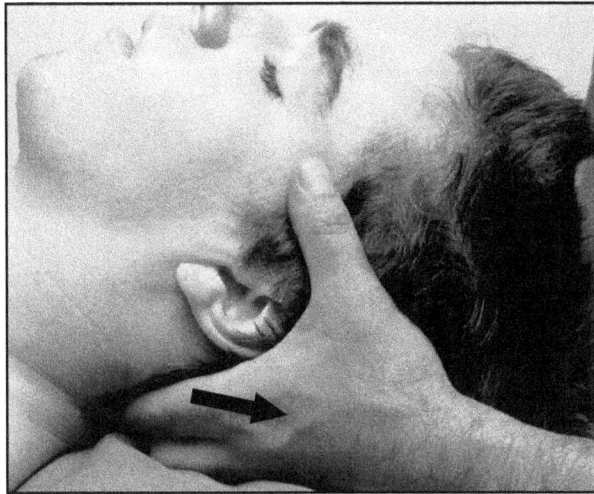

Occipital Condylar Compression Assessment

2. **Direct treatment** is performed in the same position, with the index finger of one hand drawing the condylar part posterolaterally, while the fingers of the other hand carry the squama on the same side posteromedially. In this technique, the occiput is visualized as a saucer-like structure which is rotated around a central axis, decompressing the occipital condyle from the 1st cervical vertebra in a posterosuperior and lateral direction. This position is held until a relaxation of tissue tension is felt.

   Indirect treatment may be performed if compression is more severe and unable to resolve with direct treatment. With hands along the inferior aspect of the occiput and on the midline, the restricted condylar part is carried anteromedially (exaggerating the dysfunction) by extending the upper cervical spine and side-bending toward the restricted condyle. The release is felt as anteromedial softening of the restricted condyle.

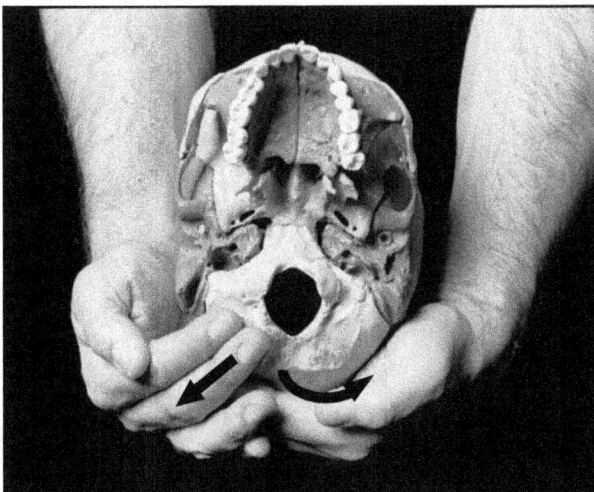

Direct Occipital Condylar Decompression

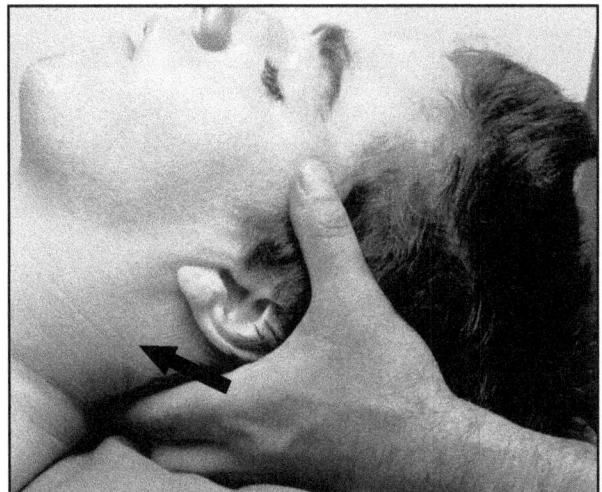

Indirect Occipital Condylar Decompression

3. **Release** of the condylar parts should be followed by restoration of normal tissue tone in the occipitoatlantal area. Slipping the middle fingers of both hands on either side of the midline of the occiput, the index fingers hold the arch of the atlas, and traction is applied between the two fingers. The thumbs should be on the mastoid portions of the temporal bones, and after applying a separative force between the index and middle fingers of both hands simultaneously, the squama of the occiput should be brought posteriorly and superiorly. The thumbs meanwhile follow the temporals as they move toward internal rotation, while the occiput releases at the atlas. To help accentuate this release, the patient may be instructed midway through the technique to gently tuck his chin and hold.

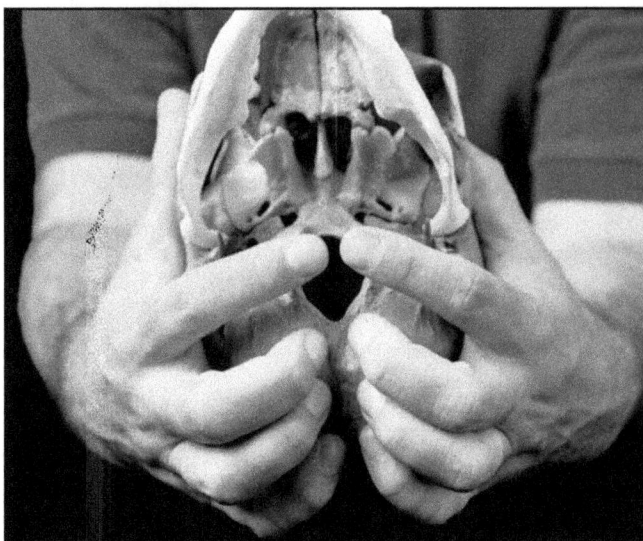

Occipitoatlantal Release

4. The **home occiput release** should be given to patients after performing this release. The exercise appears on the next page of the manual

Home Occiput Release

Purpose: This home exercise will improve the circulation of the cerebral spinal fluid and relax the membranes that cover the brain and spine. Doing this on a regular basis will aid your doctor in releasing membranous articular strains.

1. Lay on your back on the floor.
2. With feet 15" apart on the floor and knees together, bend your knees.
3. Place inches of books under the largest "bump" (external occipital protuberance) on the back of your head.
4. Lay in this position for 15 minutes once a day, preferably just before bed.
5. Roll on your side, off the books, lay quietly for 1 to 2 minutes before you get up.

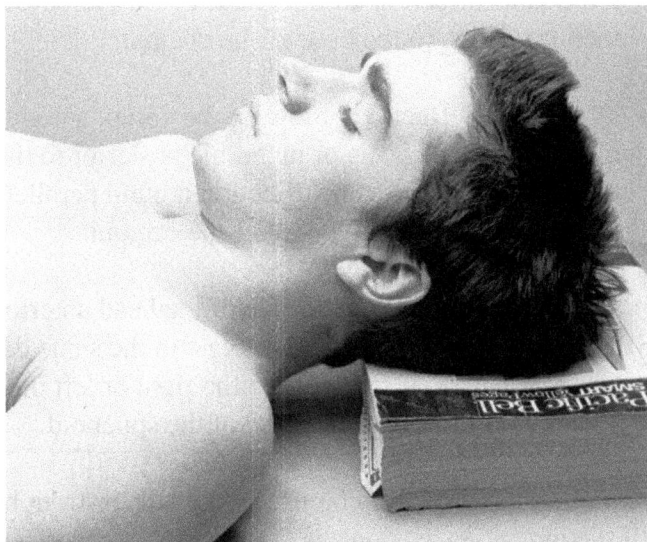

Home Occiput Release

Sphenobasilar Strain Patterns

Torsion   A response to trauma to one quadrant of the head e.g. an upward blow on the cheek. The sphenoid and occiput rotate in opposite directions around an A-P axis that extends from the nasion through the body of the sphenoid to the opisthion. The torsion is named by the higher greater wing of the sphenoid.

Side-bending Rotation   A response to lateral force at the level of the SBS inducing side-bending with convexity to the opposite side. The sphenoid and occiput: (a) sidebend in opposite directions around parallel vertical axes and (b) rotate in the same direction around A-P axes. Side-bending rotation is named by the side of the convexity.

Superior Vertical Strain   A traumatic effect of a blow on the vertex behind the plane of the SBS or inferiorly through the upper teeth anterior to the plane of the SBS. The sphenoid and occiput rotate in the same direction around parallel transverse axes carrying the base of the sphenoid superior relative to the base of the occiput.

Inferior Vertical Strain   A traumatic effect of a blow on the vertex anterior to the plane of the SBS or from below through the heels or mandible posterior to the plane of the SBS. The sphenoid and occiput rotate in the same direction around parallel transverse axes carrying the base of the sphenoid inferior to the base of the occiput.

Lateral Strain   A traumatic effect of a blow on the side of the head anterior or posterior to the plane of the SBS. The sphenoid and occiput rotate in the same direction around parallel vertical axes carrying the base of sphenoid to the right or left of the base of the occiput. Named by the direction of motion of the base of the sphenoid.

Compression   A compression of the SBS from before backwards or from behind forwards preventing full flexion and extension.

A. Torsion Strains

1. Characteristics
   a. This is a non-physiologic membranous articular strain on an A-P axis from nasion through the body of the sphenoid to opisthion.
   b. The sphenoid rotates in one direction and the occiput rotates in the opposite direction around this A-P axis. Torsion is named for the cephalad (high) great wing of the sphenoid.
   c. The anterior quadrant on the high wing side is in relative external rotation and may have a wider orbit and more prominent eyeball. On the same side the occiput is caudad (low) and that posterior quadrant is in relative external rotation.

2. Motion testing
   a. Vault hold - visualize an axle through the palm of each hand. Test motion by symmetrical rotation of each hand in opposite directions around this axle.
   b. Fronto-occipital hold - frontal hand elevates one great wing. Occipital hand elevates one side of occipital squama and lowers the other. Coordinate hands so that the great wing elevates on the same side that the occiput lowers.

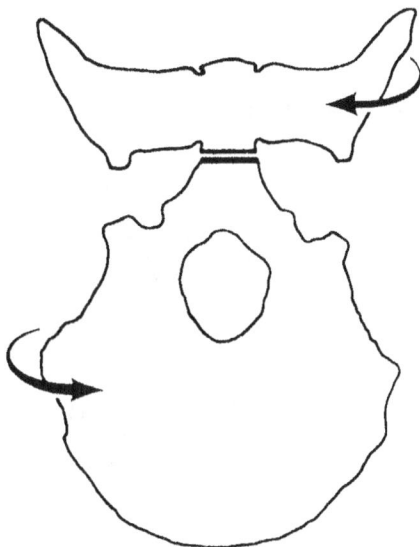

Fig. 10: Torsion Right   Torsion Right

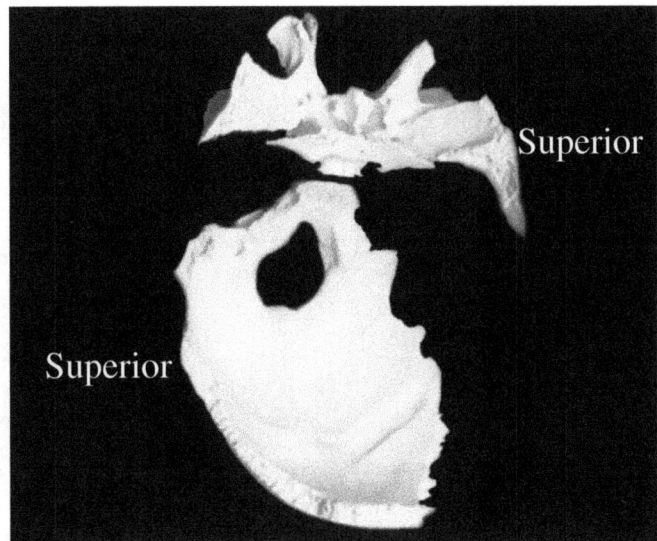

Palpatory experience: In the vault hold, one hand seems to rotate posteriorly or toward the operator (i.e., right hand in right torsion), the forefinger comes superiorly, little finger goes inferiorly , while the other hand rotates anteriorly or away from operator (forefinger goes inferiorly, little finger goes superiorly).

The experience is as if one held a pencil by its ends in each palm and turned the hands like two wheels in opposite directions. *(Note: The pencil **does not** represent the axis of motion of the bones themselves!)*

B. Sidebending - Rotation Strain

1. Characteristics
   a. This is a combined or compound motion in which rotation occurs around an A-P axis, sphenoid and occiput rotating in the same direction.
   b. Simultaneously sidebending occurs in opposite directions around two parallel vertical axes one through the center of the sphenoid body and the other through foramen magnum.
   c. In sidebending-rotation right the sphenoid and occiput move on an A-P axis with right great wing and right border of occiput moving caudad or inferiorly. Simultaneously each bone moves around its vertical axis, the sphenoid moving counter-clockwise and the occiput moving clockwise. Thus the SBS becomes convex and inferior on the right side.
   d. The sidebending-rotational strain is named for the side of convexity of the SBS.
   e. Observation
      1. One side of the head is relatively convex, the other somewhat flattened.
      2. On the side of the convexity, the anterior quadrant is in relative internal rotation with a narrower orbit.
      3. On the same side the posterior quadrant is in relative external rotation.

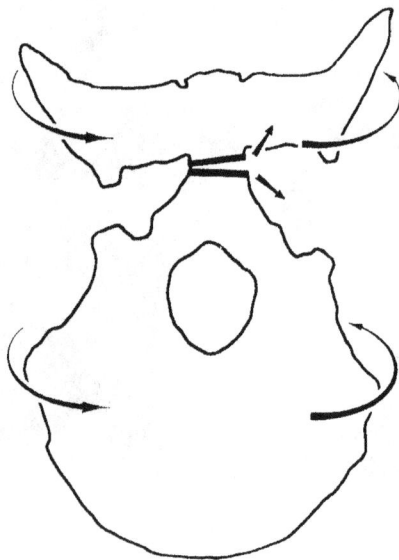

Fig. 11: Sidebending-Rotation Right   Sidebending-Rotation Right

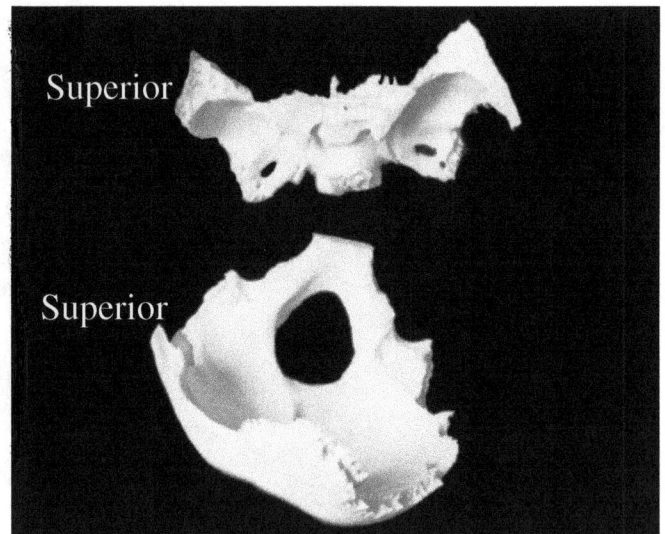

Sidebending Rotation

2. Axes: Sidebending and Rotation
    a. **Sidebending axes**: There are two vertical axes - one through the foramen magnum of the occiput and the other through the body of the sphenoid.

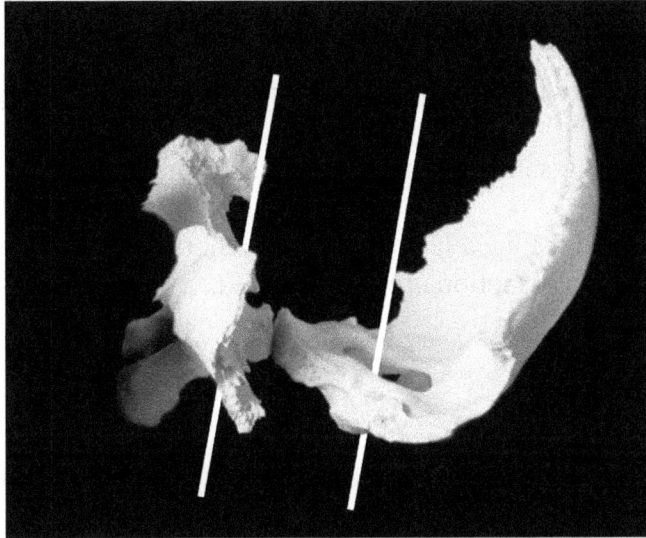

Sidebending Axes

    b. **Rotation axis**: anteroposterior axis from opisthion to nasion.

2. Motion testing
    a. Vault hold. Approximate the index and 5th fingers on one side while simultaneously lifting superiorly. Coordinate this movement with the opposite hand which spreads index and 5th fingers while simultaneously moving inferiorly.

Palpatory experience: Sidebending is experienced in the vault hold by approximating the fingers of one hand (less distance from forefinger to little finger) on the side of the concavity. Simultaneously, the other hand experiences a spreading or widening (greater distance from forefinger to little finger).

Rotation is represented by an inferior movement of the whole 'spread' hand (as in flexion) and superior movement of the whole approximated hand (as in extension).

In a right sidebending rotation the right hand is spread wider, moves inferior, and has an externally rotated temporal in its palm. There is a feeling of a 'lot more head' in the right hand.

C. Lateral Strains

    1. Characteristics

        a. This is usually caused by trauma in a lateral direction to the side of the anterior or posterior cranium.

        b. Occiput and sphenoid are moved on their individual vertical axes in the same direction (clockwise or counter-clockwise) creating a shearing strain at the SBS.

        c. The head may assume the shape of a parallelogram (infants).

        d. Basiosphenoid is forced lateralward in relation to basiocciput. The lesion is named for the direction of motion of basiosphenoid.

    2. Motion testing

        a. Vault hold - The index fingers carry the greater wings of sphenoid laterally in one direction while the fifth fingers carry the occiput laterally in the opposite direction.

        b. Fronto-occipital hold - The frontal hand carries the sphenoid laterally in one direction while the occipital hand carries the occiput laterally in the opposite direction.

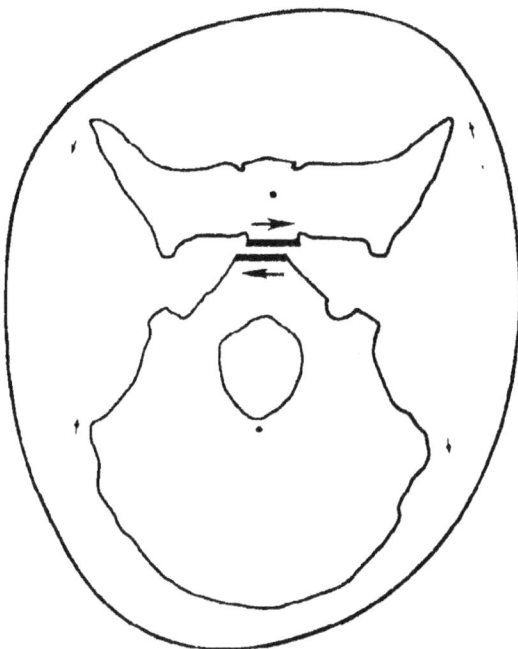

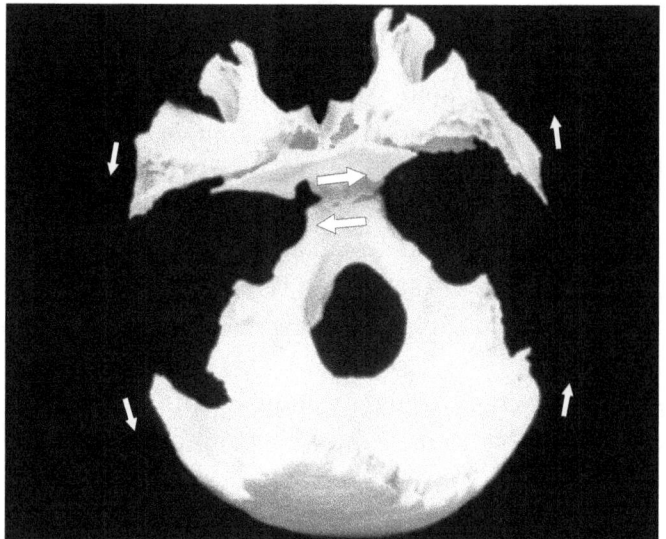

Fig. 12: Lateral Strain Right

D. Vertical Strains

1. Characteristics
   a. This is usually caused by trauma to the anterior cranium influencing the sphenoid (superiorly or inferiorly) or to the posterior cranium influencing the occiput (inferiorly or superiorly).

   b. It is a shearing strain of the SBS occurring around the transverse axis of each bone. The sphenoid is moved toward flexion while the occiput is moved toward extension or vice versa.

   c. This strain is named for the direction the posterior surface of the body of the sphenoid has been moved, i.e. vertical strain superior (high) or vertical strain inferior (low).

2. Axes: Two parallel transverse axes (as in flexion/extension):
   a. **Superior vertical strain:** A traumatic effect of a blow on the vertex behind the plane of the SBS or from below through the mouth, anterior to the plane of the SBS. The sphenoid and occiput rotate in the same direction around parallel transverse axes carrying the base of the sphenoid superior relative to the base of the occiput.

   b. **Inferior vertical strain:** A traumatic effect of a blow on the vertex anterior to the plane of the SBS or from below through the heels or mandible posterior to the plane of the SBS. The sphenoid and occiput rotate in the same direction around parallel transverse axes carrying the base of the sphenoid inferior relative to the base of the occiput.

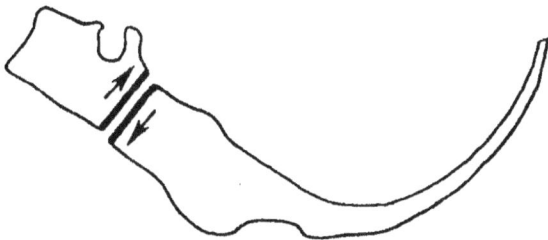

Fig. 13: Vertical Strain Superior

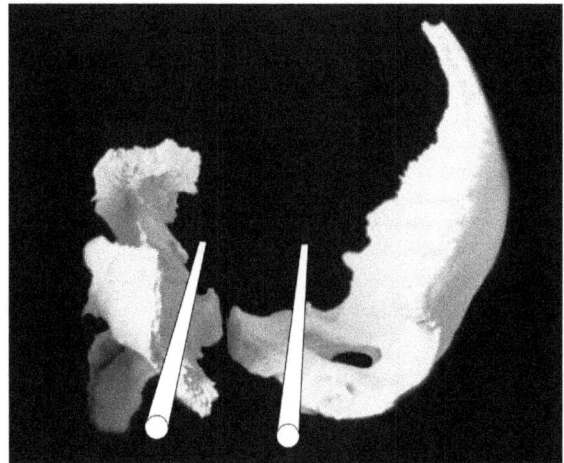

Axes of Motion- Superior Vertical Strain

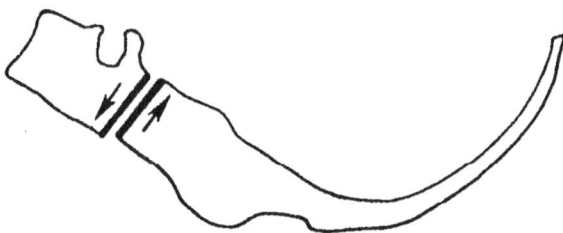

Fig. 14: Vertical Strain Inferior

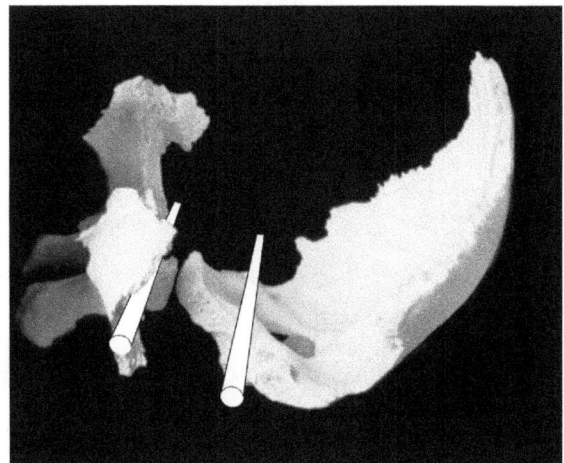

Axes of Motion- Inferior Vertical Strain

Vertical Strains

3. Motion testing

      a. Vault hold - carry great wings toward flexion with index fingers simultaneously with carrying occiput toward extension with fifth fingers. Then reverse the directions by carrying the sphenoid toward extension with index fingers while simultaneously carrying occiput toward flexion with fifth fingers.

      b. Fronto-occipital hold - this position may be easier to control for motion-testing vertical strain. The frontal hand influences the sphenoid toward flexion simultaneously with the occipital hand influencing the occiput toward extension. With hands in same position, reverse the direction of each.

Palpatory experience: In a superior vertical strain, the forefingers of both hands move inferiorly (the sphenoid base is moving superiorly). Also, the little fingers of both hands will move superiorly (occipital base is moving inferiorly).

Thus, both hands feel as if they are rotating forward in a superior vertical strain, while in an inferior vertical strain they will both rotate posteriorly.

Sacrum – in phase with occiput

54

E. Compression of SBS

1. Characteristics

   a. This strain occurs at the SBS as a result of pressure or trauma to the front of the head or face, or to the back of the head or to the entire periphery, i.e. the compression of the infant cranium during the birth process.

   b. It manifests as a restriction (mild, moderate, or severe) of any motion at the SBS. With a severe compression, the cranium feels "solid" or cement-like.

2. Motion testing

   a. This strain is recognized as the operator motion tests all of the other patterns, he is aware of limited motion or absence of motion in the SBS.

   b. compression along the anteroposterior axis (as in torsion and rotation).

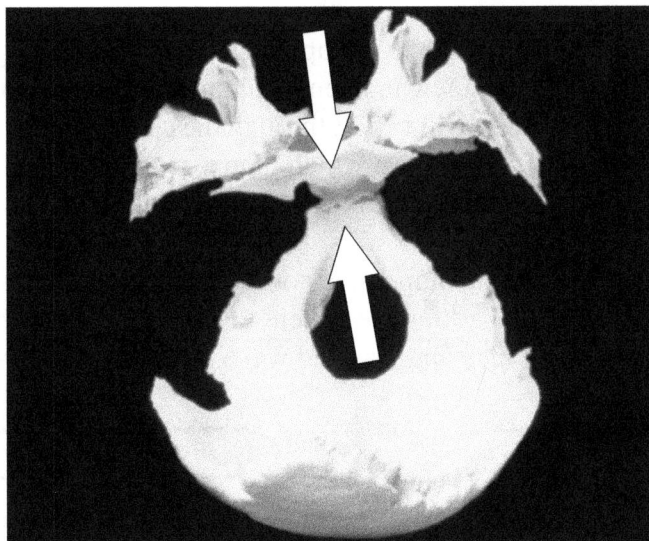

Palpatory experience: Fingers of both hands approximate. The distance between the sphenoid wings and the occipital lateral angles on both sides is reduced. Because this severely limits the resiliency of the SBS, flexion and extension are limited, and often these heads will feel hard and generally limited in movement of any kind. Occasionally, with very strong compressions, the SBS exhibits a rebound phenomena with the fingers of both hands separating.

SBS Strain Patterns- Balanced Membranous Tension

<u>Assessment</u> of SBS strain patterns is performed using the standard vault hold. Predominant SBS strains will be appreciated by the sequence of movements palpated under the operator's hands. These movements may appear in a sequence of strain patterns, one after the other, and are normally perceived as a pulling of the cranial mechanism into the configuration of one or more of the SBS strain patterns. Less dominant strain patterns can be appreciated by active motion testing. The operator induces the paired SBS strain patterns, gently holding each direction for a few moments to see if the cranial vault moves easily in the direction tested. If movement is not easily accomplished, then a strain pattern exists in the direction of easy motion testing.

<u>Treatment</u> using the point of balanced membranous tension is an indirect technique and focuses on one or more of the strain patterns identified. The focus of treatment is primarily on traumatic SBS strain patterns, including lateral strains, vertical strains and compression. The technique is performed with the vault hold into the direction of the SBS strain pattern at the neutral point of balanced membranous tension. This neutral point is a physiologic mid point between the end ranges of motion with the hands positioning the cranium in the direction of the SBS strain (*i.e.*, away from the barrier) at a point of maximal tissue compliance or minimal tension. While this position is held, stack on top any other traumatic strains present in the mechanism in the same manner. If compression exists, then the occipital and sphenoid contacts should be gently compressed together, bringing a compressive force into the compression dysfunction. After a few moments holding these strain patterns in a stacked position, a slow membranous unwinding will be felt through the contacting fingers, eventually reaching a point of no motion or a "stillpoint," at which time a gentle pulsation will be appreciated, followed by a return to normal cranial flexion and extension motion.

Frequently, unwinding occurs, but a clear endpoint is not always appreciated. Maneuvers that may help to bring about an endpoint include asking the patient to dorsiflex both of his feet or take a deep inhalation. Additionally, the operator may apply a fluid wave through the bregma by gently blowing three times.

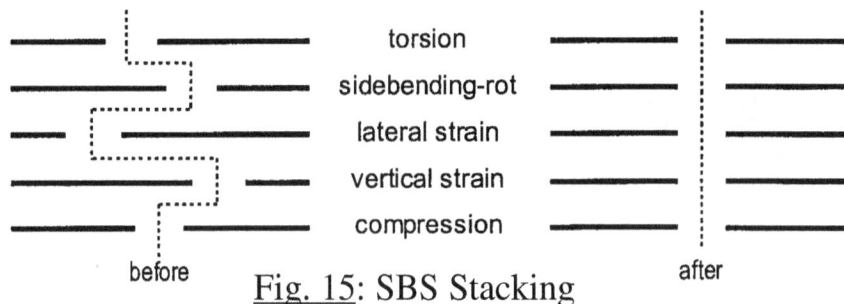

torsion

sidebending-rot

lateral strain

vertical strain

compression

before   <u>Fig. 15</u>: SBS Stacking   after

<u>Summary of Procedure</u>
-Assessment of SBS Strain
-Stacking of Individual Neutral Points
-Unwinding
-Stillpoint
-New Flexion

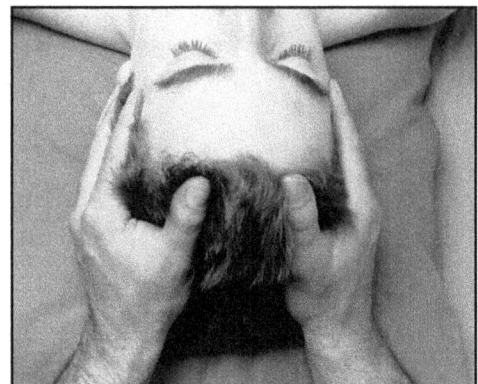

SBS Strain Treatment

Fluid Wave

Biomechanical engineering is a field that has brought new knowledge about the properties of tissue which are relevant to manual medicine, and specifically craniosacral approaches. Fluid mechanics has revealed new information regarding the properties of tissue in response to mechanical forces, both traumatic and therapeutic. All tissues in the body exist within a tissue state that ranges from solid to fluid. We know that most of the body is in fact water, and therefore most of the tissues in the body have a large percentage of water content. There is a term that describes this part-solid/part-fluid (sol-gel) characteristic of tissue, and it is referred to as colloid. Colloids exhibit properties that reflect behavior of both solids and fluids, and are the predominant constituents of the human body. Very sudden and strong forces, which are typically associated with trauma, cause the colloid to respond as a solid, with increasing tissue resistance and rigidity. However, when slow and gentle forces are used to interact with the colloid, the colloid reacts as a fluid, with yielding and flowing responses.

When we speak of a fluid wave, we are referring to a fluid movement which is initiated in the body as a result of slow, gentle but persistent forces that are introduced into the body. The fluid nature of tissue responds to these types of forces by producing flowing and rippling movements that are dispersed over a wide area of the tissue surface. Hard and sudden forces are dispersed within a very small area of the tissue, causing contracture and rigidity of the tissue.

Using this principle, we can stimulate tissue "release and flow" by directing specific forces into areas of tissue rigidity or dysfunction. In application to cylindrical and spherical objects, as in human form, a constant gentle pressure applied in an area diametrically opposite the location of tissue dysfunction serves to direct a flowing and rippling movement in the restricted tissues (i.e. sutures). In essence, we can send a fluid wave from one part of the body to treat an area of restriction in another part of the body.

V-spread and Fluid Wave Technique

This is a very simple, safe technique for releasing any peripheral suture such as frontonasal, nasomaxillary, occipitomastoid, etc.

The Technique:

Place the index and middle fingers of the ipsilateral hand on either side of the suture. (For a linear suture like the occipitomastoid use the palmar surface of the length of two fingers; for a small suture like the frontonasal use the fingertips.)

Place the palm of the other hand on the head at the other end of the longest diameter of the head from the suture; e.g. for the right occipitomastoid place the hand on the left frontal only. you will soon perceive a gentle impulse coming into the palm of this hand. Now cluster the fingers at the site of that impulse. You have thereby localized the optimum place from which to direct the potency of the CSF to the restricted suture. As long as the suture is restricted the fluid tide will bounce back but as soon as it releases you will feel a gentle, easy motion between your hands.

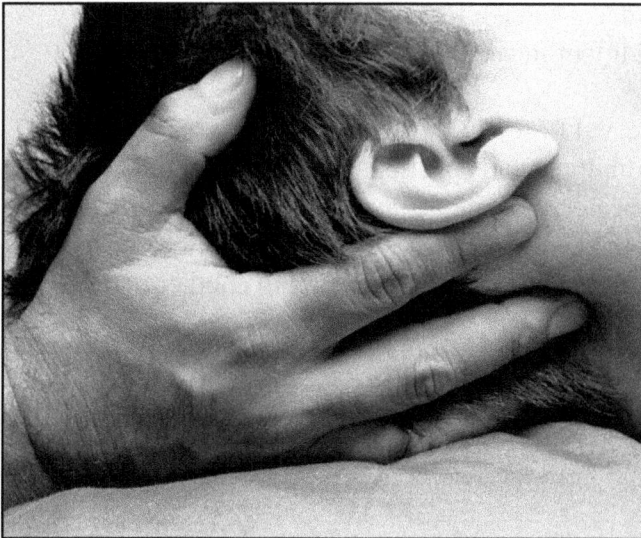

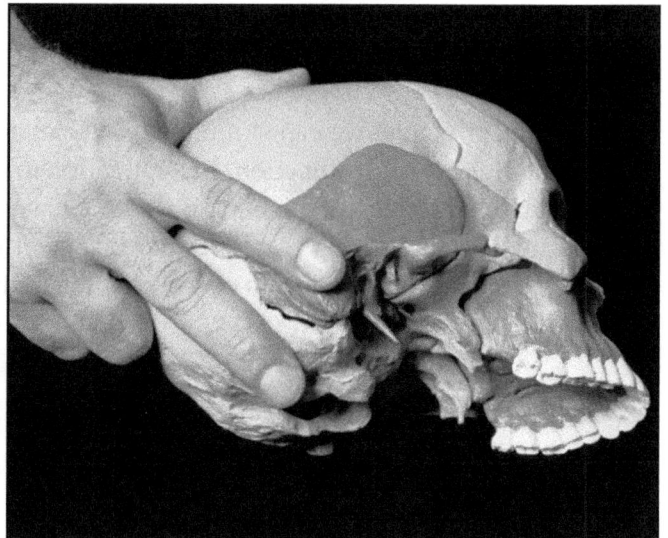

V-Spread- Occipitomastoid

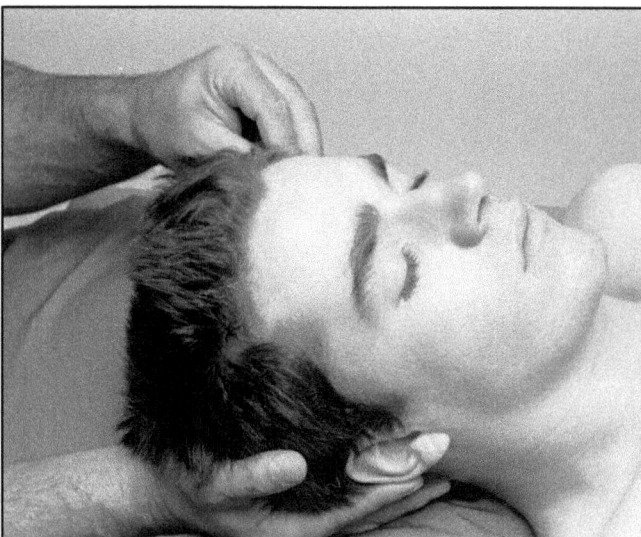

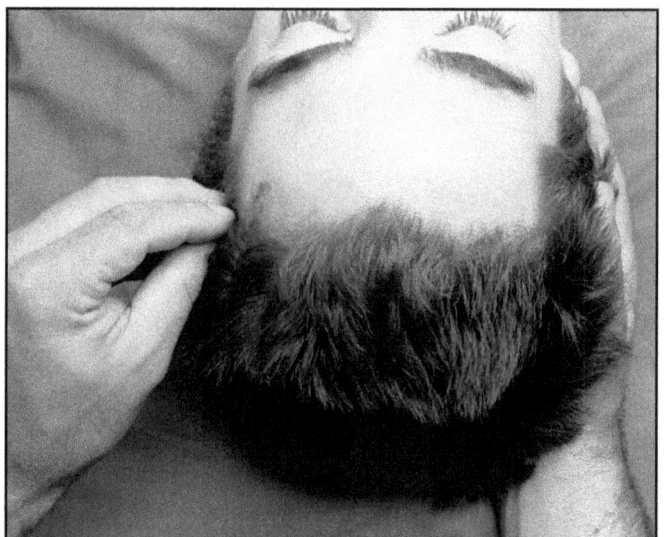

Fluid Wave- Occipitomastoid Suture

Temporal Bone Checkup

The temporal bone must be considered as one of the central factors causing cranial dysfunction. Once the peripheral articulations have been successfully treated, the temporal bone can be approached.

A general screening test for temporal bone dysfunction is a draw test, which merely applies a cephalad pressure through the mastoid process of the temporal bones to test for the relative superior compliance of this motion. A temporal bone that has dysfunction will be noncompliant in this test, and the mastoid process will not move in a superior direction. The draw test can be applied simultaneously to both sides or one side at a time.

Once the side of temporal bone dysfunction is determined, a series of tests to consider and rule out all the temporal bone dysfunctions is necessary. Starting at the posteriormost aspect of the temporal bone, we consider the temporoparietal suture and particularly the parietal notch as an initial area where dysfunction can occur. This dysfunction is assessed by doing a parietal lift, and the sensation of reduced mobility in the area of the parietal notch or temporoparietal suture can be appreciated and treated by continuing to completion the parietal lift technique.

Next we have the occipitomastoid suture as we come inferior on the temporal bone. This should be assessed and treated in the manner previously described under "V-spread".

The petrojugular region of the temporal bone can be assessed by asking the patient to take a deep inhalation and then assessing the relative movement of the temporal bones bilaterally. If there is a dysfunction of the petrojugular area, the normal external rotation of the temporal bone will not be appreciated during inhalation, and in fact an internal rotation of the temporal bone will be felt. The temporal bone is "out of phase" with respiratory motion. (if external rotation of the temporal bone is reduced upon inhalation, this is not a petrojugular dysfunction but reflects a different problem and should not be treated as "out of phase.") Internal rotation is held during a maximal exhalation, returning to external rotation upon the ensuing inhalation. Treatment should ensue in the manner described in order to bring the temporal bone motion back into phase with respiratory motion.

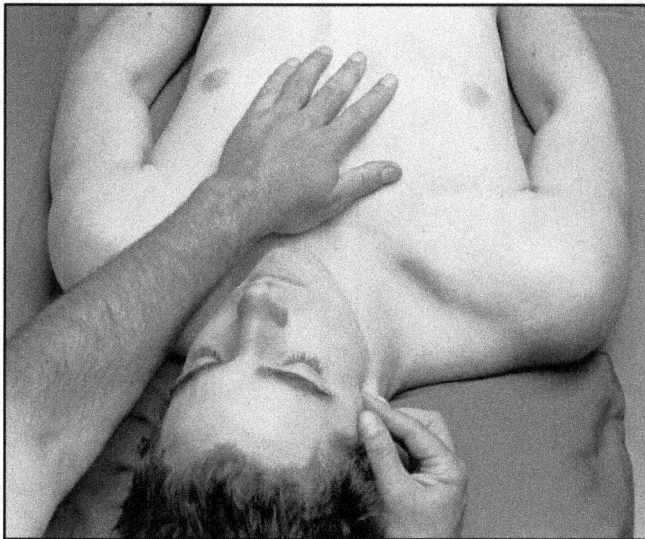

Petrojugular Treatment

Next we have the <u>petrobasilar</u> area, which is the part of the temporal bone that is affected by temporal compression, which has been previously described using the "ear pull" technique.

The <u>sphenosquamous</u> suture is next. Dysfunction of this suture can be appreciated by the operator putting his hands over the anterior aspect of the temporal bone at the pterion. The patient is asked to take a deep inhalation, the normal motion of the sphenosquamous suture will be that of expansion, with a bulging or rising sensation underneath your hands. If the suture is compressed, there will be no such movement appreciated. Treatment uses indirect intraoral technique separating and releasing the sphenosquamous articulation in the directions of flexion/extension, internal/external rotation, anterior/posterior and superior/inferior shear. When all the articulations of the temporal bone have been treated, it should be followed by temporal bone balancing technique of the dural membranes.

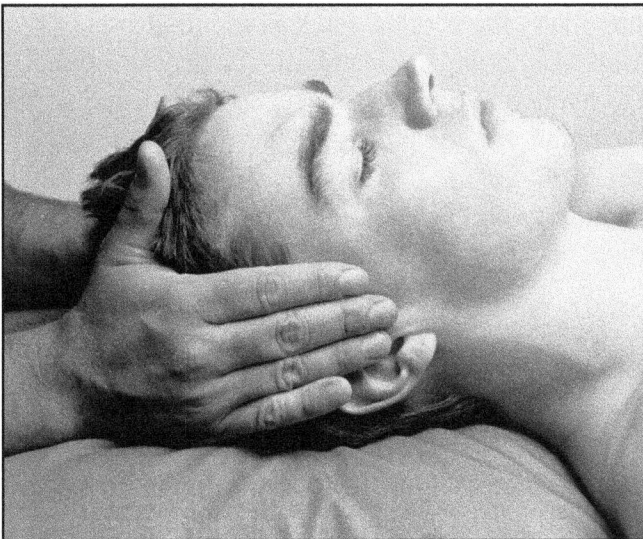

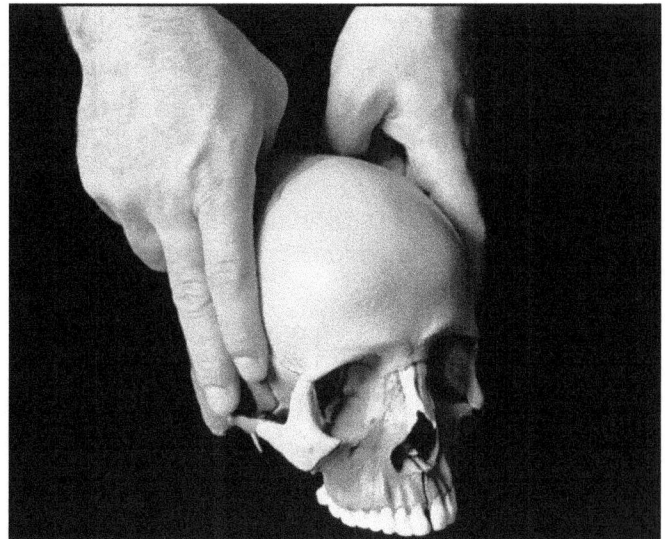

Sphenosquamous Diagnosis

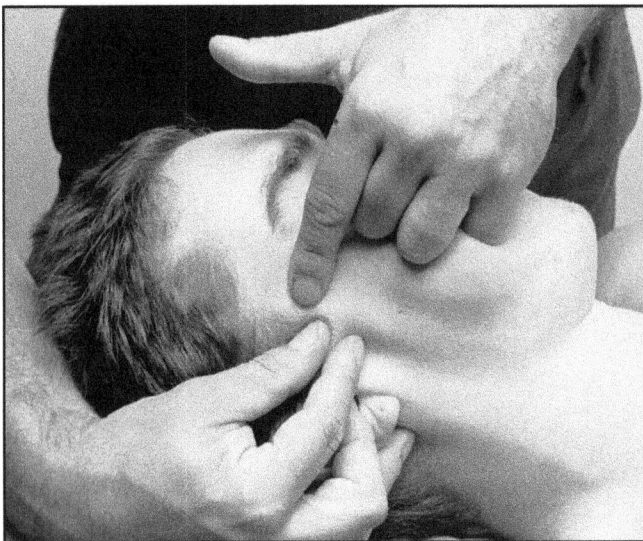

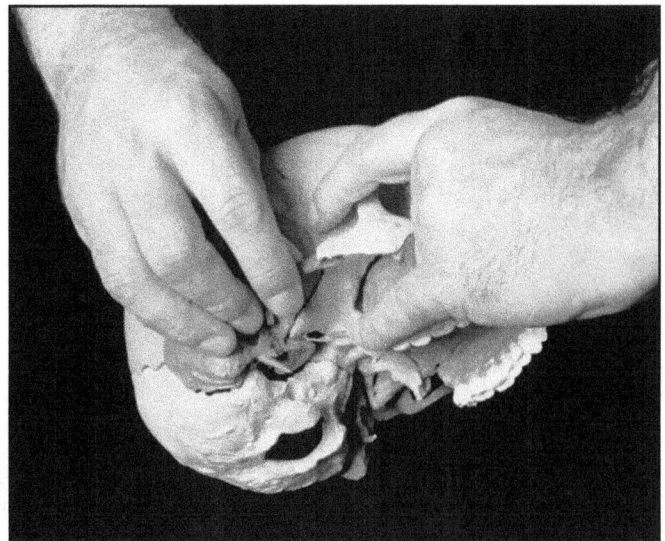

Sphenosquamous Treatment

Temporal Bone Balancing Technique

The patient is supine, the operator is at the head of the table with the temporal bone hold along the mastoid process. Temporal bone testing should be carried out by introducing cephalad/caudad and anterior/posterior translation on both sides. Position in the relative direction of ease and follow any unwinding. Next, test internal/external rotation, similarly positioning in the direction of ease.

For treatment, the directions of ease should all be held in a simultaneous fashion while unwinding is appreciated and followed until normal internal and external rotation are resumed.

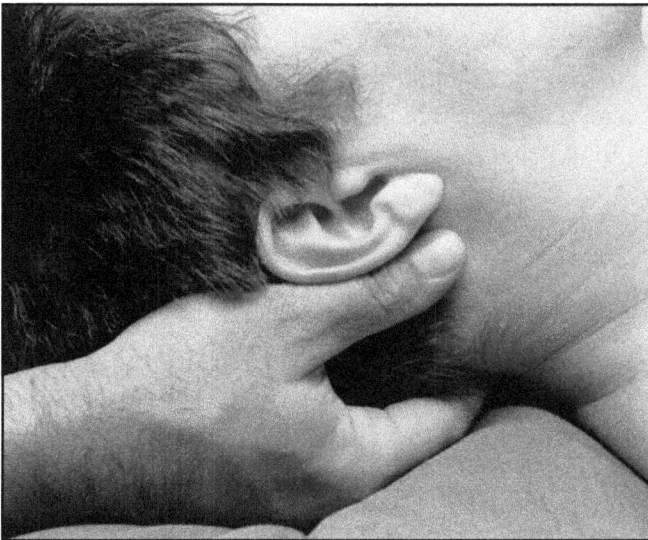

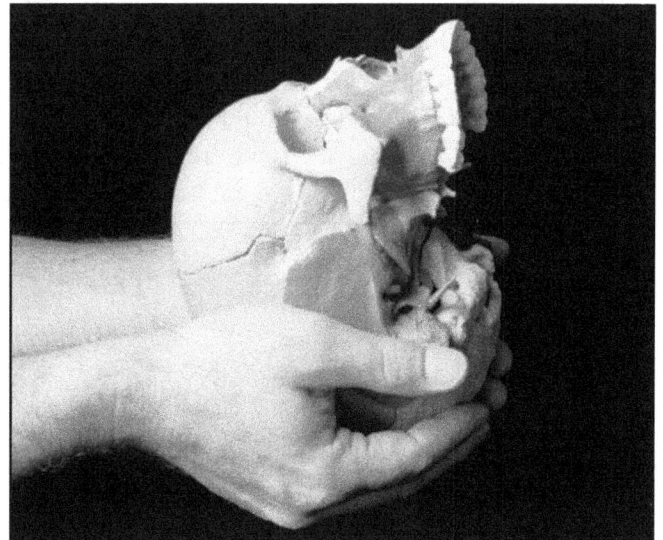

Temporal Bone Balancing

Treatment of Transverse Diaphragms Using Body Molding and Balancing Technique

1. Pelvic Diaphragm

The pelvic diaphragm is formed by the pelvic myofascial attachments circumferentially, including the levator ani group. The operator contacts the sacrum with the patient in a supine position, evaluating its motion in response to the CRI. The opposite hand is placed along the pubic rim at the pubic symphysis. Gentle compression is undertaken and the sense of movement evaluated under the influence of the CRI. A gentle swelling and contraction may be appreciated in this two-hand position. There may be a sense of unwinding present before a balanced symmetrical position of the hands is achieved.

2. Thoracic Diaphragm

The thoracic diaphragm is defined by the inferior aspects of the thoracic cage, the diaphragmatic attachments extending via the crura as far as L1 and L2. A hand is placed posteriorly spanning the area between T12 and L1 bilaterally, with the anterior hand placed at the inferior aspect of the sternum at the xiphoid process and contacting the inferior anterior rib angles bilaterally. Gentle compression is undertaken and a sense of tension appreciated for presence of asymmetry. Separating the effects of CRI from pulmonary respiration forces is difficult in this position. If necessary, the patient may be asked to hold their breath briefly to permit focusing on the effects of the CRI in this region. Once again, balancing forces between the hands culminating in a symmetrical swelling and contraction between these points should be sought. Once balanced, the cephalad-caudad rhythm of flexion and extension (coiling and uncoiling) through the central axis can be felt. Unilateral left and right thoracic hemi-diaphragms can be treated individually.

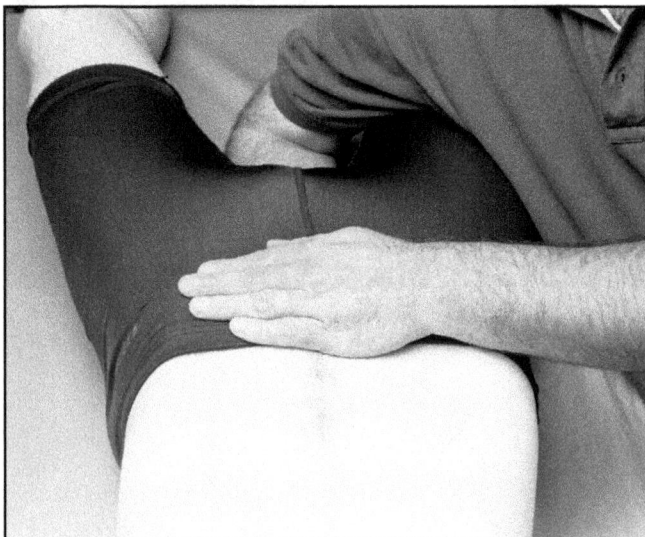

Pelvic Diaphragm Treatment

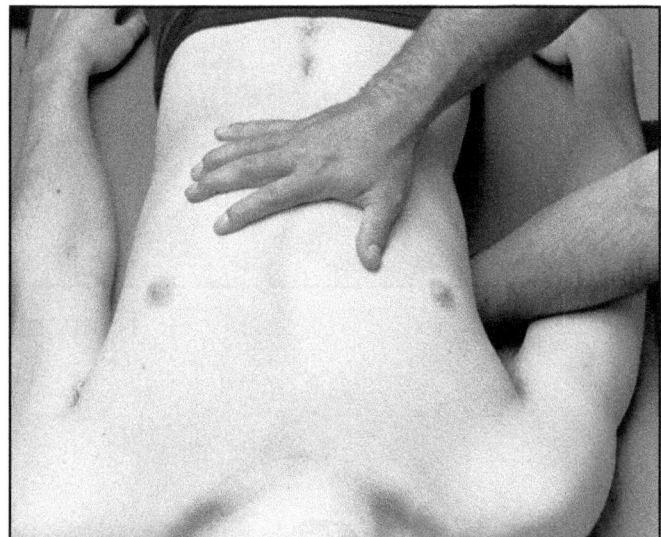

Thoracic Diaphragm Treatment

3. Thoracic Outlet

The thoracic outlet, unlike the previously described areas, does not have a well defined diaphragmatic structure, but rather is a region that behaves diaphragm-like in discriminating between major regions of the body. Contact posteriorly spans the cervicalthoracic junction bilaterally; anterior positioning includes spanning between the inferior aspects of the clavicles and the manubrium of the sternum. Again, a gentle compression is applied, with the appreciation of regional asymmetry or symmetry noted under the influence of the CRI. A balancing is sought to create a symmetrical swelling and contraction sense under the hands.

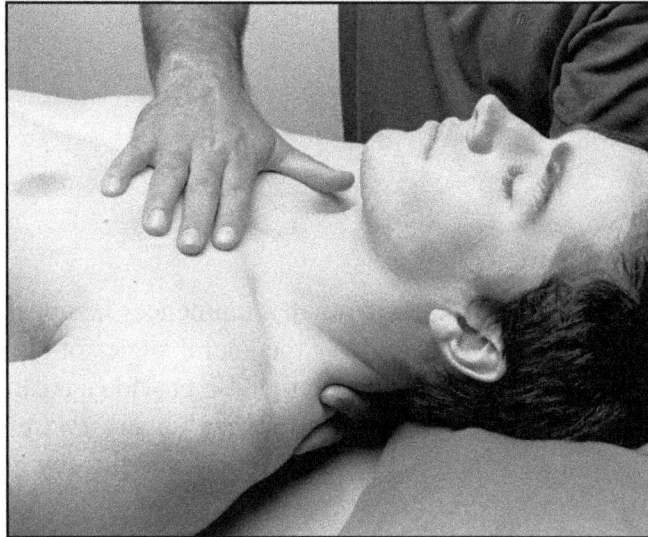

Thoracic Outlet Treatment

4. Transverse Cranial Diaphragm

The transverse cranial diaphragm describes the attachments of the tentorium cerebelli where the vault hold is contacting these structures from the side. The hand posteriorly cradles the occiput along the nuchal line posteriorly, with the anterior hand spanning the frontal bone between the two wings of the sphenoid. From this position, a flexion/extension motion of the cranial rhythm is appreciated, and a sense of symmetry or asymmetry of this motion is noted. Treatment of the tentorial components of the membrane is again addressed by gentle compression and balancing technique. Symmetrical sense of swelling or contraction of the head is sought as an endpoint for this treatment approach.

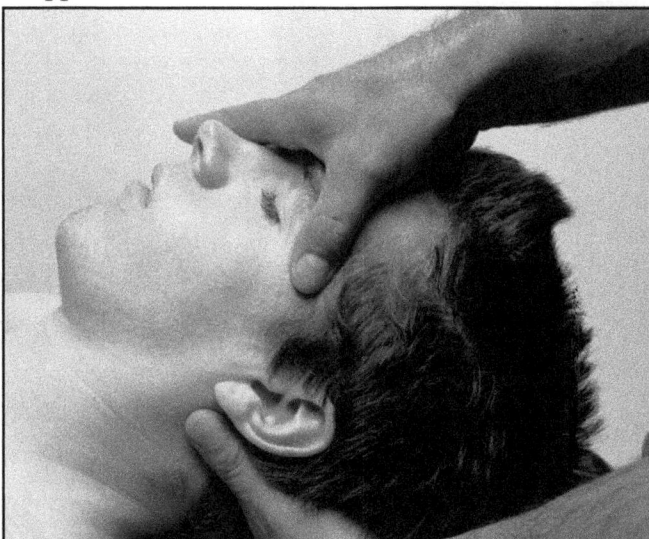

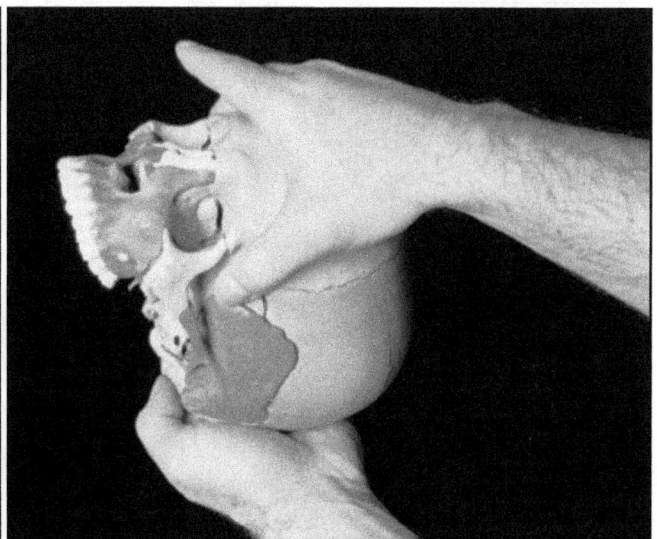

Transverse Cranial Diaphragm Treatment

63

Compression of the IVth Ventricle- Stillpoint Induction

Objective: To stimulate the body's inherent therapeutic potency to overcome whatever dysfunction is present by inducing a stillpoint.

Mechanism: By inducing extension (or internal rotation) of the primary respiratory mechanism the potency of the cerebrospinal fluid is directed from the ventricular system to the periphery of the body.

Technique:
Operator at the head of the table.
Patient supine.

1) Occipital Approach

Place one hand in the palm of the other so that the thenar eminences lie uppermost and parallel to each other. Then slip them under the head permitting the lateral angles of the occiput medial to the occipitomastoid suture to rest on them. The thenar eminences provide a cushion for the occiput which should be comfortable for the patient and operator. The fingers are free and not pressing on the neck. The weight of the head rests on the thenar eminences and thereby gently compresses the lateral angles.

Become aware of the rhythmic motion of the occiput. Follow it toward extension: i.e., as the hands rock gently toward the operator. Discourage flexion (the hands moving away). The amplitude of the motion will get progressively smaller until the still point is reached—a moment of intense activity where the therapeutic potency of the CRI is re-organizing. This passes so swiftly it may not be detected but it is followed by a sense of softening and warmth in the occiput and a gentle rocking motion like a little boat on quiet water. At the same time thoracic respiration should become primarily diaphragmatic and approximate the some rate as the CRI.

Observe the cranial activity for the inititation of a new flexion cycle and then very gently remove your hands and put the head on the table.

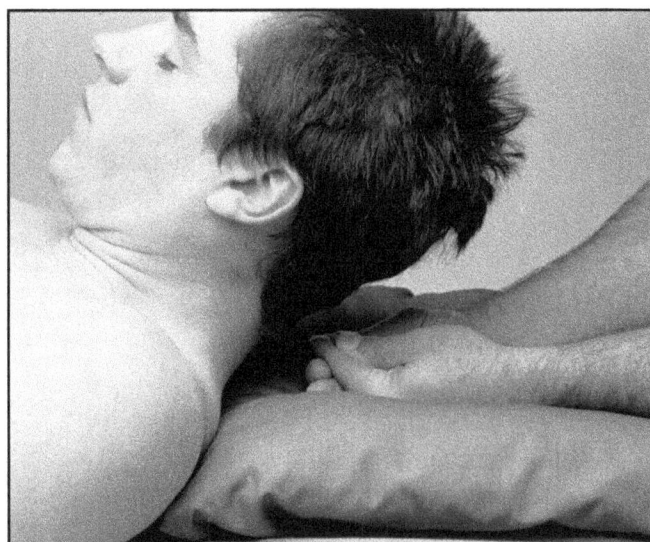

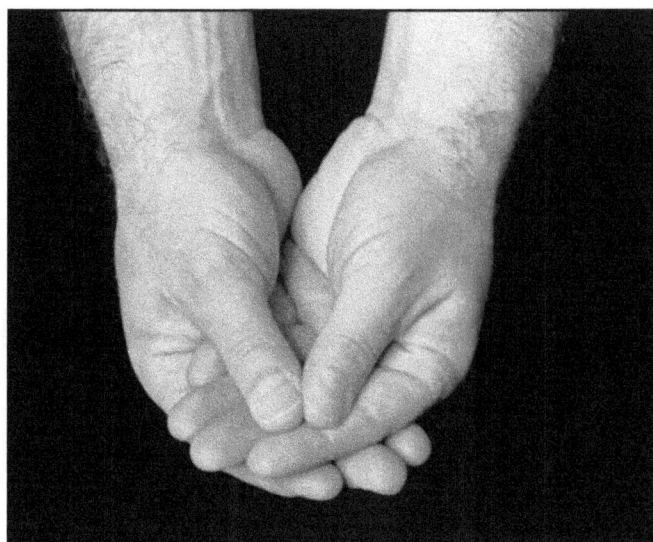

CV-IV Occipital Approach Hand Placement

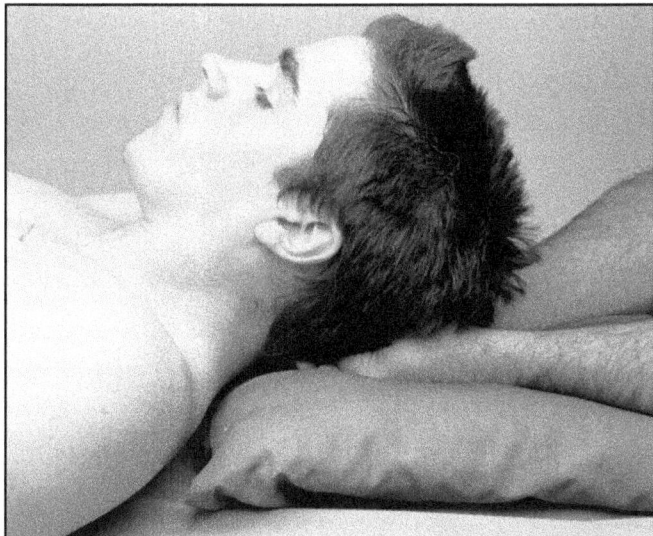
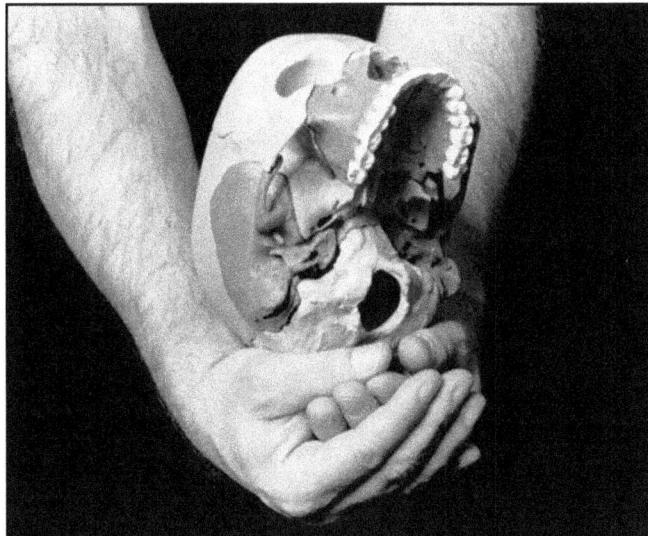

CV-IV Occipital Approach Treatment

2) <u>**Temporal Approach**</u>

The same effect can be achieved by way of the temporal bones. Cradle the occiput with crossed palms and place the thumbs along the mastoid processes. Palpate the rhythmic external/internal rotation. (In external rotation the tips of your thumbs on the mastoid process move posteromedially. In internal rotation the tips at the mastoid process move anterolaterally and the mastoid portion of the temporal bones move medially under the thenar eminence.)

Follow the rhythmic motion into internal rotation. Discourage external rotation.

The amplitude of the motion will gradually decrease until the stillpoint is reached. It will be followed by the sense of softening, warmth, and gentle motion like a little boat on quiet water. Respiration will become slow and diaphragmatic as described above.

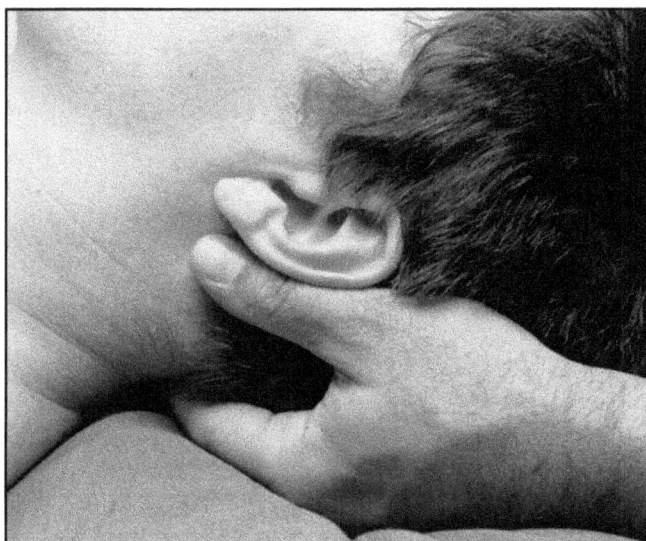

CV-IV Temporal Approach

In both techniques the CV-IV can be enhanced with respiratory cooperation. Ask the patent to hold exhalation as long as possible.

65

Principle of CV-IV Summarized:

1) Determine inherent motion under your hands.
2) Follow mechanism toward extension (internal rotation) and discourage its full range towards flexion (external rotation.)
3) You may assist this by instructing the patient to exhale and hold the breath out until they are forced to breathe.
4) Continue the above and monitor as the amplitude of the CRI progressively decreases until a stillpoint is reached. Then you will feel:
> a softening of the bone
> a sense of warmth in your hands
> a gentle, low amplitude rocking of flexion/extension.
5) Observe for the initiation of a new flexion cycle, and then remove your hands from the head very gently.

CV-IV by Sacrum:

Operator is seated to the side of the patient. Patient is supine. Operator is seated to the side of the patient's pelvis with his caudad hand under the patient's sacrum. Monitor inherent rhythm of the sacrum. Follow the sacral motion toward extension and discourage flexion. Continue to the stillpoint.

CV-IV by Parietal Bones:

Position patient and operator as in the Parietal Lift. The inherent motion of the parietals is monitored. Then internal rotation of the parietals is followed (this corresponds to extension at the SBS) while the movement into external rotation is discouraged. No 'lift' or traction is employed. Continue until the stillpoint is perceived. Then very gently remove your hands from the head.

Indications for a CV-IV

The therapeutic potency generated by the application of a CV-IV treatment stimulates the body's inherent capacity to heal itself through stimulation of increased CSF fluid production and fluctuation. Indications for the use of this treatment include the following:

1) situations of acute or chronic inflammation, including <u>fever</u>, <u>trauma</u>, <u>infection</u>, <u>swelling</u>, <u>passive congestion</u> of venous or lymphatic structures, <u>arthritic conditions</u> associated with swelling, <u>allergic reactions</u>, including skin rashes.

2) The technique helps to <u>calm an agitated patient</u> and helps the patient to more effectively process and <u>integrate changes occurring from the treatment</u> of acute and chronic dysfunctions. CV-IV is also helpful in <u>beginning or ending a treatment</u>, particularly when the patient exhibits severe dysfunction or a hard immovable cranial mechanism.

3) The <u>emptying of any body cavity</u> that has become obstructed or congested, such as constipation, the accumulation of sinus or bronchial discharge, a prolonged or difficult labor, etc.

Sequence of Treatment

1. Vault hold: assessment of the vitality of the CRI, its flexion and extension phases, and the major SBS strains without active motion testing. Diagnosis and treatment of long axis dysfunction (breath of life).

2. Lumbosacral and sacropelvic dysfunctions.

3. Transverse body diaphragms (excluding tentorium) and costal cage dysfunctions.

4. Frontal and parietal compressions.

5. Assessment and treatment of condylar compression and spinal dural stretches.

6. Temporal bone: assessment of internal and external rotation, draw test and treatment of occipito-mastoid, petrojugular, petrobasilar, and sphenosquamous dysfunctions. Temporal bone balancing.

7. Assessment and treatment of facial bone dysfunctions, including temporomandibular joint.

8. Assessment and treatment of SBS strains.

9. CV-IV, dural stretches, or tentorium release.

Goals of Treatment

1. To stimulate the inherent potency of the midline fluid membrane matrix.

2. To relieve biomechanical imbalances from articular, myofascial and membranous tissues and to optimize their mobile functions.

3. Restore autonomic balance.

4. Increase arterial, venous and lymphatic function.

Principles of Treatment

1. Direct (e.g., decompression of a compressed articulation).

2. Indirect (e.g., applying compression to a compressed articulation).

3. V-spread (e.g., directing CSF to a restricted articulation).

4. Molding (e.g., directing CSF to an area of bony distortion).

5. Fluid techniques (e.g., CV-IV, fluid wave).

6. Dural balancing (e.g., stretching, unwinding).

7. Respiratory cooperation.

Psychological Aspects of Treatment

Because treatment with craniosacral principles affects deep tissue dysfunction, it is not uncommon for emotional experiences associated with the trauma held in those tissues to be released. Release of these psychoemotional aspects of trauma are not counterproductive to treatment but in fact are additional therapeutic forces which help to resolve the deep-seated effects of trauma. The immediate effects of these releases last from minutes to hours, as do the effects of muscle soreness after such a treatment. There may be some memories that are stimulated which were associated with the trauma, and some of these memories may stimulate emotional responses in the patient. With the dysfunction being released at the tissue level, it is usually easy for the patient to accept and release these psychoemotional aspects of his trauma; however, there are occasional instances wherein the patient may benefit from follow-up with a psychological health-care professional or a revisit to your office in a few days in order to recheck the patient. It should be noted that these psychological experiences are not caused by the treatment but rather are released by the treatment. In other words, these are experiences that the patient is already carrying inside at an unconscious level, thereby unconsciously influencing pain behavior and helping to reinforce the persistence of the tissue dysfunction underlying their condition. All health care professionals are familiar with these kinds of reactions, which can occur in any therapeutic interaction, and it is for this reason that these manual approaches are only taught to health care professionals.

Cranial Exam Record

1 Rate   I   D   N   Rate   I   D   N

2 Amp   I   D   N   Amp   I   D   N

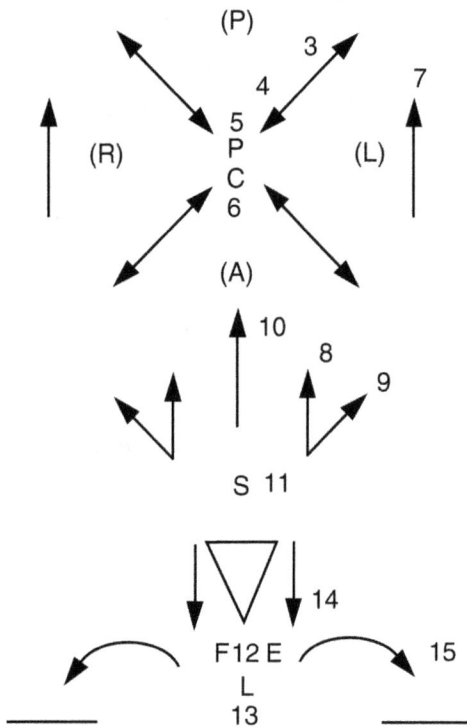

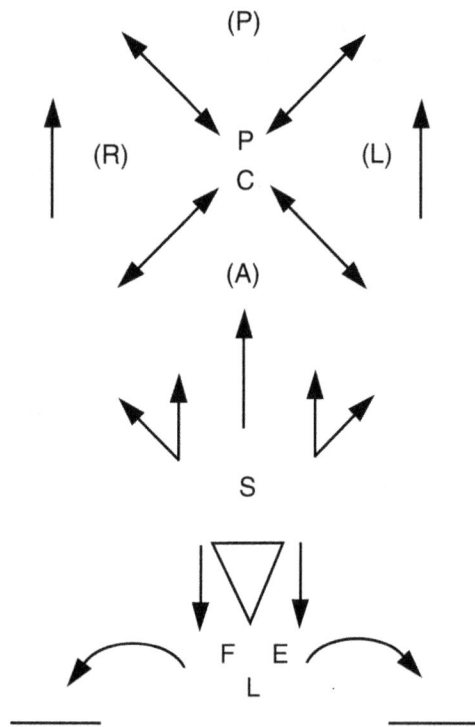

Place line in front of arrows or circle letters when restricted.

(A) Anterior   P (Posterior)   (R) Right   (L) Left

1. Is rate of CRI increased, decreased, or normal? (circle I, D, or N)
2. Is amplitude of CRI increased, decreased, or normal? (circle I, D, or N)
3. Is flexion restricted in one or more quadrants?
4. Is extension restricted in one or more quadrants?
5. Are flexion and extension out of phase with expanison and contraction (paradoxical)? (circle P)
6. Is compression of SBS present? (circle C)
7. Is temporal draw test restricted?
8. Is occipital dural tension increased?
9. Is occipital condylar compression present?
10. Is cruciate suture restricted?
11. Is diaphragm shock evident? (circle S)
12. Are flexion or extension movements of the CRI restricted in the sacrum? (circle F or E)
13. Is longitudinal (vertical) rise of sacrum absent during flexion (circle L)?
14. Is sacral traction met with resistance?
15. Is external rotation of CRI restricted in ankles? Where is most cephalad point of restriction?

Finding the Area of Primary Restriction Using the Cranial Rhythmic Impulse

Under optimal conditions, the cranial rhythmic impulse sends a wave of motion throughout the entire body, causing all the tissues in the body to expand and contract with the flexion and extension phase of the CRI. When a major restriction exists anywhere in the body, this fluctuation movement is disturbed and an associated decrease in the amplitude of the CRI can be palpated distal to the point of restriction in the body.

Diagnosis

This exercise begins with the operator standing at the foot of the table with the patient supine, hands on the dorsal aspects of the feet. In this position, a gentle fluctuating movement can be appreciated in comparing the left side to the right side. When the movement is undisturbed, there is a full rotation in the external and then internal direction of paired structures. During the external rotation phase there is a slight swelling, and during the internal rotation phase there is a slight narrowing. With a disturbance in the CRI, one side of the body will have a restriction in this movement, perceived as a dampening of the external or internal rotation movement. Moving proximally from the feet to the knees this motion is compared left to right continuing up to the upper thighs and hips, and then the pelvis, followed by the abdominal area, then lower ribs, then upper ribs and then the head, until the transition between disturbed and normal motion is perceived.

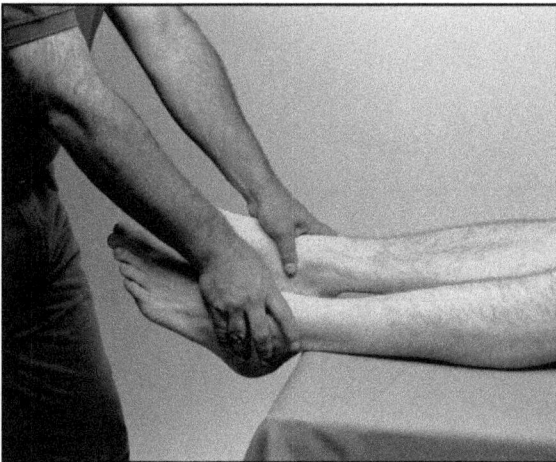

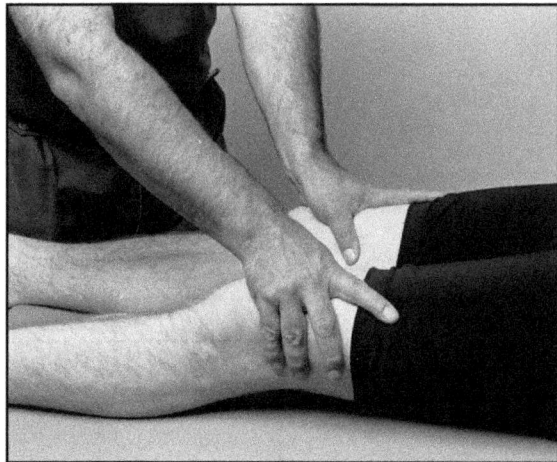

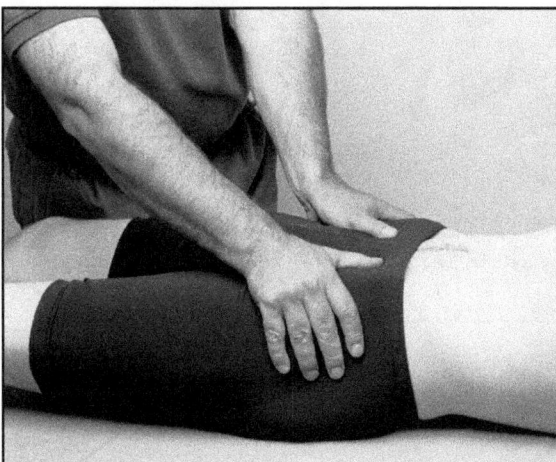

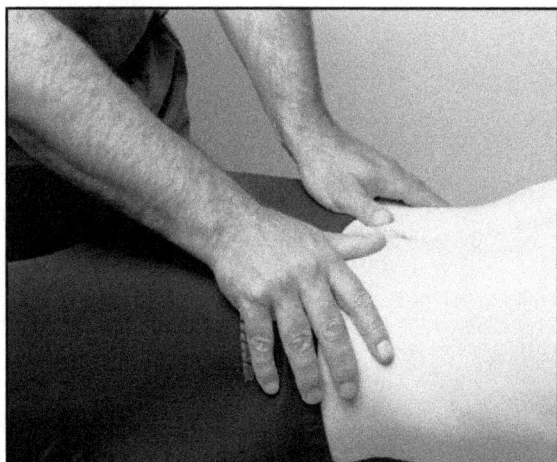

Sequence to Find Primary Restriction Using CRI

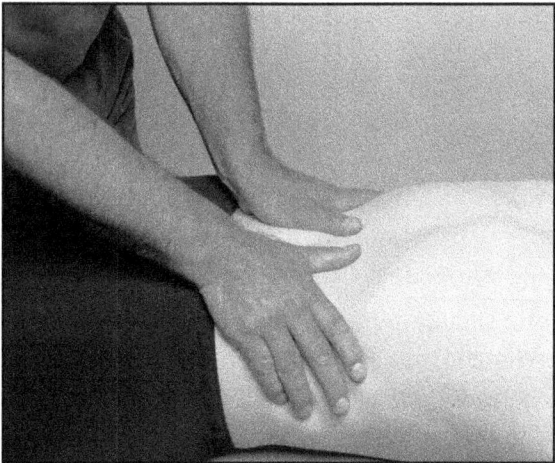 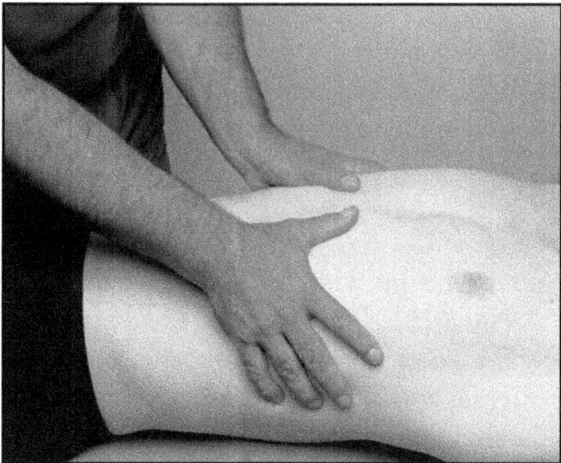

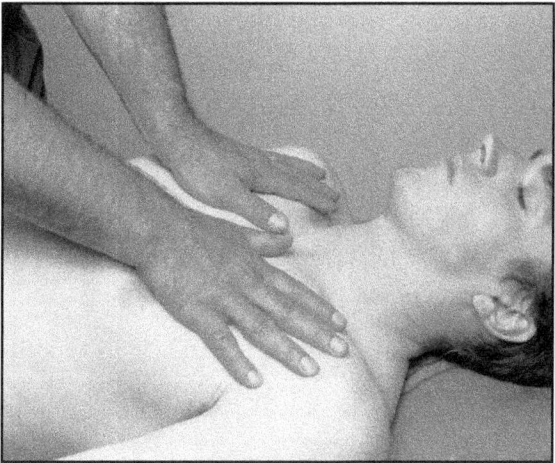 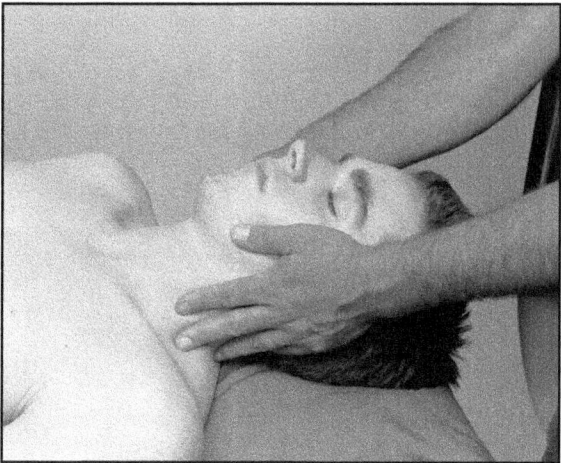

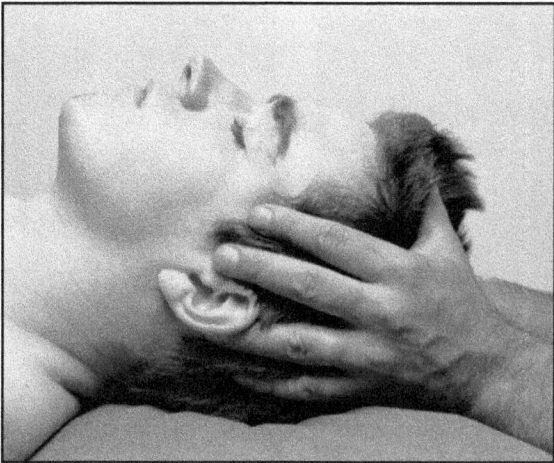

Treatment

The most proximal location where the fluctuating motion is perceived as being disturbed is the location of the primary restriction that we are interested in treating. The operator attempts to contact this area from above and below. In holding the tissue that surrounds the area in a three-dimensional manner, compression and shearing forces are introduced, taking up the tissues into the perceived tension, holding it there until a sensation of swelling moves into the area. This is a reflection of the increased fluid potency and enhanced function of the cranial rhythmic impulse and should be confirmed by recontacting the patient's feet and monitoring the distal aspects for the return of normal cranial rhythmic impulse. It may be that full return has not occurred and the operator should again recheck in the same manner, locating a point more distal than the first that may also be restricted and require treatment in the same manner.

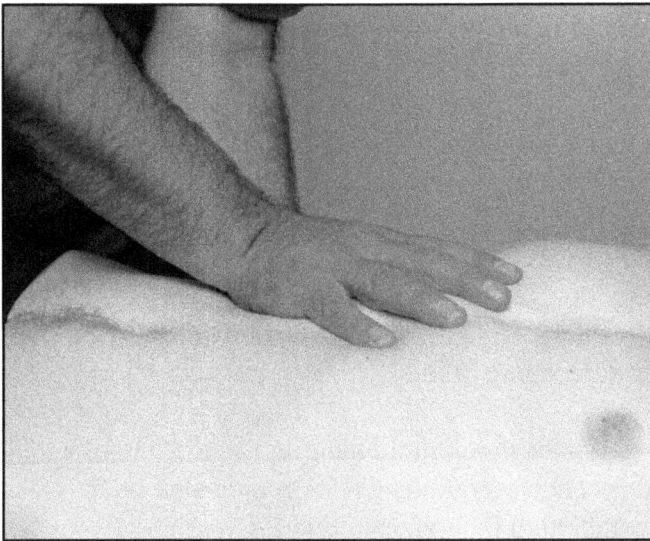

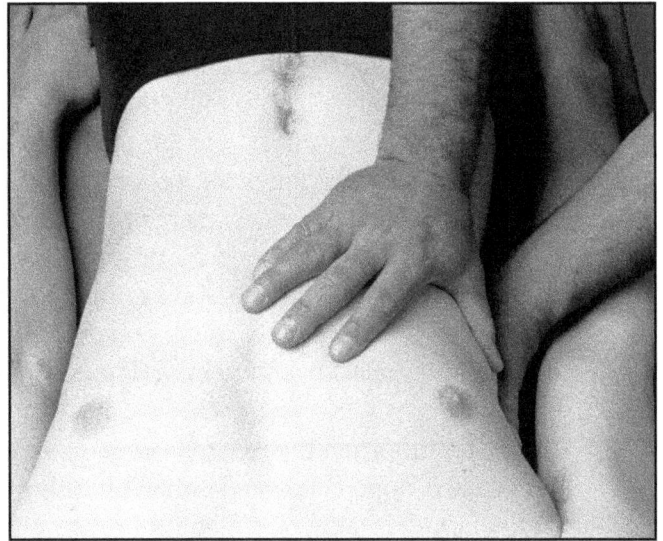

Treatment of Primary Restriction

Two-Operator Technique

Purpose. To develop more subtle palpatory skills and interexaminer reliability.

Technique. Two-operator technique with the patient supine, one operator at the head of the patient with the vault hold, the other examiner at the sacrum with the sacral hold.

1. Both examiners will focus on the CRI to identify its flexion and extension phase and any restrictions identified. An attempt should be made to correlate findings at the sacrum and at the occiput. For instance, is the occiput and sacral base restricted on the same side, the opposite side? Is there sidebending restriction of the sacrum and a correlating torsion of the SBS? (Remember, the occiput and the sacrum should be in phase, so a right SBS torsion should correlate with a sacral base on the right that is low or right side bending of the sacrum. Likewise, does the sacrum want to go off to one side or the other? A sacrum that wants to go off to the right may correlate with a left lateral strain.)

2. Attempt to stretch the dura, one operator at a time, so that the other operator can appreciate this subtle change in the tension beneath their hands. For instance, the operator on the sacrum will give a gentle traction into the sacrum, bringing the sacrum into cranial flexion. The examiner at the head should tell the examiner at the sacrum when he or she feels the pull of the dura and what they feel, i.e. accentuated flexion, a new SBS strain pattern, or a dampening of the CRI. Likewise, the person at the head should engage the dura in a dural stretch, accentuating either a superior or inferior vertical strain, whichever is more restricted. While holding this dural stretch, the examiner at the sacrum should tell the operator at the head when they feel a change at the sacrum and what they feel, for example, rotation or sidebending or accentuated flexion or extension or dampening of the CRI.

3. Progressing from the previous exercise, each examiner should hold their dural stretch until a release is appreciated and either a melting and accentuation of the CRI is appreciated or an unwinding is appreciated and followed to its completion by both examiners. Correlation should be attempted between examiners findings, i.e. the unwinding begins, the unwinding ends, a stillpoint is achieved. There should be communication between the two examiners to verify their findings.

4. Each examiner should perform a CV-4 separately, and the other examiner should just monitor and report to the operator performing the technique when they feel changes in the CRI, when they feel the still point, and when they feel a resumption to the normal flexion-extension phase.

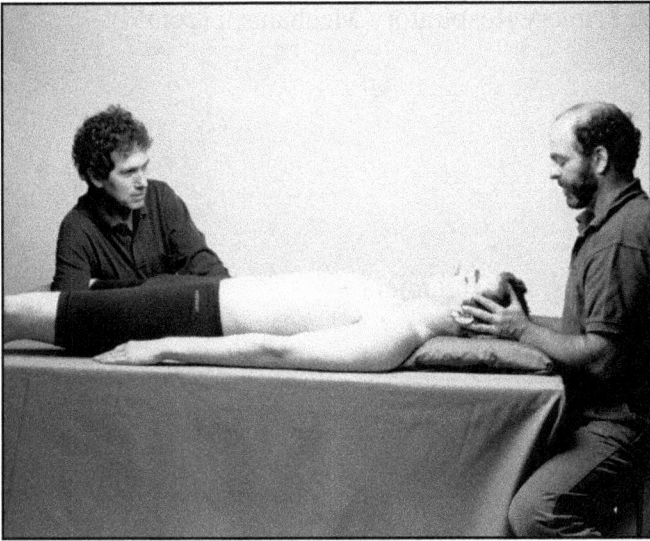

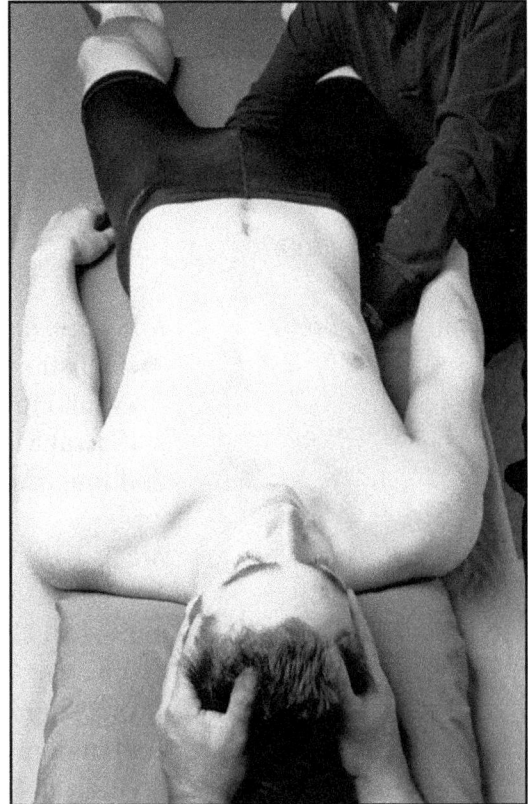

Two-Operator Technique

Level I Course Schedule- Day 1

8:00 am	(*0900*)	Introduction, Course Logistics and Objectives
8:30 am	(*0930*)	Osteopathic Philosophy and History of Cranial Osteopathy
9:00 am	(*1000*)	Components of the Primary Respiratory Mechanism •Anatomy and Physiology •Current Scientific Understanding
10:00 am	(*1100*)	Break
10:15 am	(*1115*)	Components of the Primary Respiratory Mechanism (cont'd)
12:00 pm	(*1300*)	Lunch
1:00 pm	(*1400*)	*Table Session* •Palpation of CRI •Vault Hold •Sacral Motion Testing and Treatment •Lumbosacral decompression
3:00 pm	(*1600*)	Break
3:15 pm	(*1615*)	Individual Cranial Bones •Occiput •Sphenoid •Temporals •Parietals •Frontal •Ethmoid •Vomer
4:30 pm	(*1730*)	Demonstration of Technique •Frontal Lift •Parietal Lift •Temporal Bone Motion Testing and Decompression
5:00 pm	(*1800*)	Adjourn

Level I Course Schedule- Day 2

8:00 am   (*0900*)   *Table Session*
          •Frontal Lift
          •Parietal Lift
          •Temporal Bone Motion Testing and Decompression

10:00 am   (*1100*)   Break

10:15 am   (*1115*)   *Table Session*- Direct Membranous Release
          •Evaluation of Pelvic Motion
          •Treatment of Dysfunction
          •Evaluation of Occipital Condylar Motion
          •Treatment of Occipital Condylar Compression
          •Direct & Indirect Approaches

12:00 pm   (*1300*)   Lunch

1:00 pm   (*1400*)   SBS Strain Patterns
          •Torsion
          •Sidebending/Rotation
          •Lateral Strains
          •Vertical Strains
          •Compression

3:00 pm   (*1600*)   Break

3:15 pm   (*1615*)   *Table Session*
          •Diagnosis and Treatment of SBS Strains Using Point of
            Balanced Membranous Tension Technique

5:00 pm   (*1800*)   Adjourn

Level I Course Schedule- Day 3

8:00 am	(0900)	*Table Session*-Fluid Wave and V-Spread
9:15 am	(1015)	Demonstration: Temporal Bone Check-up
		•Petrojugular dysfunction
		•Sphenosquamous dysfunction
9:45 am	(1045)	Break
10:00 am	(1100)	*Table Session*- Temporal Bone Checkup
12:00 pm	(1300)	Lunch
1:00 pm	(1400)	Transverse Body Diaphragm Molding and Balancing
2:45 pm	(1545)	Break
3:00 pm	(1600)	*Table Session*- Fluid Fluctuation Technique
		•CV-IV
		•Home Exercise
4:30 pm	(1730)	Sequence and Principles of Treatment
		•Indications and Complications of Treatment
		•Psychological Aspects of Treatment
		•Cranial Screening Exam
5:00 pm	(1800)	Adjourn

Level I Course Schedule- Day 4

8:00 am   (*0900*)   *Table Session*
- Course Review

10:00 am   (*1100*)   Break

10:15 am   (*1115*)   *Table Session*
- Course Review

12:15 pm   (*1315*)   Lunch

1:15 pm   (*1415*)   *Table Session*- Palpatory Exercises
- Finding the Area of Primary Restriction Using the CRI
- Two Operators Monitoring CRI Changes at Head and Sacrum

3:15 pm   (*1615*)   Break

3:30 pm   (*1630*)   *Table Session*
- Palpating the Fluid Membrane-Matrix and the Breath of Life

4:30 pm   (*1730*)   Concluding Remarks

5:00 pm   (*1800*)   Adjourn

Notes:

**SFIMMS SERIES IN
NEUROMUSCULOSKELETAL MEDICINE**

OSTEOPATHIC MANIPULATIVE MEDICINE APPROACHES TO THE PRIMARY RESPIRATORY MECHANISM

Level II
Embryology, Newborns, Trauma, and the Rest of the Body

OMM Approaches to the Primary Respiratory Mechanism

Level II
Course Objectives

Enhance integration of the material from the basic course by sharing clinical experiences, asking pertinent new questions, and performing a complete table review of diagnostic and therapeutic approaches

Introduce cranial concepts regarding embryology, birth, infant anatomy and pediatric case management

Introduce osteopathic concepts regarding breathing and diaphragm function and their importance to whole-body functioning

Learn evaluation and treatment approaches for breathing and diaphragm function

Introduce cranial osteopathy as it applies to the face and its related anatomy and physiology

Learn evaluation and treatment approaches for the face and jaw

Introduce and learn osteopathic approaches to the face and dura incorporating two operators

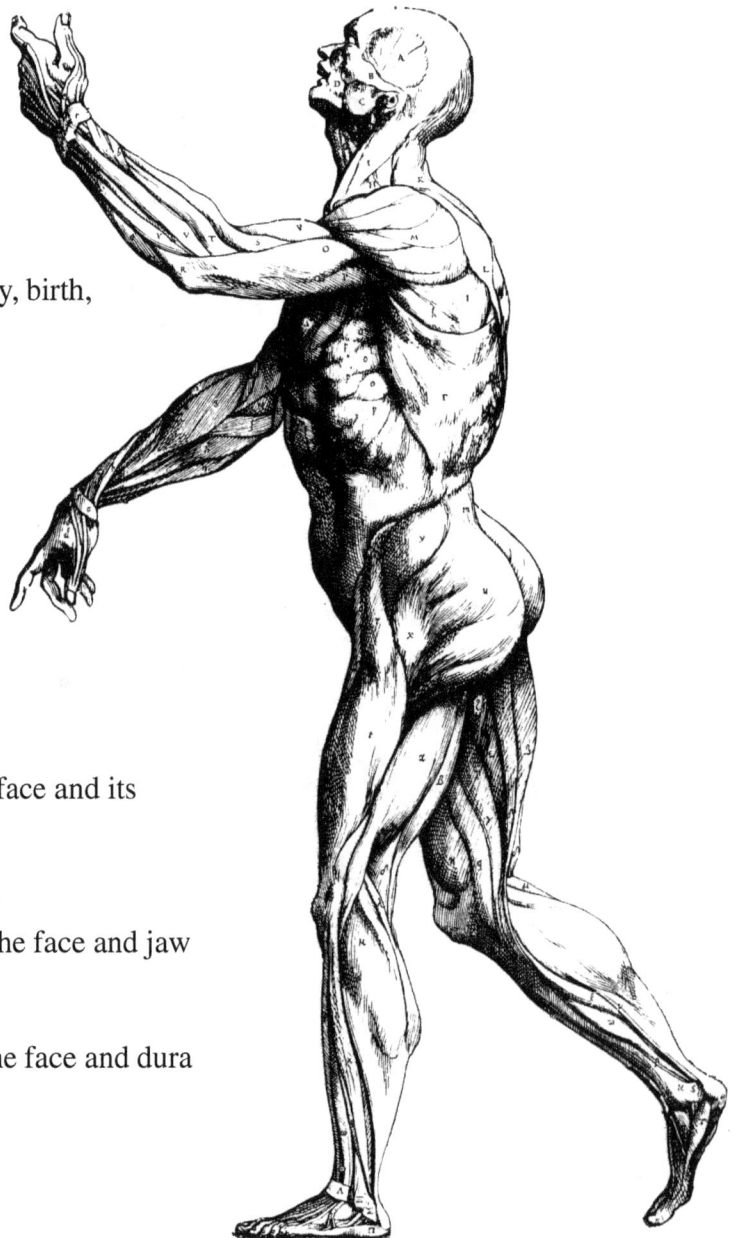

Basic Course Table Review Supplement

1. Integration of **other manual medicine techniques** is an important idea to keep in mind. Oftentimes cranial dysfunctions will resolve when the rest of the body is treated with whichever approaches might be appropriate for the patient's presentation.

2. **Not everyone is a cranial patient**. It should be remembered that cranial dysfunction and treatment affect deep releases, both physically and psychologically, and some patients are not able or are not ready for this kind of treatment. If a patient presents some question about their physical and/or psychological stability, you can attempt to initiate cranial treatment, but it should be done extremely slowly, if at all. Never go through the entire sequence of treatment in one session. This is even true for "healthy patients." The sequence of treatment that has been suggested is merely a guideline and one that should be followed slowly over six to ten treatments, not all at once in one treatment.

3. A note regarding **unwinding**: many times a stillpoint will be achieved; however, a new flexion and extension does not ensue, and instead another process of unwinding follows. You must be certain that flexion and extension have returned; otherwise, you are still in an unwinding process. The unwinding can be interrupted momentarily by a stillpoint and then resumed, so you should be careful to continue following the unwinding until its absolutely completed.

4. Principles of the indirect technique for **lumbosacral decompression** include the following: in addition to compressing the two hands together, remember to test the relative compliance for mobility between the two hands in a side-to-side or translatory direction, in a rotatory direction, and in a sidebending direction. All these different opposite motions should be paired together in the direction of ease to enhance the release.

5. Regarding **frontal and parietal lifts**: We have originally taught that the lifts should be performed in a direction 90 degrees perpendicular to the plane of the frontal or parietal bone. In actuality, the tension should be assessed and a slight angulation of the force vector applied into the direction of ease, so that if lifting on the frontal bone with a little angulation toward the operator seems to be more restricted, then the treatment should be applied with a slight angulation away from the operator and with rotation either to the right or to the left, depending on which way the bone seems to move more easily. The same principle would be applied to the parietal bone, adjusting the superior force of the lift slightly anterior or posterior and adding a rotation adjustment in order to bring the mechanism into the direction of greatest ease.

6. There are some distinctions of **temporal bone dysfunctions** that should be understood. There are temporal dysfunctions which are restricted, and others which reflect a "locked" mechanism. The locked temporal bone does not move at all in one direction, and has a strong feeling of being stuck in either the internally or externally rotated position. The restricted temporal bone has movement in both directions; however, the movement in one direction is noticeably less. The temporal bone which is locked is understandably of more greater clinical importance than that which is restricted.

7. With respect to **SBS strain patterns**, a vertical or lateral strain present in a patient should be observed to note whether there is a flexion and extension component present. As the CRI begins moving into flexion, there is a noticeable shift as the mechanism goes into a vertical or lateral strain pattern. This is a vertical strain without SBS compression. If SBS compression is present, there will

be no flexion or extension of the mechanism appreciated. The finger contacts over the sphenoid and occiput will just go immediately into a vertical strain pattern without the initiation of a flexion or extension movement. Vertical or lateral strain patterns may present in this manner, and those which have no flexion and extension movement are obviously of greater concern than those that have some flexion and extension in their presentation.

8. In treating **SBS strain patterns**, the pathological strains are the most important to treat (vertical, lateral strains and compressions). These are the patterns in which the sphenoid and occiput move in the same direction (as opposed to opposite directions) about their disturbed motion axes. (e.g. vertical strains move around two parallel transverse axes in the same direction) It is not necessary to stack all the physiologic strain patterns (torsion and sidebending-rotation) unless they are the only patterns which have any motion.

9. Application of sufficient forces is essential to produce a resolution in the dysfunction palpated. At the start of any procedure, forces are minimal, increasing as the tissues require, to a point where the force applied "matches" the force within. At this point the force held within the patient's tissues pushes back and the operator senses an expansion between their hands. Tissue reorganization and unwinding will follow immediately.

Osteopathic Approach to Infants

Osteopathic Embryology

Embryologic development proceeds along electrochemical gradients within a fluid membrane matrix. Within this matrix lies the inherent potency for the expression of life. Embryonic movements establish a longitudinal midline within the fluid membrane matrix from which all tissues develop a midline relation. This original fluid membrane midline has clinical significance in the osteopathic approach to patient care.

The organization of embryonic structure and function occurs within an electromagnetic fluid matrix that forms a midline process or potency from which all other structures develop and function throughout life. It takes four or five million sperm lining up around the unfertilized egg to find its electromagnetic midline which, when penetrated, quickly grows into an embryonic plate, where in the midline becomes the notochord. The notochord elongates and forms the basic nervous system structure around which all other systems will develop. As this neural system develops it forms a tube that has an opening at the top and the bottom. The amniotic fluid is the cerebral spinal fluid of the embryo. This neural tube eventually closes off at the lamina terminalis at both ends. The nervous system then begins a process of coiling (bending), which occurs around a fulcrum within the hypophysis during its early development. This is also the place where the neural tube ends. As this coiling occurs, the heart sac and cavity develop, hanging down from the inferior aspect of this same fulcrum. The pericardial and pleural sac are continuous with the urachus and the peritoneal cavity, and they all hang from this fulcrum beneath the developing nervous system.

The first six weeks of life are considered the embryonic stage and are essentially pregenetic and preimmunologic. Embryos as this stage look quite similar from species to species. It is after the embryonic stage when genetic expression stimulates differentiation and the various fetuses develop into different looking species. At about this time, there are primordial germ cells that find their way from the yolk sac into the developing fetus, which simultaneously initiates the beginnings of the immune system, differentiating the self from not-self.

As the nervous system develops, the role of the ventricular system is significant from the beginning. Amniotic fluid is surrounded by the neural tube, becoming the ventricular system which transmits the fluid impulses governing the growth and development of the nervous system and its coiling and uncoiling movements. During embryonic coiling of the nervous system, the neural tube encloses the fluid matrix, and fluids are directed through the ventricular system in a longitudinal and lateral wave. As embryonic coiling proceeds, midline tissue emanating from the neural tube folds in on itself, forming all the various body cavities of the head, neck, thorax, and abdomen.

Fetal development is directed toward maturation of organ systems established in the embryonic period. This maturation includes uncoiling of the central nervous system as the fluid membrane matrix is directed anteriorly, superiorly, posteriorly, inferiorly, laterally, and filled with central nervous system tissue. These embryonic and fetal movements reflect potencies which are active throughout life. Osteopathic management allows a fuller expression of these potencies, identifying midline disturbances and restoring midline function of the fluid membrane matrix.

Table 4: Overview of CNS Embryology: Theory and Function

Ectoderm (16 days - 6 weeks) influenced by notochord

Ectodermal germ layer (2-3 weeks)

Neural folds fuse to form a neural tube (22-27 days)

By day 27, both ends of tube close

Narrow caudad portion becomes spinal cord

Broader cephalic portion with several dilations becomes brain

Central canal continuous allowing CSF to fluctuate between brain and spinal cord

Rapid growth of CNS causes a cephalo-caudad flexion (folding)

Disproportionate growth of ectodermal tissue

Cervical and cephalic flexure

CSF system of connected ventricles can be recognized

Continuous growth of prosencephalon (forebrain) in anterior, dorsal, posterior, inferior, and lateral direction

After 3 months, disproportionate growth of mesodermal tissue (vertebral column)

Embryology of skull

Cranial base laid down in cartilage (occiput, sphenoid, temporal ethmoid)

Vault laid down in membrane

Growth of skull follows growth of CNS within

Inherent motion of CNS

Birth Mechanics

The consequences of birth through the vaginal canal have a number of important considerations. Most importantly, the compression of tissues in response to contractile forces in the maternal pelvis causes a subsequent expansion of tissues associated with the initiation of cardiopulmonary function. Similarly, fluid membrane relations within the central nervous system and its associated structures are stimulated by this expansion to function properly. After birth, primary respiratory function or the CRI is fundamentally linked to and influenced by secondary or cardiopulmonary respiration. The forces of labor are also associated with the introduction of asymmetrical forces into the musculoskeletal system, including the fluid membrane matrix. The assessment and subsequent treatment of these asymmetries comprises the basis of the osteopathic approach to infants.

In a study of 1250 newborns, Dr. Viola Frymann, DO, FAAO, demonstrated that strains to the head could be observed by trained osteopathic physicians in 90% of subjects. By observing clinical responses to osteopathic treatment, it would appear that many common problems of the neonatal period are associated with these membranous-articular strains. Difficulty suckling or swallowing, vomiting, irritability, muscular tension, poor coordination, and irregular breathing are often overcome as soon as these strains are corrected.

Just before birth, the infant in utero is positioned for delivery by presenting the smallest head diameter to the largest diameter of the mother's pelvis: this is the position of full head flexion. As contractions continue, the infant is conducted by the inclination of the maternal pelvic floor into the midline for delivery around the pubic symphysis by a process of extension of the head.

This descent in full flexion, progressing to birth by extension of the head, is of profound significance to the initiation of cardiopulmonary respiration. The respiratory activity associated with the expulsion from the birth canal combines with the vigorous vocal activity of the newborn, expanding the cranial mechanism and stimulating motion of the bony and membranous structures. Healthy sequential development of the central nervous system within can then be optimized.

Ideal circumstances seldom occur in our modern, civilized world. Owing to such factors as poor nutrition of the mother, structural inadequacies before and during pregnancy, drug abuse, inadequate preparations for labor, and, sometimes, the mechanical or artificial acceleration of labor by an impatient obstetrician, only a relatively few infants are born without undue strain or cranial trauma.

Structural inadequacies of the maternal pelvis may cause the fetus to assume a degree of extension (and lateral cervical flexion) greater then the ideal; the result will be a presentation of a portion of the head greater than the minimum occipitobregmatic diameter. This can range from a moderate extension to a posterior occiput, a transverse arrest, a brow presentation, or even a complete extension in which the face itself presents and in which vaginal delivery is impossible. In such a circumstance, cesarean section is necessary if the baby is to survive. But the compressive forces will have already traumatized the head as the uterine contractions force it progressively towards the birth canal. Prominence of the base of an anterior maternal sacrum may obstruct descent of the head on one side, and such asynclitism can distort the cranial mechanism. The presence of large twins, both striving to present the head at the same time, may cause cranial stress to one or both even before the active labor begins. These are only a few of the mechanical insults that may occur before birth.

During false labor, during a long hard labor when there is cephalo-pelvic disproportion, or when dilation of the cervix is slow delaying descent of the presenting part, the infant is compressed from crown (if the head is somewhat extended) or occiput (if the head is well flexed on the chest) to rump. The cranial mechanism is compressed by the confines of an unyielding birth canal while the infant is being propelled by unrelenting uterine contractions. At the same time the infant's pelvic mechanism is compressed through the sacral units and the lumbosacral area by the expulsive uterine contractions because it cannot advance rapidly enough in response to the propelling forces.

The lumbar spine may respond to such forces by sidebending. If the situation is further aggravated by delay as the lumbar spine curves around the maternal sacral promontory the lumbar curve may not spontaneously resolve after birth.

These three factors:
   1) cranial compression – particularly through the occiput
   2) sacral compression
   3) lumbar sidebending
may lay foundations for the so-called "ideopathic" adolescent spinal scoliosis. Prevention of this deformity begins in infancy or early childhood.

Infant Anatomy

The vault of the newborn skull is a membranous structure. Plates of bone are enveloped in two layers of membrane, which are in apposition at the anterior and posterior fontanelles and sometimes at the pterion and asterion. These plates of membranous bone are designed to telescope into each other as the skull passes through the birth canal—the parietals overriding the frontal at the coronal suture, and the occiput at the lambdoidal suture. The degree of this overriding is controlled and limited by the investing dural membranes.

The bones of the base develop from the cartilaginous chondrocranium. At birth, development is still incomplete. The occipital bone is in four parts, united by intraosseous articular cartilage. The sphenoid is in three parts, the temporal in two, the maxilla in two, and the frontal frequently in two. The adult cranial suture is designed for a very small but vital degree of motion. With such incomplete bone formation encased in membrane, how much greater is the potential motion of the bones of the developing newborn skull! At this time each part of each of these bones functions virtually as a separate bone, moving in relation to its other parts.

Let us consider the occiput. It is most commonly the presenting part, and therefore the part that may take the brunt of the trauma of labor. The four developmental parts surround the foramen magnum. The base articulates anteriorly with the base of the sphenoid. Posterolaterally, it articulates with the lateral masses. The hypoglossal nerve, which innervates the muscles of the tongue, passes out of the skull between the base and the lateral mass, through the intraosseous cartilage in the space that will become the condylar canal. The occipital condyle, which articulates with the atlas, spans the intraosseous cartilage; its anteromedial third is found on the base, the posterolateral two-thirds on the lateral mass.

Immediately anterolateral to this condylar area is the jugular foramen, a space between the condylar part of the occiput and the petrous portion of the temporal. This foramen gives passage not only to the jugular vein but also to cranial nerves IX, X, and XI (glossopharyngeal, vagus, and accessory, respectively). The vagus nerve provides innervation to the gastrointestinal and cardiorespiratory systems.

The supraocciput formed in cartilage fuses with the membranous interparietal bone to form the occipital squama. Compression transmitted through the squama to the condylar part on one side may disturb the function of the vagus and/or hypoglossal nerve, causing vomiting, irregular respiration, and difficulty in sucking. If this compression is transmitted further to the base, the relationship of the base of the occiput to the base of the sphenoid may be distorted, causing a lateral strain of the sphenobasilar articulation and a parallelogram deformity of the cranium. Bilateral condylar compression may cause a buckling type of strain of the cranial base, producing a vertical strain between the occiput and the sphenoid at the sphenobasilar articulation. This may be associated not only with vagal dysfunction but also with symptoms of tension, spasticity, opisthotonic spasms, sleeplessness, and excessive crying due to the irritation of the pyramidal tracts on the anterior and lateral aspects of the brain stem in the foramen magnum. This may be considered as a precursor of the spastic type of cerebral palsy.

The sphenoid bone is in three parts at birth: the central body bears the lesser wings, with the greater wings (from which the pterygoid process subtends) on either side. The greater wing-pterygoid unit articulates with the body by an intraosseous cartilage. This is situated immediately beneath the cavernous sinus, through which pass cranial nerves III, IV, and VI, innervating the extraocular muscles, and the ophthalmic division of V, which is sensory to the orbit, upper face and scalp. The body of the sphenoid articulates with the base of the occiput posteriorly and is therefore distorted by the lateral or vertical strains resulting from condylar compression. Anteriorly the body carries the lesser wings, which enter into the formation of the orbit. The orbit is approximately pyramidal in shape; the apex is at the optic foramen, where the root of the lesser wing connects to the body. Its anatomic integrity is dependent on the relationship of the greater wing to the lesser wing, which is in fact the relationship of the greater wing-pterygoid unit to the body.

In the event of a lateral strain at the base due to unilateral condylar compression of the occiput, the orbit will be distorted by rotation of the base of the sphenoid carrying the lesser wing anterior on one side and posterior on the other. In the parallelogram head due to lateral compression, the greater wing is compressed medially and carried forward on one side and posterior on the other. In either event, lateral muscle imbalance of the eyes is commonly found in varying degrees ranging from mild esophoria or exophoria to severe strabismus.

The temporal bone is in two parts at the time of birth—the petromastoid portion, developed in cartilage that projects obliquely between the occiput and the greater wing of the sphenoid to articulate at its apex with the body of the sphenoid, and the squamous portion, developed in membrane that forms the greater part of the lower lateral wall of the skull. The tympanic portion is not yet a bony canal but resembles a horseshoe adherent to the inferior posterior aspect of the squama. These two parts, the squamous and tympanic, unite just before birth. The petromastoid portion contains the auditory and the vestibular apparatus. The auditory apparatus consists of the bony eustachian tube emerging between the petrous and squamous portions, from which the cartilaginous tube extends to the fossa of Rosenmuller. The eustachian tube is susceptible to distortion, which may impair hearing if lateral stress compresses the squamous portion. Laterally the eustachian tube opens into the middle ear, which, by the ossicular mechanism, transmits the auditory vibrations received from the tympanic membrane to the internal ear. The vestibular apparatus includes the semicircular canals, precisely related to each other and geometrically balanced with those of the opposite side. Distortion of the axis of the petrous portion may disturb this delicate mechanism of equilibrium.

Infant Evaluation

1. Gestational and perinatal history

2. Visual observation of symmetrical form and function of the head (especially the eyes), face, thorax (respiration), upper and lower extremities, including:
   - deformities
   - curvatures
   - muscle tone
   - motion symmetry

3. Presence of infantile reflexes
   - Babinski
   - grasping
   - light
   - startle (sound)
   - stepping

4. Assessment of mobile function in the following areas:
   - lower extremity (ankles, knees, and hips)
   - sacropelvic region (rotation, side-bending, and sacral nutation)
   - thoracolumbar region (costal cage translation)
   - cervical/thoracic region (costal cage compression)
   - craniocervical junction (occipital side-bending and flexion)
   - upper extremity testing (shoulder abduction and clavicular compliance)
   - head (cranial base mobility through the temporal bones, and SBS flexion/extension movements)

Table 5: Birth History

_____ Maternal Illness or Medication During Pregnancy

_____ Prolonged Labor

_____ False / Ineffective Labor

_____ Fetal Distress

_____ C-Section

_____ Umbilical Cord Around The Body

_____ Cyanosis

_____ Low APGAR Scores

_____ Placenta Abnormality

_____ Neonatal Jaundice

_____ Internsive Care or Other Extended Hospital Stay

_____ Breech or Other Abnormal Presentation

_____ Forceps / Suction Delivery

_____ Head Deformity

_____ Pre-Maturity

_____ Post-Maturity

_____ Unwanted Pregnancy

Table 6: Developmental History

_____ Chronic Infections/ Illness

_____ Breast Fed

_____ Difficulty Swallowing

_____ Spitting Up

_____ Irritable

_____ Throwing Head Back

_____ Irregular Bowels

_____ Poor Speech

_____ Poor Hearing

_____ Poor Vision

_____ Poor Eye Movements

_____ Poor Muscle Tone

_____ Poor Coordination
-Crawling
-Creeping
-Walking

_____ Head Injury/ Other Falls

_____ Surgery

_____ Orphaned/ Adopted

_____ Marital Problems at Home

Principles of Newborn Treatment

The first assessment should be of the overall vitality in the system. This can be accomplished either by contacting the head in the vault hold or by contacting the lower extremity and feeling for the bilateral cranial rhythmic impulse.

Knees are often dysfunctional due to twisting in the birth canal during the latter stages of delivery. Alignment of tibia with patella should be noted as well as mobile function. Gentle myofascial release is usually adequate to restore full motion.

Symmetrical movement of the pelvis can be assessed and treated simultaneously with bilateral contact of anterior pelvis with the fingertips in the sacral sulci. Direct fascial release of restricted side-bending, rotation, flexion, and extension elements can be easily applied.

Sacral mobility is an essential goal of treatment, both in relation to the lumbar spine, as well as the bilateral pelvic bones, and the rest of the spinal mechanism. Tension of the dural tube can be influenced through the sacrum. Sacral decompression from the lumbar spine as well as from the ilia can be carried out using direct or indirect approaches.

Lumbar spine can be treated simultaneously with the pelvis by inducing side-bending and rotation.

Thoracolumbar junction compliance can be assessed and treated along with the lower costal cage using gentle myofascial releases incorporating rotary and translatory forces into the lower costal cage elements.

Upper thoracic cage compliance can be assessed in a similar fashion using rotation and translation into the upper anterior costal cage elements.

Clavicle and shoulder dysfunction may also be important due to birth and developmental strains and can be assessed and treated with bilateral contact over the clavicles or with unilateral contact over the shoulder and scapular mechanism. Directions of reduced motion are identified and treated with myofascial or fascial ligamentous release.

In evaluation of the occipital bone, condylar compression and dural tension can often be treated together by using direct stretching or indirect compression.

The rest of the vault can be appreciated and treated where the restrictions might lie, i.e., temporoparietal or frontoparietal sutures. This would include assessment and treatment of overlapping sutures and temporal bone dysfunctions.

Hard palate molding may enhance treatment of vault dysfunction, particularly in relation to release of deep facial structures such as the ethmoid and vomer or suture compressions.

SBS dysfunction can be assessed and treated in combination with midline occipital and bilateral greater wing contact releasing the Sutherland fulcrum and stimulating the fluid membrane matrix and the tidal body.

Craniofascial Exam

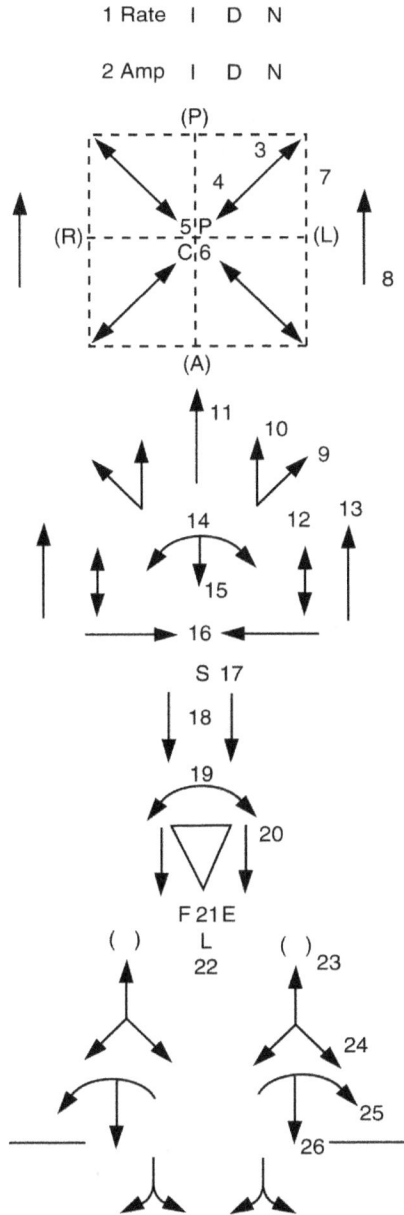

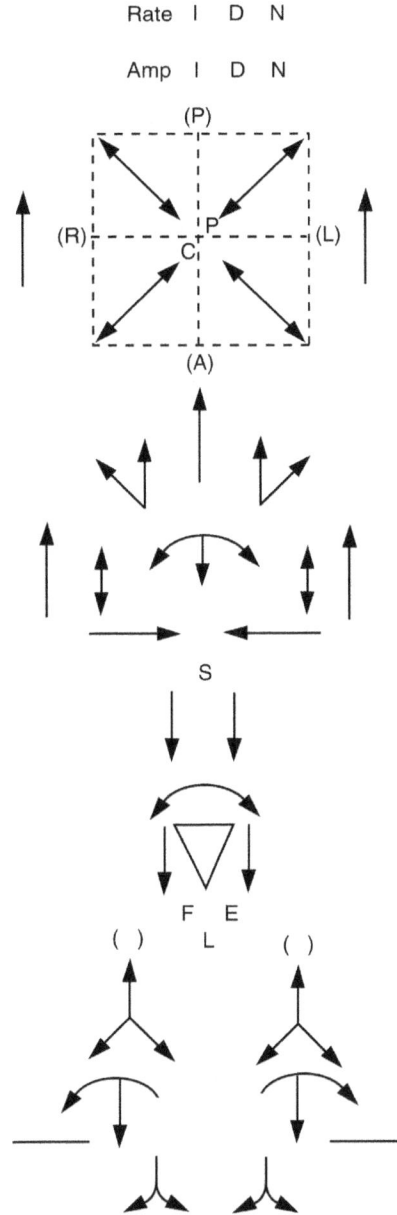

1 Rate I D N   Rate I D N

2 Amp I D N   Amp I D N

1. Is rate of CRI increased, decreased, or normal? (circle I, D or N)
2. Is amplitude of CRI increased, decreased, or normal? (circle I, D or N)
3. Is flexion restricted in one or more quadrants?
4. Is extension restricted in one or more quadrants?
5. Are flexion and extension out of phase (paradoxical) with expansion and contraction? (circle P)
6. Is compression of SBS present? (circle C)
7. Are sutural compressions present? (mark with an x)
8. Is temporal draw test restricted?
9. Is occipital condylar compression present?
10. Is occipital dural tension increased?
11. Is cruciate suture restricted?
12. Is clavicular "wiggle" restricted?
13. Is shoulder abduction restricted?
14. Is upper costal cage compression restricted?

15. Is sternal compliance restricted in response to compression?
16. Is lateral costal cage translation restricted?
17. Is diaphragm shock evident? (circle S)
18. Is lumbar sidebending restricted?
19. Is pelvic rock test restricted?
20. Is sacral traction met with resistance?
21. Are flexion and extension movements of the CRI restricted in the sacrum? (circle F or E)
22. Is longitudinal (vertical) rise of sacrum absent during flexion? (circle L)
23. Does tibial tuberosity bisect patella?
24. Is tibial varus or valgus present?
25. Is external rotation of CRI restricted in ankles? Where is most cephalad point of restriction?
26. Is traction test restricted in leg?
27. Is inversion/eversion restriction of ankle present?

93

Effects of Trauma on Breathing and Diaphragm Function

Breathing is a vital force which is essential to all body systems and is influenced greatly by musculoskeletal function. In addition to powering the air pressure gradient for the oxygenating function of the cardiopulmonary system, the diaphragm provides the intrathoracic pressure changes necessary for proper fluid return to the heart. Specifically, this refers to venous and lymphatic return from peripheral tissues. Proper delivery of arterial blood to metabolizing tissues also depends on this pressure gradient. Dr. Robert Fulford, DO is credited with many of the approaches to breathing and diaphragm function covered in this text. Dr. Fulford stressed the importance of breathing disturbances in many clinical syndromes and traced such disturbances to insufficient tissue expansion associated with the first breath of life.

During inhalation, the thoracic diaphragm descends, expanding intrathoracic volume and creating negative pressure in the chest. This provides a pressure gradient for fluid return to the thoracic cage. During exhalation, positive pressure is restored by diaphragmatic elevation into the thoracic cage, decreasing intrathoracic volume. If diaphragmatic motion is compromised, intrathoracic pressure gradients will be altered and will compromise proper fluid return to the heart.

Musculoskeletal elements associated with diaphragmatic function include:
- The thoracolumbar spine and lower costal cage, thoracic and extrathoracic muscles and their fascial interconnections.
- Functional relations to the lower extremity and pelvis through direct muscular attachments as well as forces transmitted through the lumbodorsal fascia and pelvic diaphragm.
- Neural innervation of the diaphragam from C3, C4, and C5 (phrenic nerve).
- Myofascial elements within the diaphragm itself that can become compromised during circumstances of traumatic or emotional shock. This is mediated through both local tissue response and supra-segmental reflex mechanisms.

When respiration is impeded suddenly, as with the often audible sigh accompanying the inhalation burst that results from a traumatic or shocking stimulus, the diaphragm's gamma feedback system may be short-circuited by the extreme acceleration force and adrenaline response generated. Recovery may take several minutes to hours. In the interim, hyperventilation may occur from asynchronous diaphragm contraction and vocalization may be absent or significantly altered. The diaphragm demonstrates altered motion even after the adrenaline response has subsided, held in the inhalation phase by resulting muscular and fascial restrictions. The diaphragm's pull on the xyphoid process will cause a slight depression laterally, usually to the left of the xyphi-sternal joint due to the dampening effect of the liver on the right.

Release of these myofascial elements may cause a return to normal diaphragmatic (and cardiorespiratory) function, as well as exerting a profound influence on physiologic and psychologic phenomenon related to breathing, diaphragm function and the shock of trauma. When optimal respiratory mechanics are in place, the midline fluid function of the CRI is more easily stimulated and maintained. The following costal cage approaches focus on direct engagement of restrictions involving larger myofascial structures. While indirect methods may be applied, they are often insufficient to match the force held within these unique structures.

Shock Release Technique

Diagnosis is performed while patient is supine, operator stands to the side; left side if the patient is female, right side if patient is male. Run your fingers lightly along the left medial costal margin towards the xyphoid process. A depression of the soft tissues medial to the costal margin and lateral to the xyphoid process can be palpated when shock is present in the body.

Treatment: Operator places hands side-by-side, all fingers in a line, with a little finger at each end. Gently and slowly the operator introduces these eight fingers into the abdomen in the midline between the umbilicus and the xyphoid (interlocking thumbs provide stability). Continue downward with each exhalation, deep into the subdiaphragmatic fascia until a firm resistance is met. Keep holding tension at this point of resistance until a melting sensation occurs under your fingers and you feel a softening of the tissues—a gentle rocking, bobbing motion—this indicates that a stillpoint has been achieved. This procedure takes two to three minutes and can be quite uncomfortable (test abduction of the shoulders before and after this procedure to note any difference). As shock is released, often the memory of its cause will be retrieved and the psychological stress released.

For infants and children, clump three fingers together and allow them to sink slowly into the abdomen below the xyphoid process, with the other hand cupped above the vertex of the head, proceed as above to the point of resistance and hold for the release.

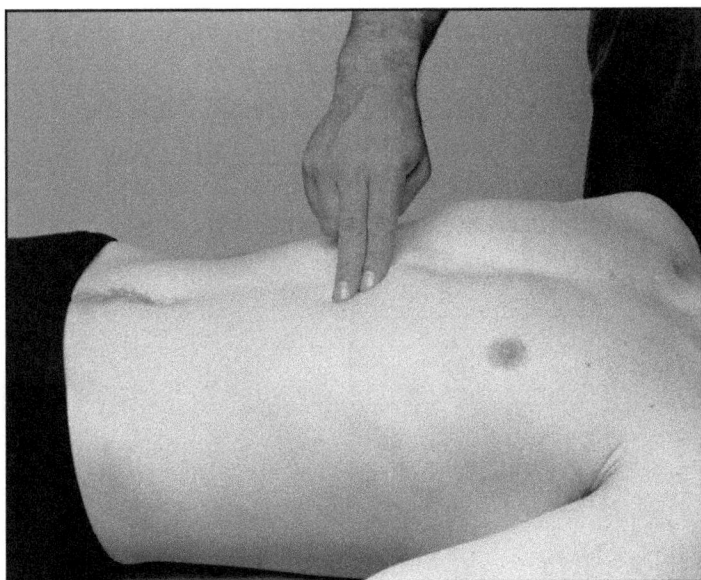

Diagnosis for Shock Release Technique

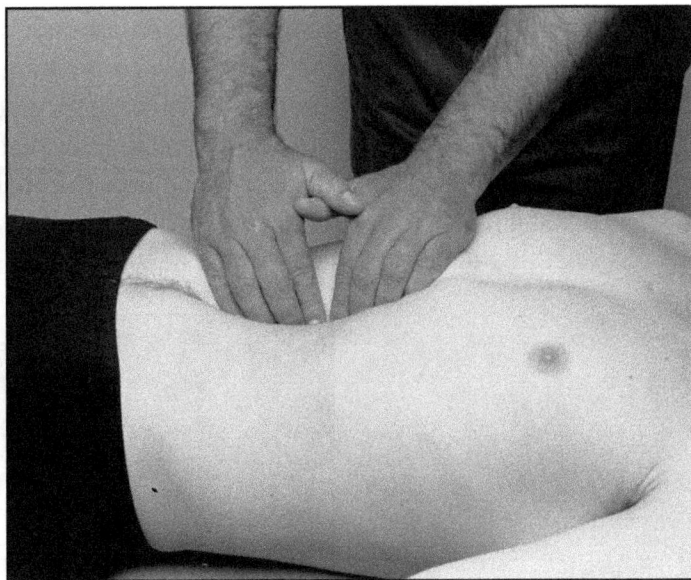

Shock Release Technique Treatment

Rib Cage Release

Diagnosis is made with patient supine and operator to the side as before. Test for medial compression and lateral translation of the inferior costal cage for areas of restriction.

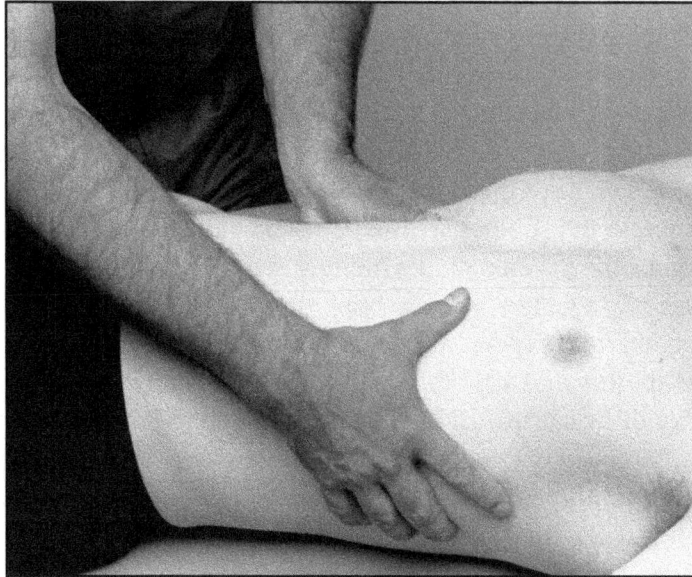

Rib Cage Release Diagnosis

Bilateral **treatment** is performed with operator's hands over the anterior lateral rib cage components. The thumbs come together along the costal margins parallel and just lateral to the xyphoid. The operator strongly compresses the rib cage medially with internal rotation into the xyphoid while the patient holds their breath deeply inhaling through their nose. The release at the xyphoid will occur just before the patient feels a strong urge to exhale. Patient may assist medial compressive force by placing hands over operator's. Recoil inhalation can be stimulated after patient exhales by quickly releasing hands at the start of the next inhalation.

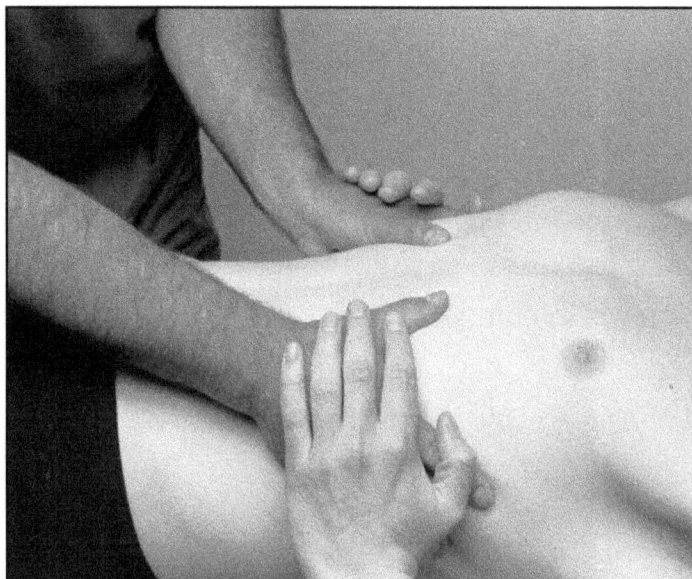

Rib Cage Release Treatment

Anterior Diaphragm Release

Diagnosis of an anterior diaphragm restriction is made with the patient supine, the examiner standing on either the left or the right of the patient. A gentle pressure is exerted underneath the anterior costal margin bilaterally. Resistance to pressure should be tested just underneath the rib cage at the anterior attachment of the diaphragm from the sternal notch to about the area of the anterior axillary line.

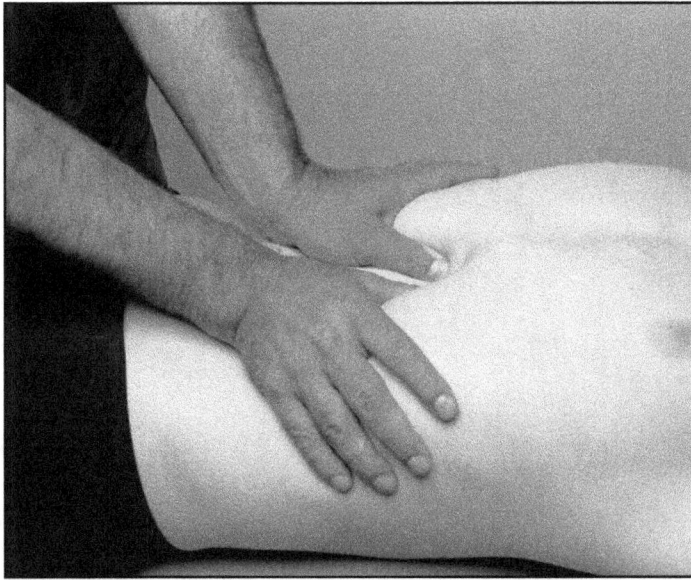

Diagnosis for Anterior Diaphragm Release

Unilateral treatment of any tissue resistance assessed should be made by direct myofascial engagement and release using one hand to compress underneath the rib cage, the other hand gently compressing the ipsilateral costal cage to help increase the depth with which the fingers are engaging the diaphragm. The patient should be instructed to breathe as normally as possible and the tissue compressed further with each exhalation of the patient. The treatment is completed when a release is felt under the fingers in the tissues being compressed.

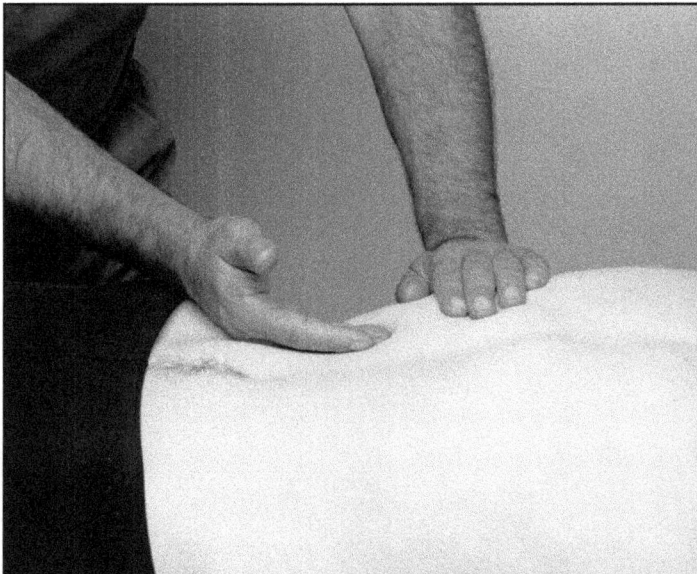

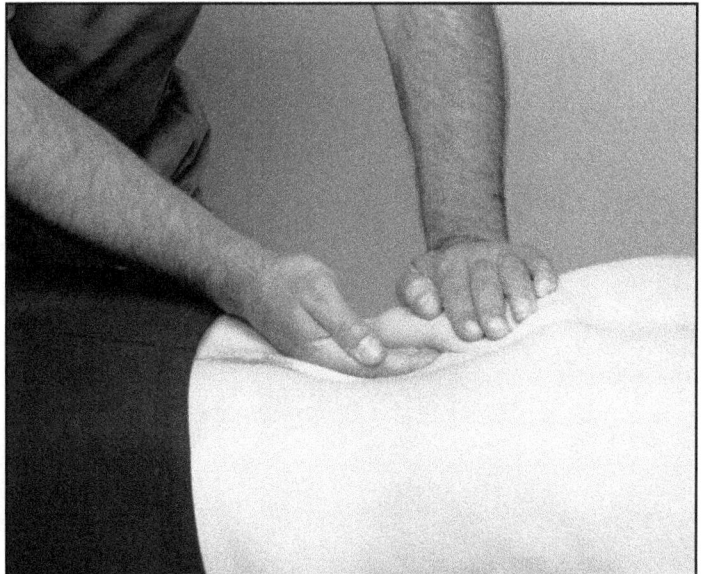

Anterior Diaphragm Release- Unilateral Treatment

Bilateral treatment can be carried out by placing the thumbs medially and exerting lateral and superior pressure beneath the costal margins. Maintaining this pressure, thoracic cage side bending and rotation are added in a direction which allows further laterosuperior penetration of the thumbs into the areas of subcostal tension. Inhalation and exhalation modulation can be added until a release of tension is palpated.

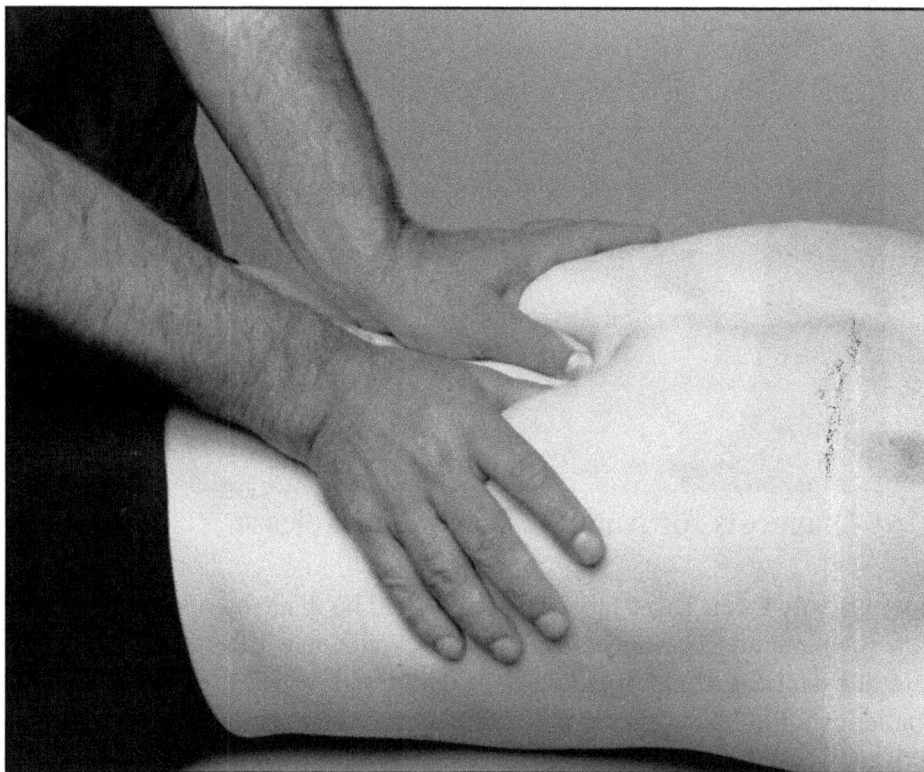

Anterior Diaphragm Release- Bilateral Treatment

Sternum

Diagnostic testing for compliance of sternum is done by introducing a posterior compressive force through the sternal midline.

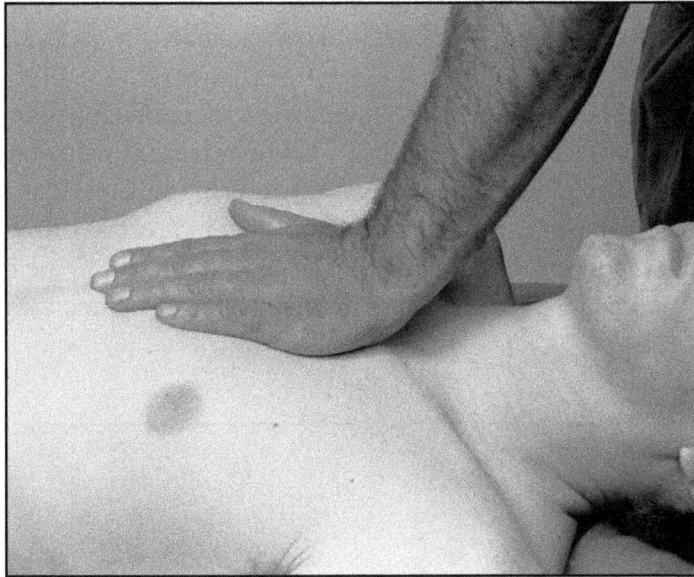

Sternum Diagnosis

Treatment with thumb contact. Contact is with the patient supine, operator at the side, as before. Gently rock the sternum with thumbs on either side of the sternal angle, above and below. Tension will build and then release with an increase in sternal compliance after 6-9 cycles.

Treatment with hands is accomplished by pushing simultaneously on either side of the sternal angle, using the thenar/hypothenar aspects of both hands in a gentle pumping motion.

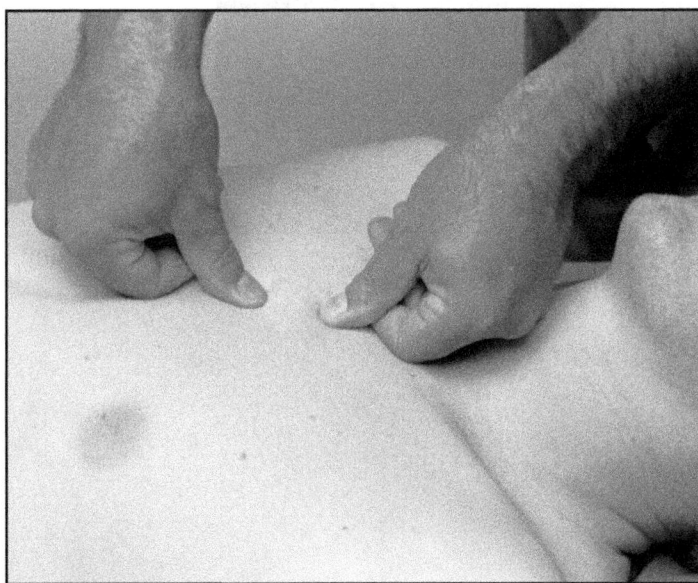

Sternum Treatment- Thumb Contact

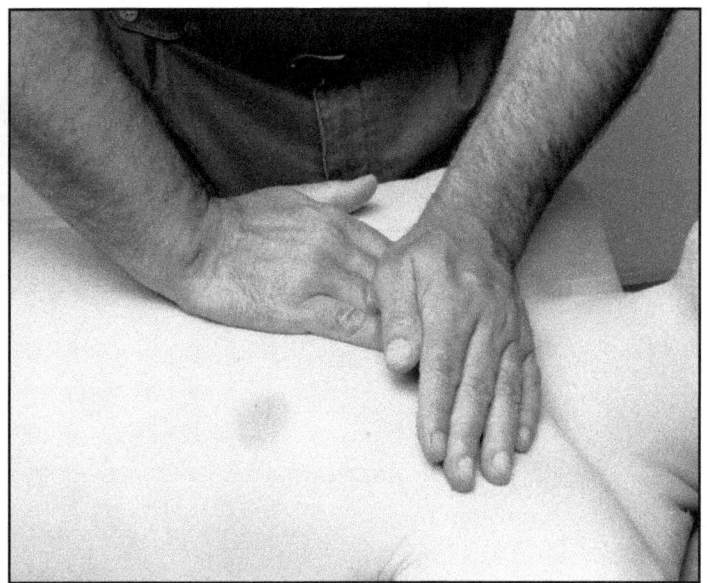

Sternum Treatment- Hand Contact

Clavicle

Diagnosis is performed with the patient supine, operator sits at the head of the table, holding onto the medial third of the clavicle, one in each hand, between the thumb and index finger. Diagnosis of the side that is restricted is performed by carrying out the "wiggle" test by gently moving each clavicle superiorly and inferiorly, testing for decreased compliance.

Bilateral treatment is carried out by placing the thumbs in the supraclavicular space over the area of greatest tissue tension. Inferior traction is held until a gentle release is palpated. Fine tuning for this release is achieved by gently accentuating membrane tensions in the directions of ease in a medial/lateral and internally rotated/externally rotated direction. This indirect positioning helps to focus the inferior traction forces into the tissue disturbances posterior and inferior to the clavicle. After completion of the technique, the "wiggle" test should be repeated to appreciate any change.

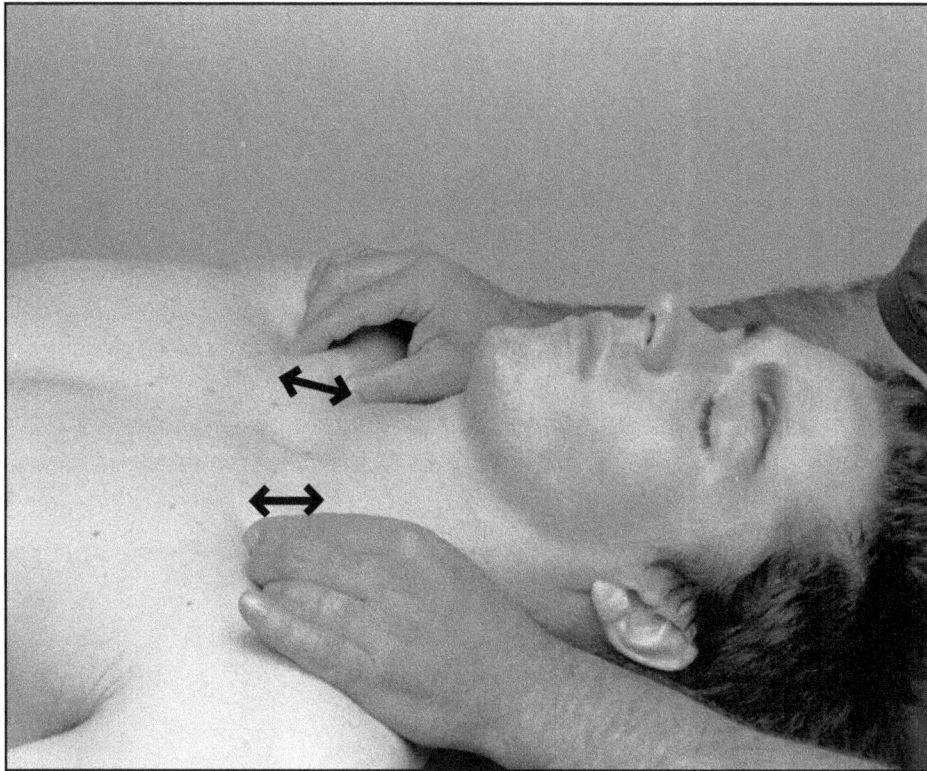

Clavicle Diagnosis and Treatment

Shoulder

Diagnosis is performed with the patient supine, the operator stands at the head of the table with each hand placed over the lateral trapezius, with firm contact against the lateral aspect of the clavicle. Diagnosis of shoulder dysfunction is achieved through sidebending the thoracic girdle one side at a time to determine the side that has reduced compliance, not necessarily reduced range.

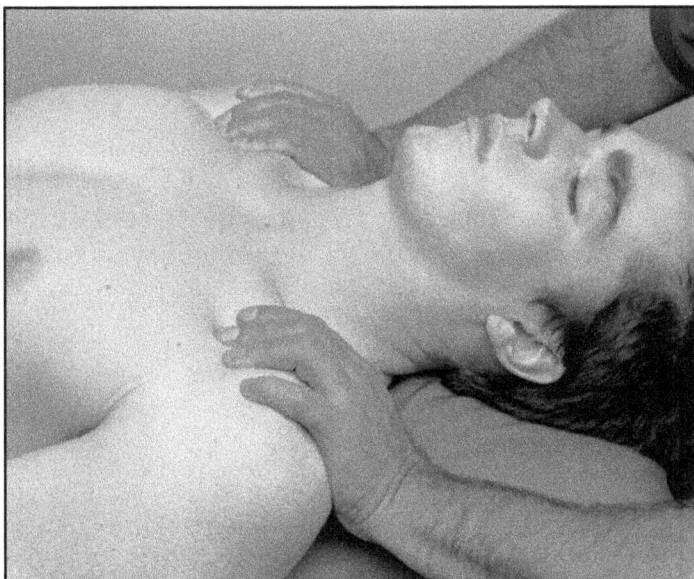

Shoulder Diagnosis

Treatment is then carried out with the operator sitting on the side of the dysfunction facing the head of the patient, with one hand cupping the inferior angle of the scapula, the other hand contacting the acromion and clavicle in one motion. The patient's arm rests in the groove created by the operator's arm and flank. The scapula, clavicle, acromion, and shoulder are all gently compressed and translated into their directions of relative ease and held until a gentle release occurs. Sidebending of the shoulder should be repeated to access any change. This is the only indirect treatment in this sequence because of the multiple articulations converging on the scapula. Direct technique can also be applied, however.

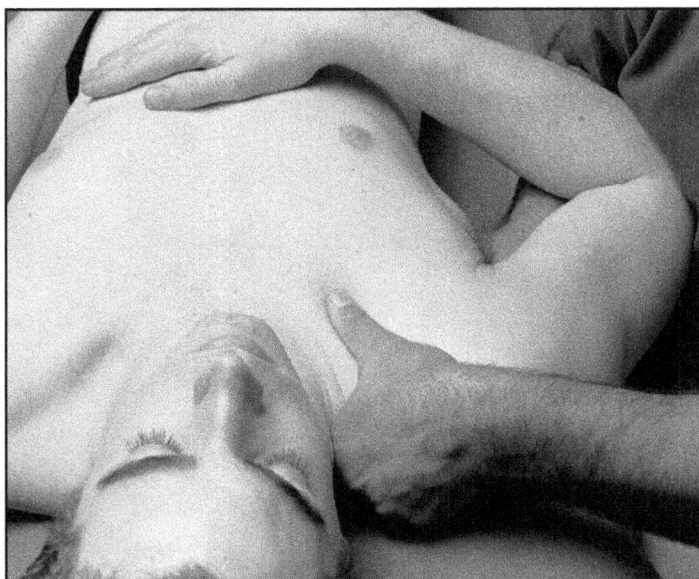

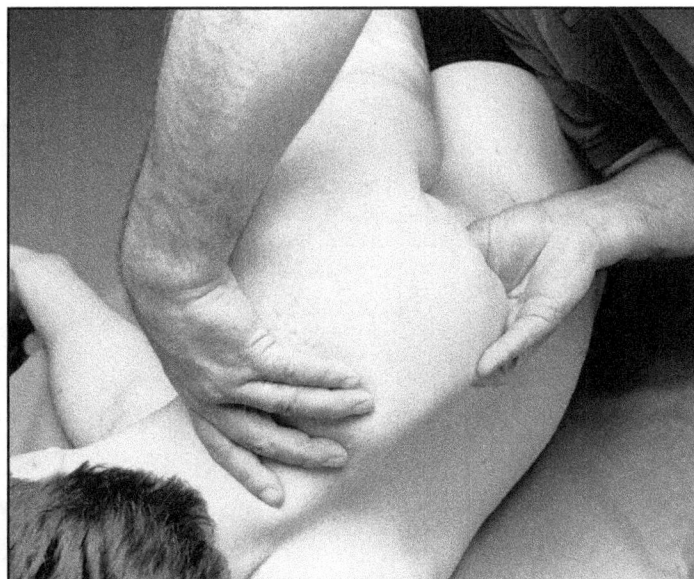

Shoulder Treatment

Daily Supplemental Exercises

These exercises were developed to maintain and augment the vital force within. Done daily, these exercises will assure that the beneficial effects brought about by your treatments are maintained. Though these exercises are straightforward and simple, they have a profound effect. Doing these daily and properly will help assure you of better health and increased vitality.

Breathing

Sitting up straight and comfortably, place the tongue behind the two front teeth on the roof of the palate. Close mouth and inhale through your nostrils, fully expanding your lungs and hold for the count of seven. Exhale through the mouth at your own rate, keeping the tongue touching the palate.

Do this for seven breaths twice a day.
*This is considered the most important exercise.

Arm-Raising From Horizontal

1. Stand with your feet shoulder width apart, with arms extended out to the sides shoulder height.
2. Left palm should face upward and the right palm should face downward.
3. Hold this position for as long as possible, breathing full deep breaths. The ideal length of time is 5-10 minutes.
4. At the end of the exercise, keeping the arms straight, slowly raise them up and out to the sides of the body and above the head, not letting the arms come forward.

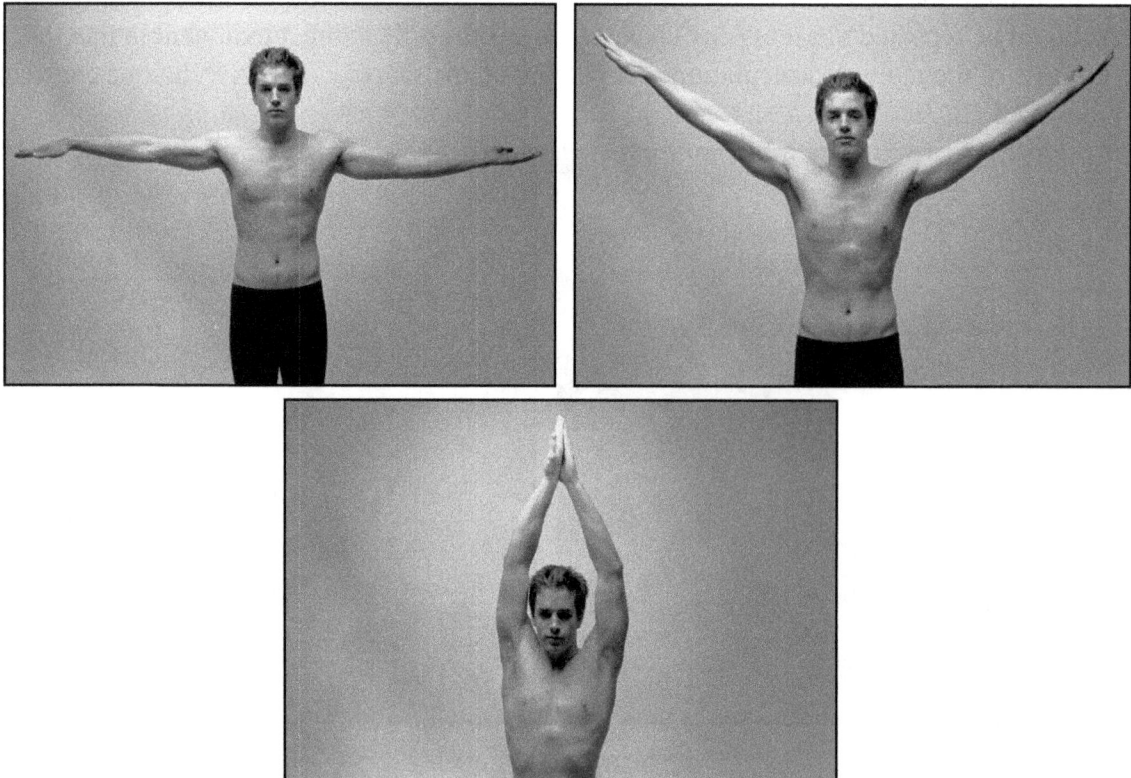

Arm-Raising From Horizontal

Hip Twist

1. Lie on your back with your arms stretched out to your side at shoulder level (like in the previous excercise) with the left palm facing up and the right palm facing down. (not shown in picture)
2. Bring the feet together with knees straight.
3. Lift the right leg off the floor, keeping the leg straight and roll the right hip and right leg over the left leg, keeping the lumbar spine on the table as much as possible.
4. Keep both shoulders on the floor and breathe fully while holding the position for up to 5 minutes or until you feel pain.
5. Bring the leg back to its original position and do the same procedure for the left leg.

Hold the positions for 5 minutes or until pain, on each side once per day. Ideally the excercise should be done without experiencing pain.

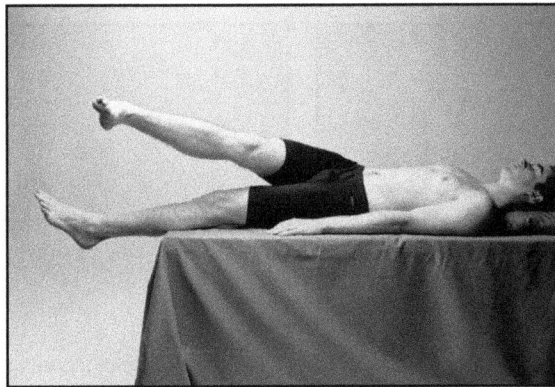

Hip Twist

Spinal Stretch

1. Sit upright in a chair so that your thighs are parallel with the floor and the lower part of the leg is perpendicular to the floor.
2. Bend forward, moving your head first, then the thoracic spine, then the lumbar spine to place your elbows on the inside of your knees and hands on the floor.
3. Let your spine fully relax and stretch in this position.
4. Breathe slowly and fully for up to 5 minutes. Do one time a day.

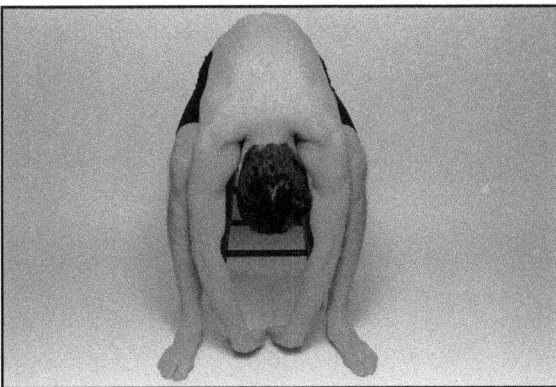

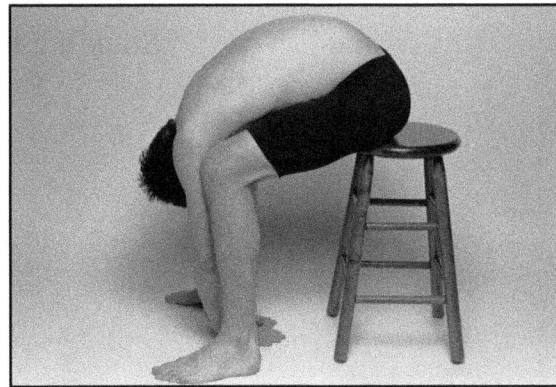

Spinal Stretch

Standing Full Arm Raise

1. Stand against a wall so that your heels, lower back, the spine between your shoulder blades and the back of your head touch the wall.
2. Raise your arms straight out in front of you. Then, with a deep inhalation slowly raise them straight above your head, finally touching the wall.
3. Then lower the arms out and down to your sides as you exhale.
4. Remember to breathe slowly and fully.

Do this 2 times, once per day.

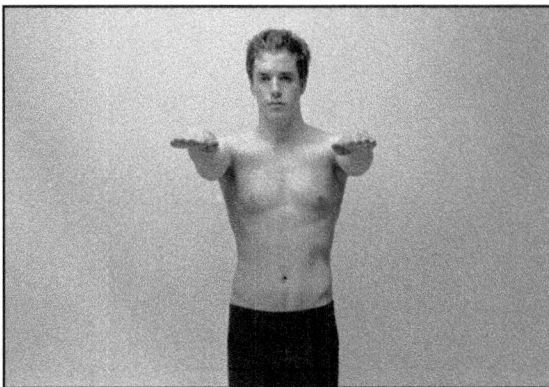

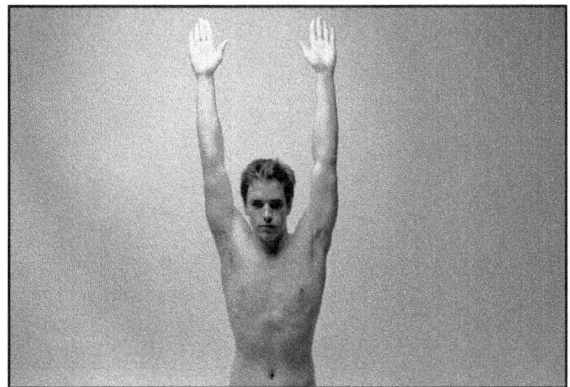

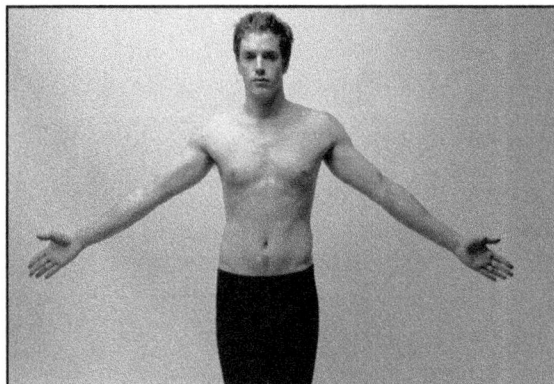

Standing Full Arm Raise

Technique to Bring the Three Diaphragms into Phase

Synchronous movement of the body's functional diaphragms should be assessed and restored to optimize respiratory and midline function. Inhalation is associated with expansion and caudal movement of the body diaphragms. Exhalation is associated with cephalad movement.

I. Tentorium Cerebelli/Thoracic Diaphragm Synchrony

Hold the temporal bone with the little and ring fingers on the mastoid process, middle finger in the external auditory meatus, index finger and thumb grasping the zygomatic arch. The other hand reaches over the thorax so that the fingers rest below the costal margin on the same side as the temporal bone. Let the head rest in the curve of the elbow of the thoracic arm.

Ask the patient to take one deep inhalation. Note the direction of motion of the thoracic diaphragm. (Physiologically it should descend.) Note the direction of motion of the temporal bone. (Physiologically it should externally rotate.) If the temporal bone moves into internal rotation the following treatment is used. (If external rotation is restricted this is not the proper treatment, the temporal bone must move into internal rotation for this treatment.)

As the patient takes a deep inhalation the temporal is carried by the inherent mechanism into internal rotation. Hold it in that position while the patient fully exhales. This action brings the thoracic diaphragm into its exhalation phase. Thus, both temporal bone and thoracic diaphragm are being held in the exhalation phase while the patient maintains the exhalation to the limit. At the moment when the inhalation cannot be resisted any longer there is a swing of the temporal into external rotation. Recheck on deep inhalation.

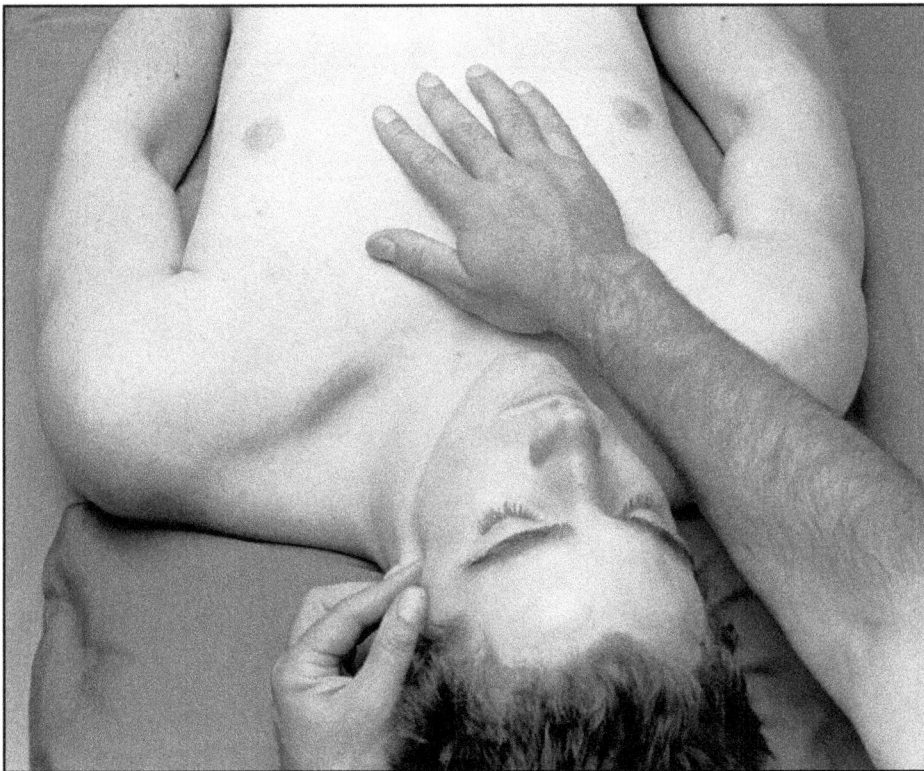

Balancing the Tentorium Cerebelli and the Diaphragm

II. Pelvic Diaphragm/Thoracic Diaphragm Synchrony

To approach the pelvic diaphragm the patient should be supine with the operator seated at the side of pelvis to be treated, facing the patient's head.

Flex the patient's knee and hip on this side. Identify the ischial tuberosity. Introduce the index and middle fingers medial to the tuberosity, letting the pads of the fingers keep contact with the medial surface of the ischium. The examiner's fingers are now in the ischiorectal fossa, the inclined roof of which is the pelvic diaphragm. As the patient inhales the pelvic diaphragm should press down on the examiner's fingertips. If, however, the pelvic diaphragm is unable to descend, i.e., it is held in the exhalation phase of its cycle, the following technique is used.

With the hand closest to the patient the operator introduces two fingers as described above into the ischiorectal fossa. The other hand is placed just below the costal margin on the same side to monitor movement of the thoracic diaphragm. The patient is instructed to take a deep inhalation, then exhale to the limit and maintain the exhalation until forced to breathe. The operator accentuates the cephalad position of the diaphragm with upward pressure of the fingers. At the moment of forced inhalation or a moment before, the pelvic diaphragm descends. Recheck. Always evaluate both sides!

If the pelvic diaphragm is in an inferior position and will not ascend into exhalation, instruct the patient to hold his breath to the limit in inhalation and the pelvic diaphragm will begin to ascend a moment before forced exhalation occurs. The operator accentuates the inferior position with slight pressure above the pubes downwards. Repeat on the other side.

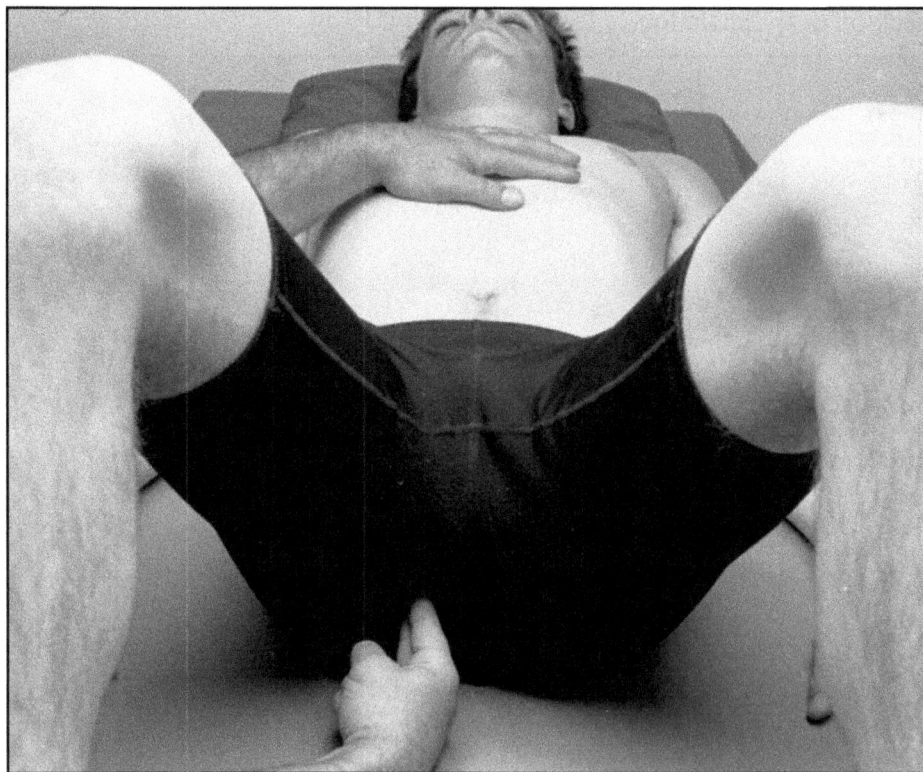

Balancing the Pelvic Diaphragm and the Diaphragm

(Reference: "Core Link and the Three Diaphragms." AAO Yearbook 1968, pp 13-19)

Diagonal Vector Release

Forces entering the body as the result of injury may take on spiraling or diagonal vectors. Myofascial structures involved in total body balance and counter-balance may be effected by the torquing strain pattern introduced into the body. Both dural and extra-dural tissues are involved in these diagonal vector injuries. Often you will see a sacroiliac restriction and an occipital restriction on opposite sides of the body. Usually, the temporal bone and zygoma on the same side of the occipital restriction will also be involved.

Simple techniques which engage the diagonal vector with gentle compressive forces along the spiraling axis of restriction produce releases affecting total body balance and counterbalance.

Diagnosis. Contacting the supine patient on the bilateral ASIS determines which sacroiliac joint is restricted. Then contacting the cranium determines if there is an occipital or temporal bone dysfunction, i.e., condylar compression, occipital mastoid compression, or positive temporal draw test.

Treatment. Standing along the supine patient, the operator contacts the ASIS of the hemipelvis where the restriction was assessed and the other hand rests on the mid chest at the sternum. An alternating, pumping, rocking force is introduced in an AP direction, first the pelvis then the sternum. The feeling of chest cage and pelvic resistance will increase to a point and then resistance will decrease at the point of diagonal vector release. Hand contact can also be situated in other locations, for example, on the zygoma and the ASIS, with posterior compression through the zygoma.

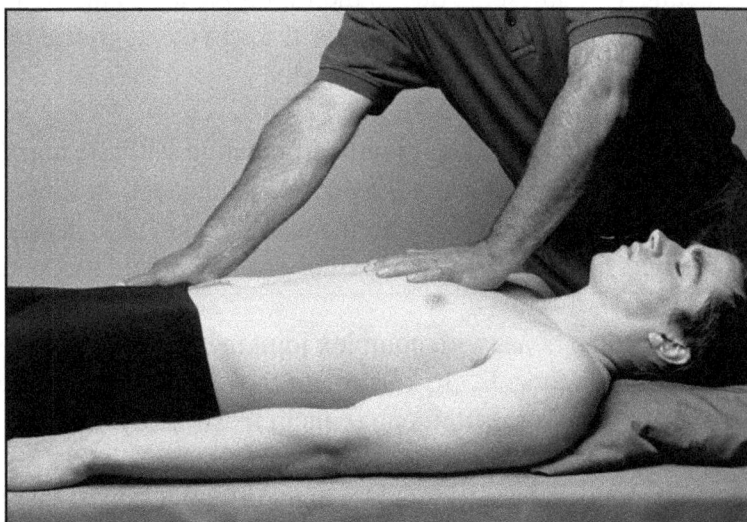
Diagonal Vector Release Treatment

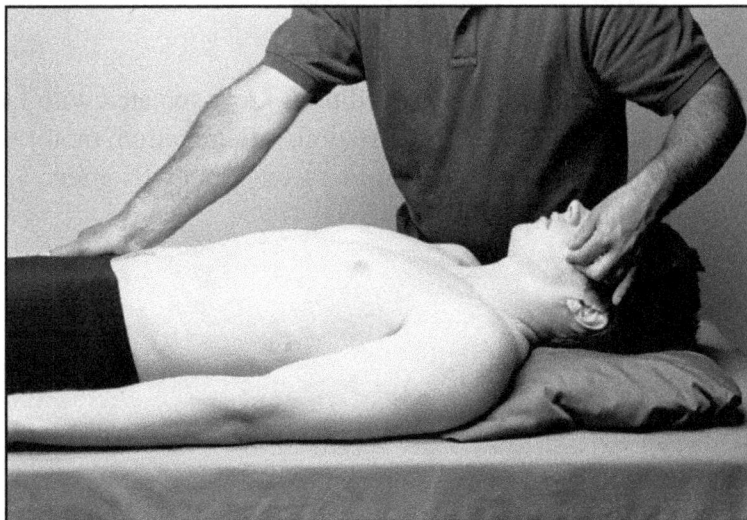
Alternate Diagonal Vector Release Treatment

Facial Trauma

Anatomic relations of the facial bones and their associated movements deepen our understanding of the cranial concept. Contrary to its appearance as a static structure, the face contains innumerable and complex articulations with functionally dynamic properties resembling gears, tracks, hinges, grooves and movable plates. Due to torsional, shearing and compressive forces associated with micro and macro trauma, these dynamic articular functions may be compromised. Only through proper understanding of these articular mechanics can traumatic disturbances be properly assessed and the appropriate therapeutic forces applied.

Basic physiologic movements of the SBS, in its respective flexion and extension phases, are intimately linked to the associated physiologic movements of all the facial bones. The two midline bones attached to the sphenoid are the **vomer** and **ethmoid**, both of which move in a gear-like fashion, in a direction opposite to that of the sphenoid. Though both bones are protected by their maxillary armor, both are equally vulnerable to disturbances introduced through the maxillary bone. Making up the prominence of the cheeks, the **maxillae** and **zygomae** are frequent recipients of head-on and lateral blows. Dental procedures, such as difficult tooth extractions, as well as orthodontic appliances, can cause disturbances of their normal articular relations and associated movements. The zygomae are particularly troublesome due to their multiple articulations with the frontal, temporal and maxillary bones. Shearing compressive forces through the zygomae obstruct the physiologic movements of these bones, and usually occur unilaterally.

At the posterior end of the hard palate of the mouth, articulating with the maxillary bone, is the equally troublesome **palatine** bone. Like a brake pad, it simultaneously directs and restrains motion of the sphenoid bone through its articulation with the lateral and medial ptyergoid processes. This track-like relation is easily disturbed by faulty maxillary or sphenoidal mechanics.

The **mandible** is the last midline bone, with complex joint mechanics due to its discogenic, ligamentous, articular and muscular components. Its relation to the temporal bone is of fundamental concern, as well as its role in conjunction with the maxilla in masticatory and oratory functions.

Contributions to orbital anatomy are contributed by eight different bones, therefore making this particular region susceptible to disturbances of anatomic relations of the face. Physiologic functions associated with the face and eyeball reflect integration of mechanical, motor, neural and fluid properties.

Numerous clinical syndromes and pathologic conditions are associated with facial bone disturbances. They may include neuropathies, neuralgias, congestion, inflammation, motor dysynergies of the eyes, mouth and face, tinnitus, cephalgia, learning disorders, emotional disorders, as well as disorders of sensation related to the skin, nose and tongue.

Intraoral Technique

1. Cruciate Suture: Screening Test of the Facial Mechanism

The vomer provides a valuable diagnostic and therapeutic communication between the accessible hard palate and the inaccessible sphenobasilar synchondrosis. The rostrum on the inferior surface of the sphenoid is received into the superior articular surface of the vomer as the hull of a ship is received into a dry dock. The body of the sphenoid has a movement here like that afforded by a universal joint, but at the same time it transmits its inferior or superior motion of flexion or extension, respectively, through the vomer to the hard palate. The vomer is a significant factor in depressing the palate in flexion and elevating it in extension provided that its articulation with the horizontal plates of the maxillae is intact.

Diagnosis: Standing on the right side of the patient's head, place the pad of the tip of the right index finger on the cruciate suture where intermaxillary and interpalatine suture bisects the maxilla-palatine in the roof of the mouth. Place the left thumb on the glabella just superior to the frontonasal articulation and the middle finger on the sagittal suture. (Bregma contact can also be used.) If the mechanism is moving physiologically, slight pressure on the cruciate suture will produce elevation of the sagittal suture and slight prominence of the metopic suture, as in sphenobasilar extension. Conversely, slight pressure with the vault contact will depress the cruciate suture.

Treatment: Gently accentuating this rocking motion will encourage drainage of the ethmoid sinuses. If motion of the hard palate is restricted, maintain gentle steady pressure until it "softens" and begins to move, and increased motion is observed by the vault contact.

In some instances, when the hard palate is markedly elevated and the alveolar margins form a very narrow dental arch, i.e. extreme extension of the sphenoid and internal rotation of the maxillae and palatines, the vomer may not provide the usual transmission of motion between the sphenoid and the palate. Pressure on the cruciate suture does not produce extension and elevation of the sagittal suture, and pressure on the glabella or sagittal suture does not produce descent of the cruciate suture.

Additional testing should be carried out on each of the four bones of the hard palate to observe if cephalad forces are transmitted to the glabella. Treatment should be carried out on the maxilla and palatine bones demonstrating poor compliance to this motion, as follows.

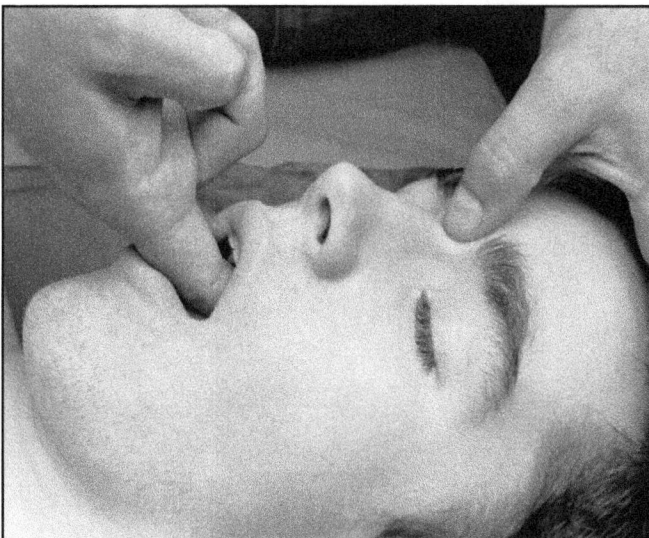

Diagnosis and Treatment of
Cruciate Suture

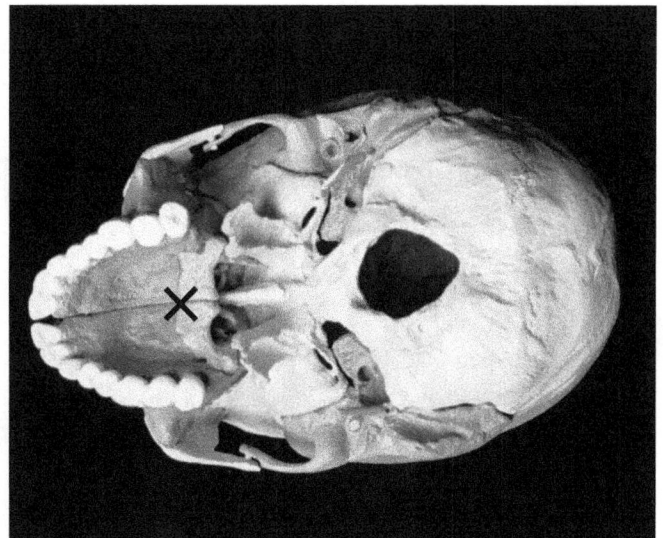

Location of Cruciate Suture

2. Maxilla.

In the adult there are two maxillae with the intermaxillary suture between them. Developmentally each maxilla has two parts. The premaxilla is a small, somewhat rectangular portion bearing the upper incisor teeth of that side and extending to the anterior inferior margin of the nasal cavity. The body of the maxilla carries all the other teeth and enters into the formation of the roof of the mouth, the floor of the orbit, lateral wall of the nose and the anterior wall of the sphenomaxillary fissure.

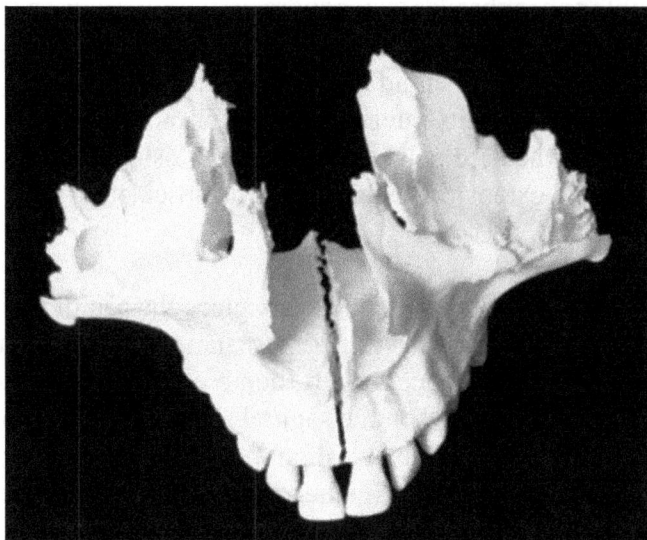

Maxilla

Unilateral Treatment. The palatine process of the maxilla is bevelled superiorly where it articulates with the horizontal plate of the palatine bone. This articulation is frequently locked by orthodontic procedures. To restore physiologic motion, it is necessary to lower the articular surface of the maxilla while elevating that of the palatine. The operator stands on the right side of the patient and introduces the index finger immediately posterior to the right upper incisor teeth. By gently lifting the anterior part of the maxilla, the posterior part descends. At the same time the tip of the middle finger is placed on the horizontal plate of the right palatine and gently lifts it in a cephalad direction. Meanwhile the thumb of the left hand monitors the motion of the perpendicular process of the maxilla just lateral to the right nasal bone. The procedure is completed when there is restoration of motion of the palatine at the suture; there is a sense of "softening" the patient feels the tenderness leave and the vertical process assumes a more transverse motion. Repeat on the other side. An alternate treatment approach introduces one finger from each hand, with the pinky finger on the palatine bone.

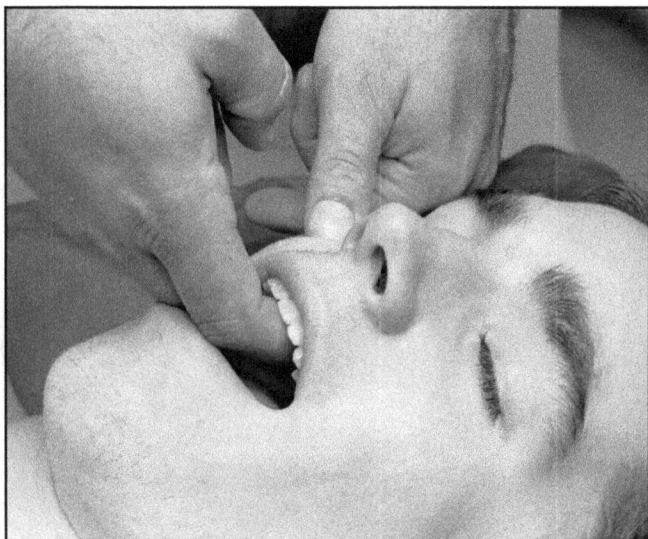

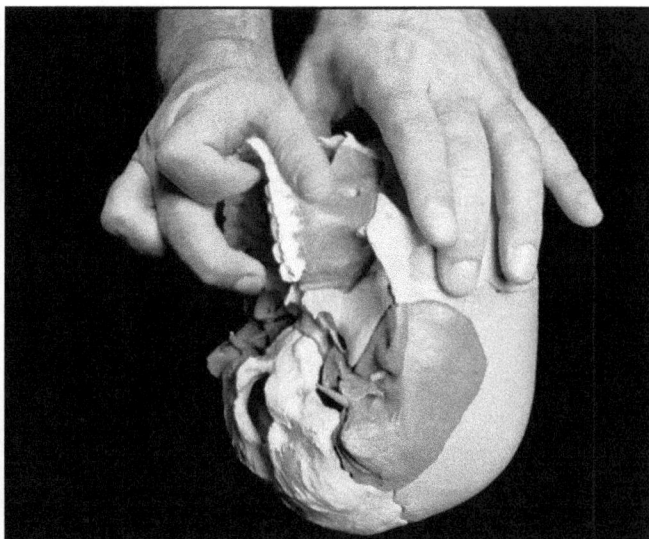

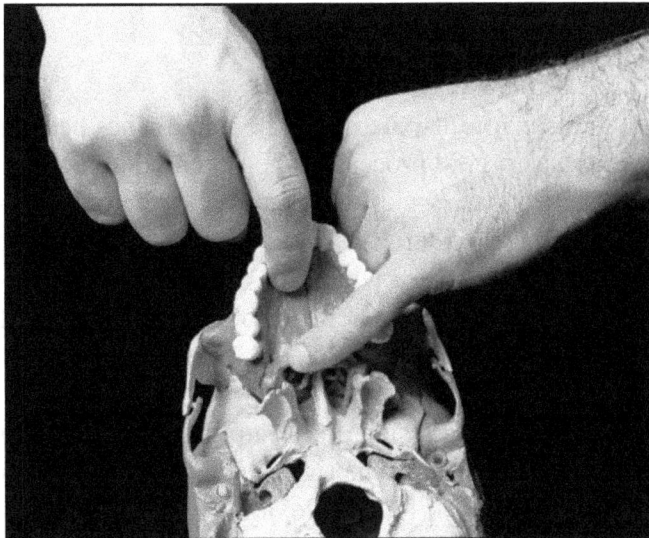

Alternate Unilateral Maxilla Treatment

Bilateral Treatment. The intermaxillary suture permits a small degree of shearing motion such as occurs when biting a hard morsel on one side of the mouth. It is possible to create a strain at this articulation by such asymmetrical chewing or by some orthodontic procedures. Stand at the head of the table, lay the pads of the two index fingers on the inferior surfaces of the palatine processes of the maxillae, right finger on right maxilla, and left on left. Gently test the relative vertical motion of one relative to the other. Follow in the direction in which they move more freely, apply a slight lateral traction to decompress the suture and await the "softening" and restoration of physiologic motion.

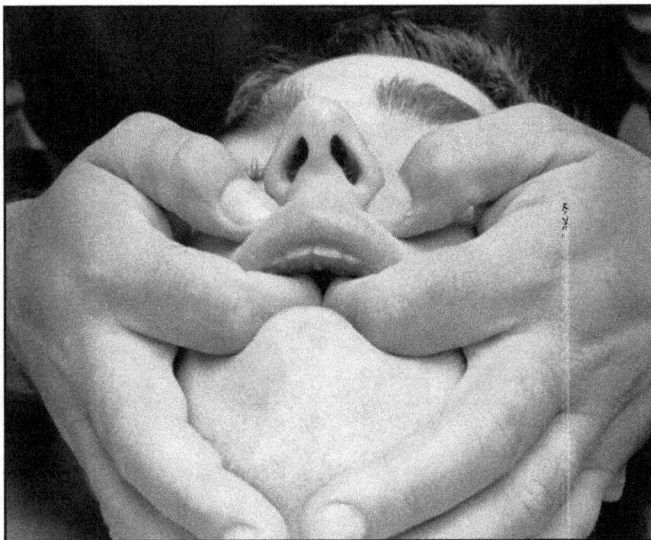

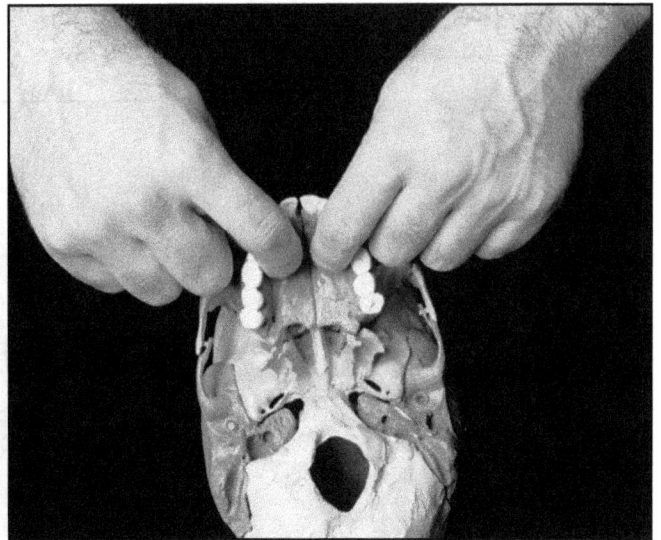

Bilateral Maxilla Treatment

3. Palatine

Inferior fixation. The relationship of the palatine to the maxilla has been considered. Posteriorly the palatine articulates with the pterygoid process of the sphenoid bilaterally. The medial and lateral pterygoid plates are separated by a narrow cleft which provides "a track" in which the pyramidal process of the palatine can glide. The posterior articular surface of this pyramidal process is divided into two concave articular surfaces by a crest which runs between the two pterygoid plates like the "foot" of an electric train within its track. This delicate articulation may be disturbed in traumatic lesions of the sphenoid or during a difficult upper dental extraction.

Diagnosis: The operator stands at the right side of the supine patient and introduces the pad of the right index finger onto the horizontal plate of the right palatine. The left hand gently grasps the sphenoid by the greater wings and rocks it toward flexion. If motion is unimpaired at the articulation, sphenoidal flexion should occur without difficulty as the intraoral finger holds the palatine in internal rotation.

Treatment: If motion is restricted, maintain the slight cephalad contact on the horizontal plate of the palatine, with gentle medial or lateral deviation (whichever is easier) maintain the sphenoid toward flexion and await the "softening" and restoration of physiologic motion. Repeat on the opposite side.

Superior fixation. If the palatine bone is positioned superiorly, it may not resolve with the treatment described above. When the pyramidal process of the palatine is compressed superiorly into the pterygoid plates, then the palatine bone has to be brought down inferiorly to separate it from the pterygoid plates of the sphenoid. To accomplish this, the sphenoid is brought into flexion as before; however, the operator's finger is positioned on the palatine process of the maxilla instead of the palatine. With a superior pressure applied to the moveable maxilla, the palatine can be fixed in a relatively inferior position. Next, the sphenoid is brought back up into extension through the greater wings gently articulating back and forth into flexion and extension to tease loose the restriction between the sphenoid and the palatine.

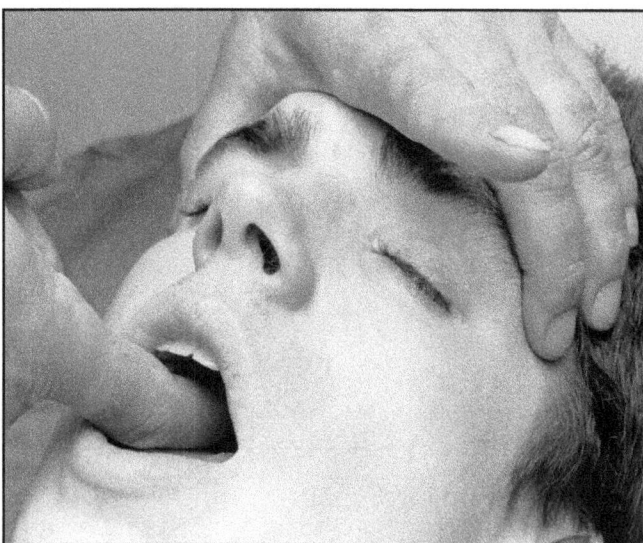

Palatine Treatment

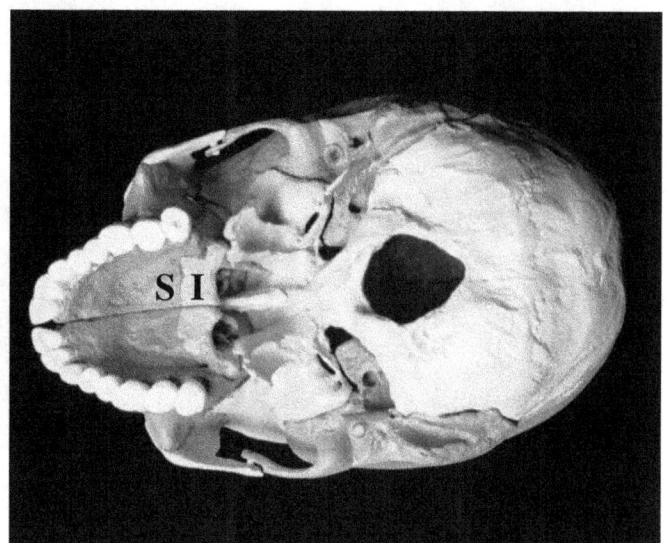

Finger Placement for Superior (S) and Inferior (I) Fixation

4. Zygoma

Diagnosis: Cephalad traction through the inferior aspect of the zygoma tests for the relative compliance of these articulations.

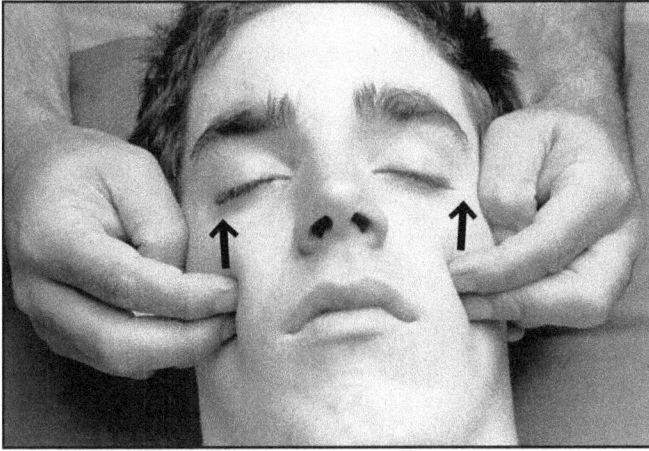

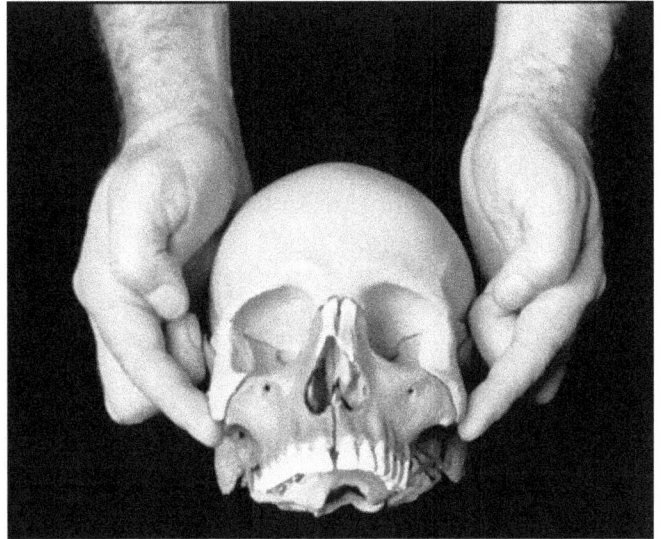

Zygoma Diagnosis

Treatment: A three-point zygoma technique can be carried out while sitting at the head of the patient. With single-finger contact on each of the bones that articulate with the zygoma (frontal, maxilla, and temporal), exert a slight compressive force of that bone into the zygoma. With one addition finger, the inferior edge of the zygoma is palpated and lifted superior and lateral to test its internal rotation function and compressed medially and inferiorly to test its external rotation function. The direction of greatest movement or least restriction is assumed in conjunction with the three-point compression through the adjacent bones. This position is held until a softening release is appreciated and the bone begins to move in its normal external/internal rotation.

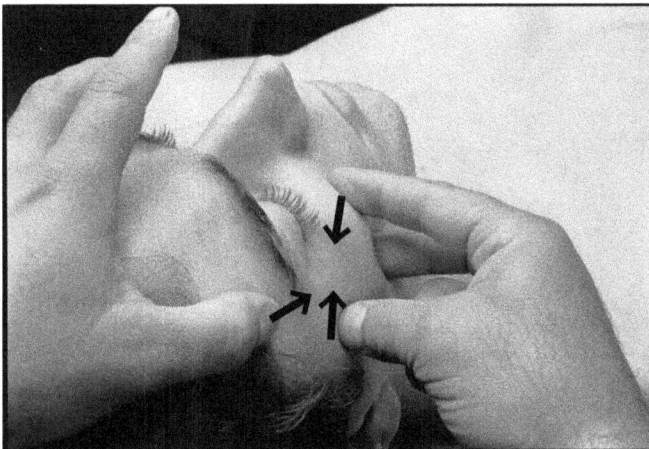

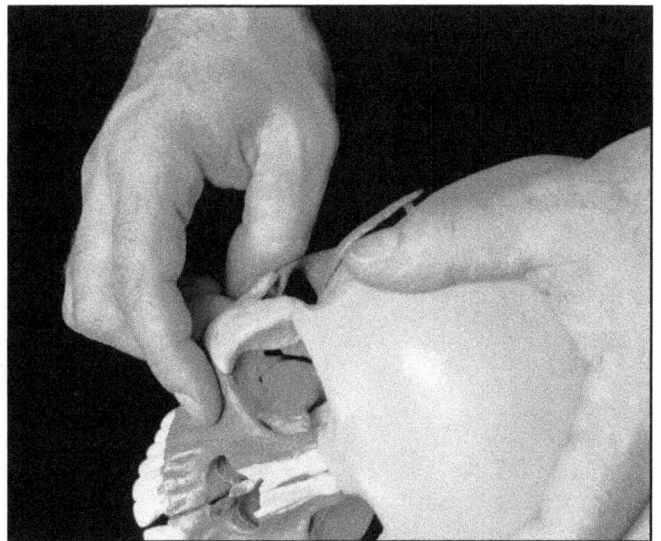

Zygoma Treatment

5. Vomer

Now the maxillae are ready to receive the vomer into its relationship at the intermaxillary suture. Stand on the right side of the supine patient. Rotate the maxilla into external rotation by placing the index finger on the lingual (medial) surface of the left third molar, and the middle finger on the lingual surface of the right third molar. Gently separate these two fingers while the left hand rocks the sphenoid into flexion by the greater wings. The moment of restitution of the vomer may be determined by a palpable click, or by a sudden freedom of motion of the sphenoid toward flexion. Then re-evaluate the motion of the vomer using the cruciate suture. An indirect approach to the vomer compresses the maxilla into internal rotation by cephalad pressure on the cruciate suture or by contacting the upper teeth laterally and squeezing medially while bringing the sphenoid into extension and awaiting the fluid "softening" and expansion release.

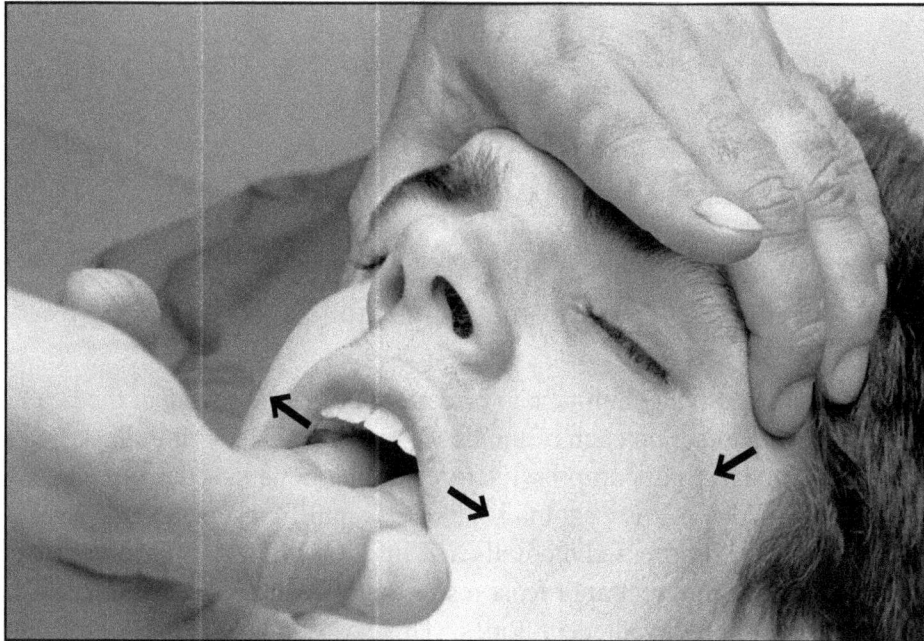

Vomer Treatment

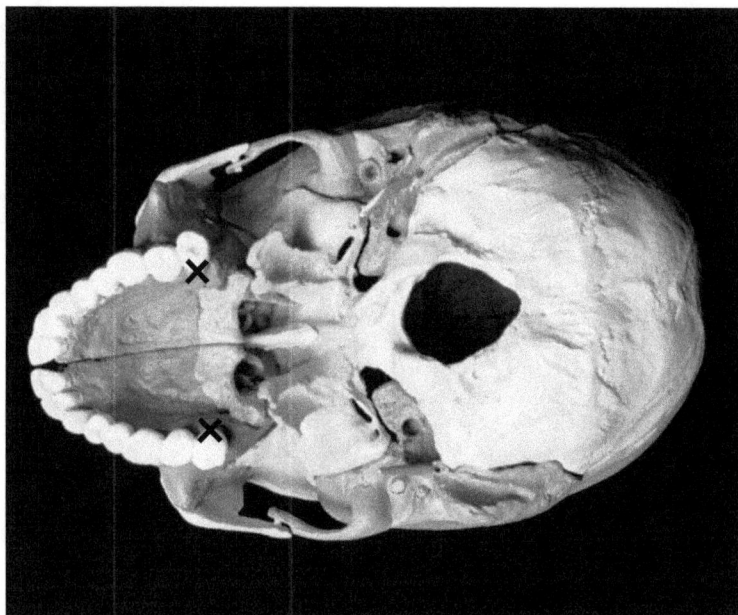

Finger Placement for Vomer Treatment

6. Ethmoid (Fronto-Maxillary)

Extraoral treatment. Operator stands to the side of the patient with the index and thumb of both hands assuming a pinching position at the base of the nose on either side of the frontomaxillary articulation. A compressive force is introduced between the frontal and maxillary bones, and proceeding in an indirect fashion, following the translatory and rotary forces surrounding the ethmoid. This three-dimensional tension is balanced and held until a gentle softening release is appreciated.

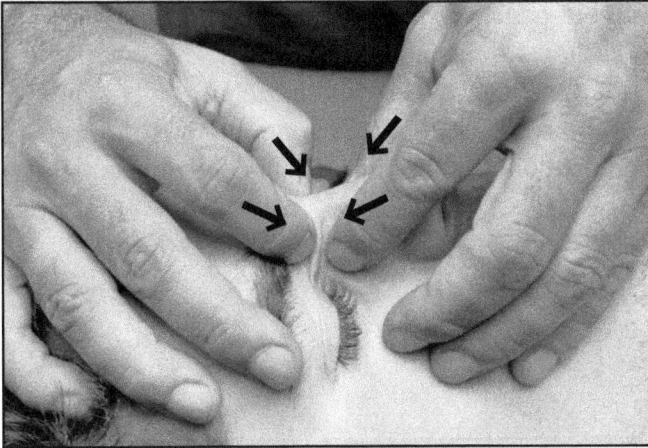

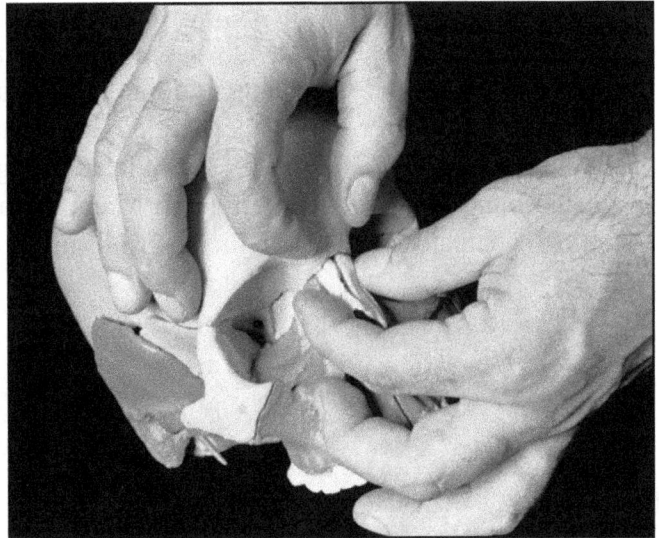

Extraoral Ethmoid Treatment

Intraoral treatment. Treatment is the same as above with maxillary contact inside mouth, just under the lips on the anterior maxilla.

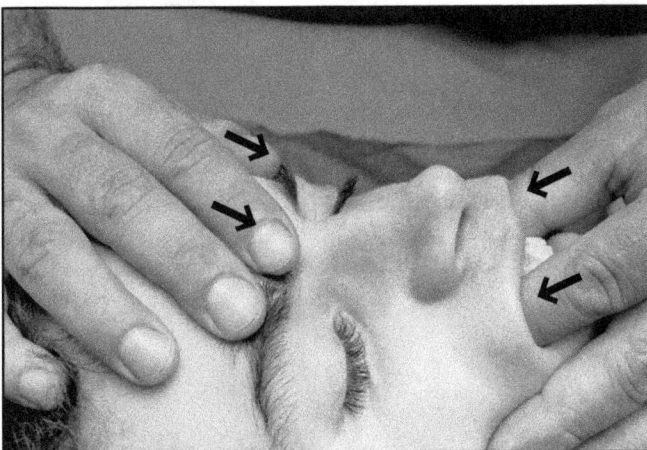

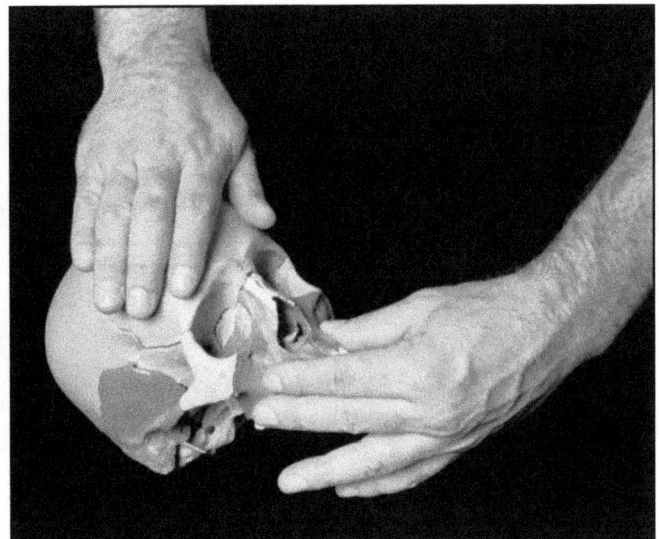

Intraoral Ethmoid Treatment

7. Sphenopalatine Ganglion

Diagnosis: To test for the necessity of treating the sphenopalatine ganglion, fronto-sphenoid, and sphenosquamous articulations, refer to #9. Sphenosquamous pivot.

Treatment: Operator stands opposite to the side being treated. The pad of the (right) little finger is placed on the outer side of the upper teeth on the (left) side of the mouth. Being careful not to pinch or stretch the cheek or lip, the finger is slipped posteriorly on the buccal surface of the teeth, and continue around the tuberosity of the maxilla to the lateral pterygoid plate. It can be identified by its flatness in contrast to the curved maxilla. This is a sensitive area. BE GENTLE. The space between the mandible and the maxilla may be very narrow, ask your patient to laterally shift their jaw towards the side being treated. Direct the little finger cephalad as toward the lateral angle of the eye, but the distance transversed will be dependent on the spasticity of the lateral pterygoid muscle. Apply gentle inhibitory pressure to the soft tissue while directing cerebrospinal fluid from the midpoint of the right coronal suture with the left hand. Maintain the contact until "softening" occurs and physiologic motion is palpated. Repeat on the opposite side.

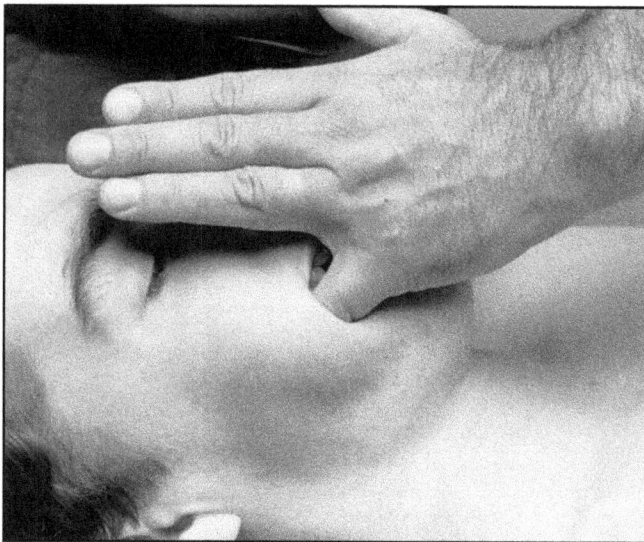

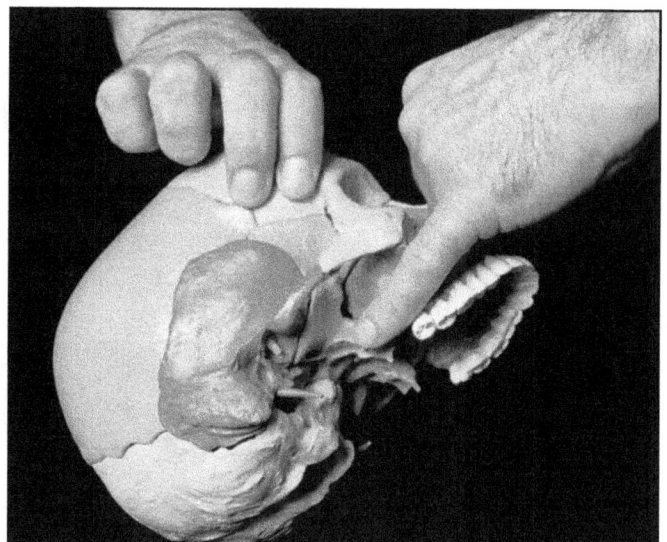

Sphenopalatine Ganglion Treatment

116

8. Frontosphenoid Articulation

This large L-shaped articulation may be compressed by trauma from above or below, and is not infrequently the maintaining factor in a torsion pattern. Introduce the little finger on to the lateral aspect of the lateral pterygoid plate as in #7 above. Place the index finger of the same hand on the external aspect of the greater wing of the sphenoid which is located in the depression posterior to the outer canthus of the eye. Place the thumb of the right hand on the left greater wing and the middle finger on the right lateral angle of the frontal bone. Maintaining the thumb as the fulcrum, lift the right lateral angle cephalad off the right greater wing of the sphenoid which is stabilized by the little finger on the pterygoid process and the index finger on the greater wing. Maintain this traction between the two hands until a "softening" and a restoration of physiologic motion is palpated. If there is a long-standing severely compressed condition at this articulation, reverse the approach using an indirect technique to gently compress the frontal into the sphenoid until a ballooning sensation occurs as they begin to decompress. Then proceed with the direct decompression. Repeat on other side.

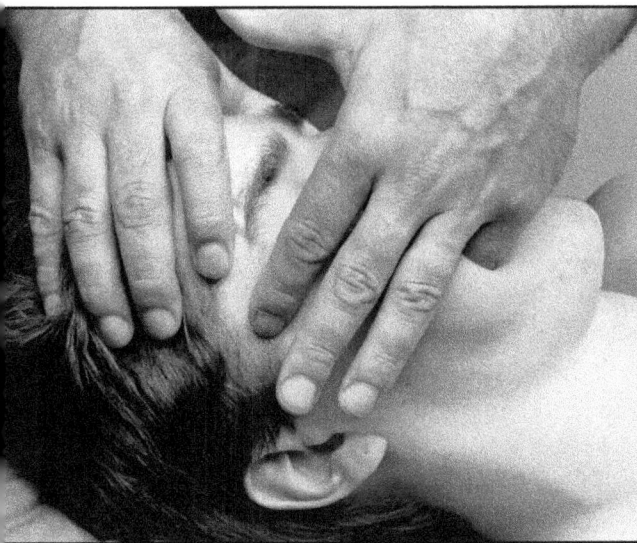

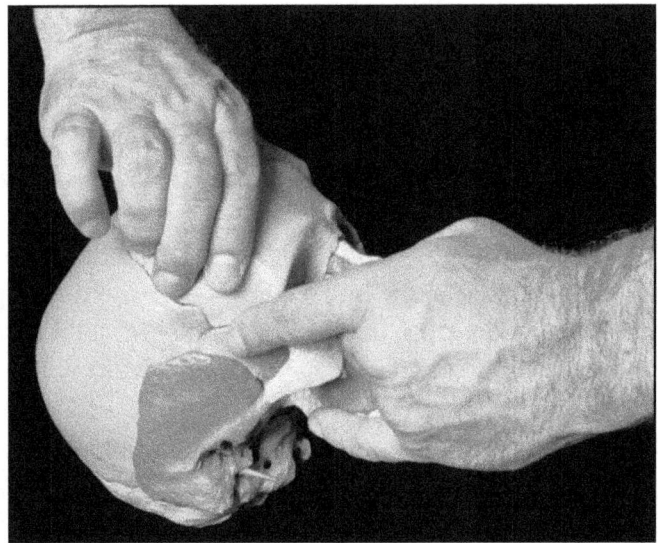

Frontosphenoid Articulation Treatment

9. Sphenosquamous Pivot

Diagnosis: Contacting the sphenosquamous portion of the pterion, the operator palpates for symmetrical external rotation (a sense of expansion) of the anterior temporal bone with a deep inhalation by the patient.

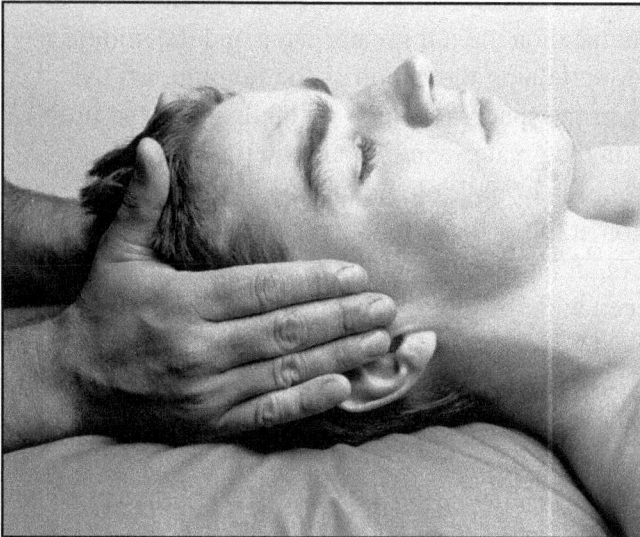
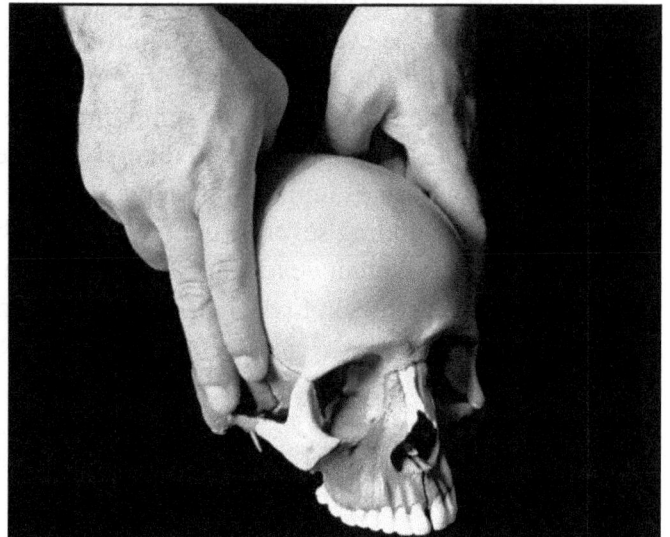

Sphenosquamous Diagnosis

The sphenosquamous pivot is situated at the point where the bevels of the temporal and sphenoid bones change, where the vertical and horizontal portions meet. To decompress this, place the little finger on lateral pterygoid plate and index finger on the greater wing as in #8 above. Place the other hand on the temporal bone, little and ring fingers on the mastoid process, middle finger in external auditory meatus, index finger and thumb hold the zygomatic arch. Evaluate flexion, extension, external and internal rotation, anterior/posterior and superior/inferior shear, and hold in the direction each bone moves more freely. Start with A/P and lateral shearing forces and add flexion/extension and rotational directions which will follow more easily. Ask the patient to inhale deeply and hold, assisting the decompression of the "gills of the fish." While performing this technique be sure to support the opposite side of the head with your shoulder or knee to stabilize the sphenoid. Sphenosquamous anatomy is complicated by two changes in the direction of bony opposition. Direct technique is not recommended due to the clinically labile character of this articulation.

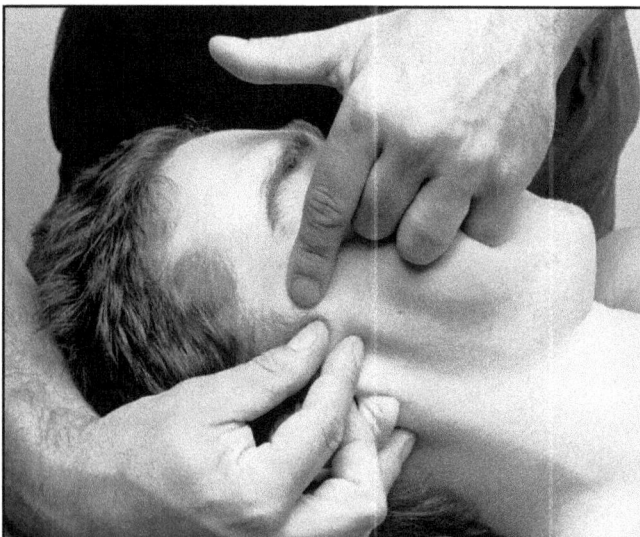
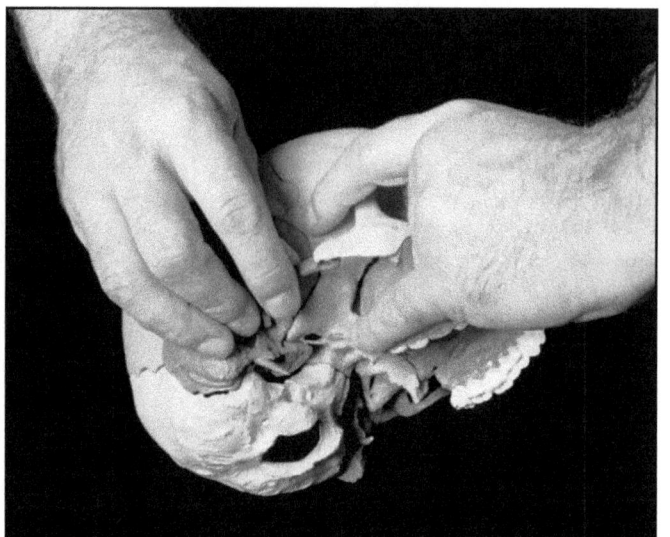

Sphenosquamous Pivot Treatment

Orbital Techniques

It has often been said that the eye is the window of the soul, but there is certainly no question that the orbit is an important key to the whole cranial mechanism. Review the anatomy.

Roof	Frontal	-Frontal has an extensive articulation with the Sphenoid.
	Lesser Wing of Sphenoid	
Lateral Wall	Zygoma	-Provides lateral stability to face and temporal bone anteriorly
	Greater Wing of Sphenoid	
Floor	Zygoma	
	Maxilla	-Each maxilla is related to the other. It is related to the vomer. It articulates with the nasal.
	Palatine	-The palatine is a transmitter of sphenoid motion to the maxilla.
Medial Wall	Maxilla	
	Lacrimal	
	Ethmoid	-Provides anterior superior pole of attachment for the falx cerebri.
	Body of Sphenoid	
	at Root of Pterygoid	-Articulates with occiput at sphenobasilar synchondrosis.

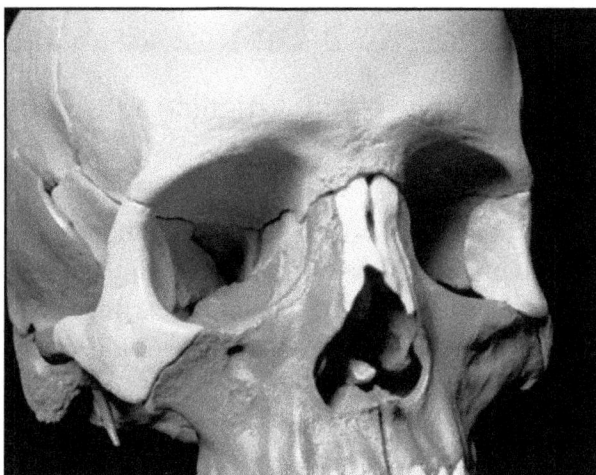

Orbital Structures

The extraocular muscles are attached by fascia to the wall of the orbit and are inserted into the eyeball. The recti muscles take origin from the margins of the optic foramen, i.e., the roots of the lesser wing and from the fibrous annulus of Zinn which provides a connection between the developmental parts of the sphenoid, the body and lesser wings medially and the greater wing/pterygoid unit laterally. The frontal and the maxilla provide origin to the superior and inferior oblique muscles respectively.

Thus, cranial trauma may have profound effects on ocular function, and extraocular muscle imbalance may cause, maintain or result from membranous articular strains of the cranial mechanism. The eyeball is a fibrous, fascial, fluid structure whose shape is subject to distortion as in astigmatism, which is measurable, or in dimensions which can be deduced by changes in acuity. Superior or inferior vertical strains compromise visual acuity. A superior strain is accompanied by a decrease in the antero-posterior dimension of the orbit, and increased hyperopia. An inferior vertical strain increases that orbital dimension and is associated with increased myopia. A lateral strain or side-bending rotation may contribute to a lateral ocular imbalance such as eso- or exophoria. The ocular imbalance may, conversely, sustain the lesion of the cranial base. Optimal function of the sinuses is also enhanced by orbital treatment.

1. Compression of the Fronto-Nasal Articulation

Diagnosis is by testing for sutural compliance by distracting the second and third fingers across the suture. Compare both sides for symmetry.

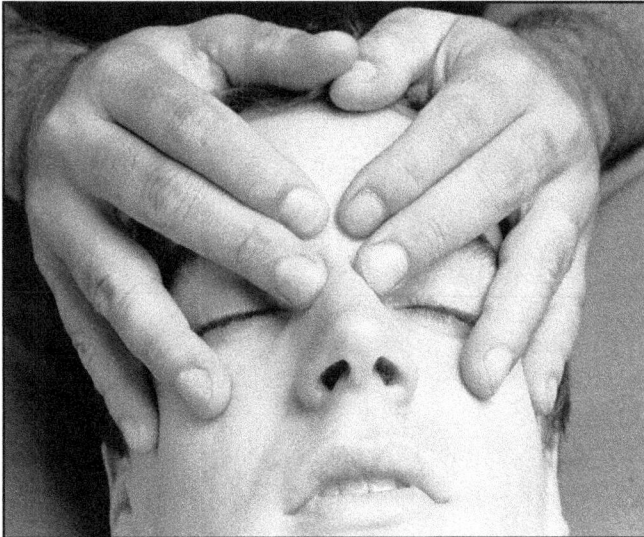

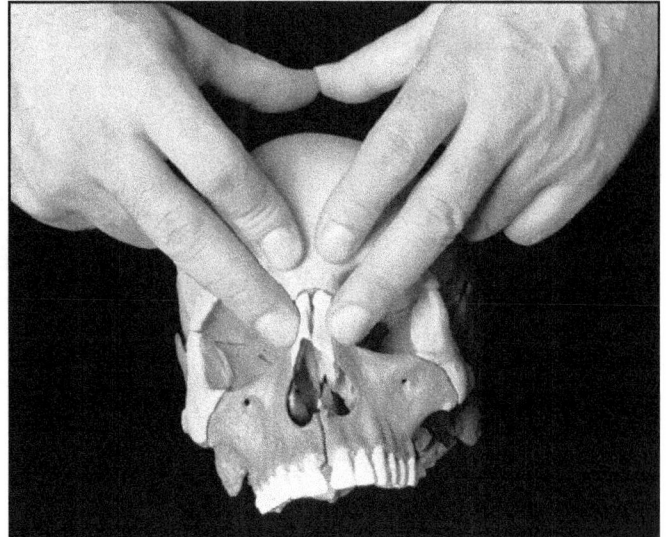

Diagnosis of Fronto-Nasal Articulation Compression

Treatment. For the left fronto-nasal articulation, cradle the right hemi-occiput in the right hand and direct cerebrospinal fluid from the margin of the foramen magnum just to the right of the midline with the index or middle finger to the V created by the left index finger on the frontal bone and the middle finger on the nasal in close approximation to the edges of the suture. Maintain slight separation of the nasal and frontal fingers while fluid is directed until a sudden "softening" and inherent motion are palpated between the nasal and the frontal. Repeat on the right side.

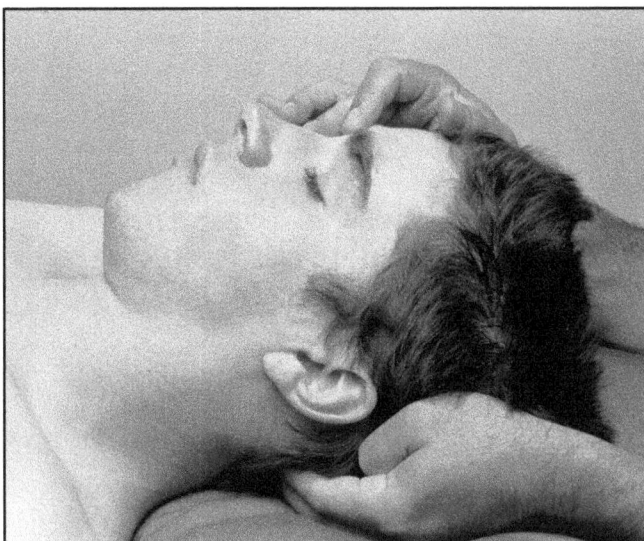

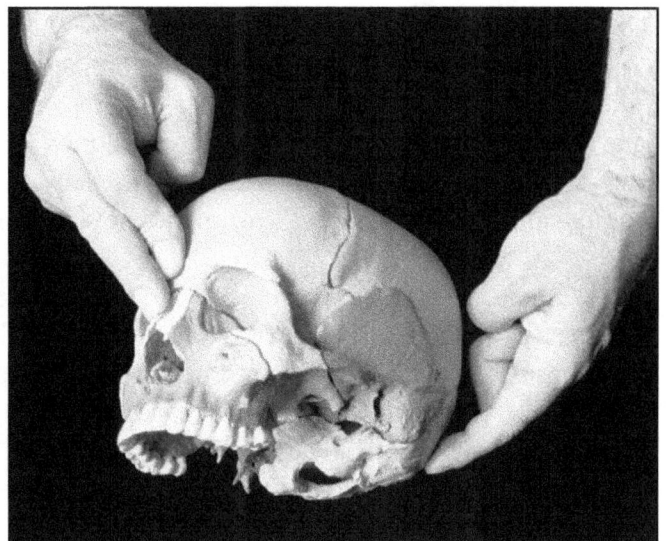

Treatment of Fronto-Nasal Articulation Compression

2. Compression of the Naso-Maxillary Articulation

Diagnosis is by testing for sutural compliance as in (1) above.

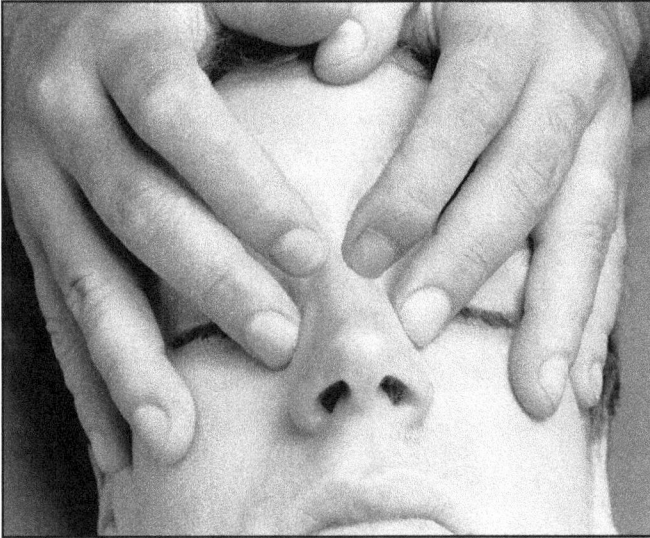

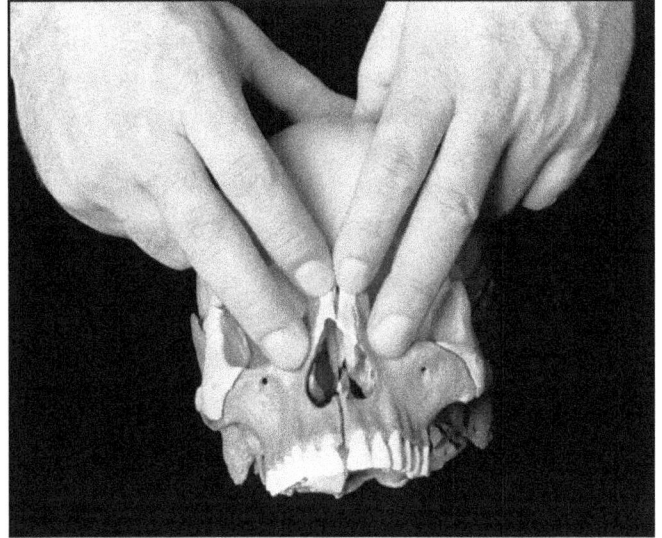

Diagnosis of Naso-Maxillary Articulation Compression

Treatment. Release this with a V-spread as in (1) above; the index finger on the nasal, middle finger on the ascending process of the maxilla and fluid direction from the occipital squama just to the opposite side of the midline.

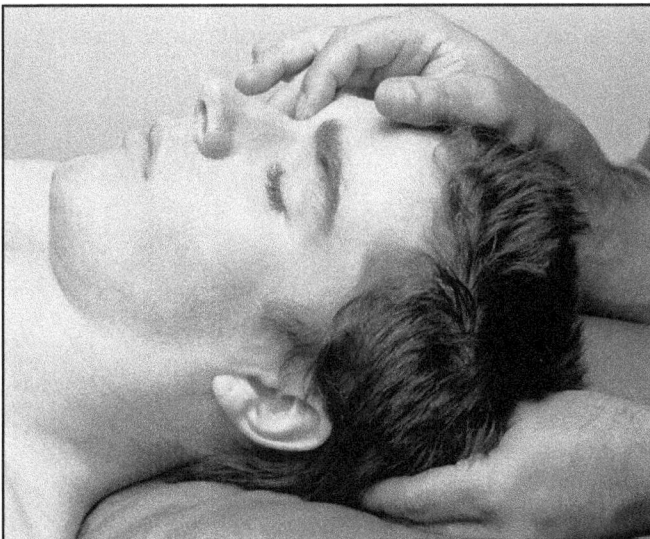

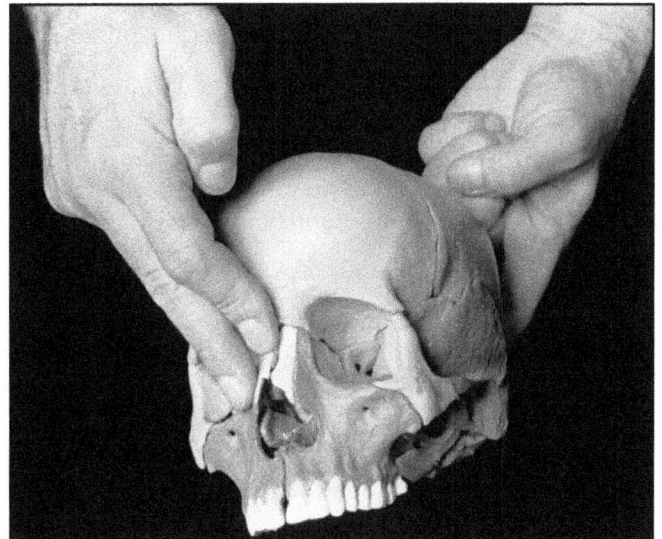

Treatment of Naso-Maxillary Articulation Compression

3. The Orbit

The orbit is then approached as a unit, like an upside-down cone, the circumference of the base of the cone being accessible to the palpating fingers and the apex of the cone projecting in a line to the opposite occiput.

Diagnosis. When evaluating the orbits, group the fingertips of the hands on the borders of the circumference of the orbit, e.g., the thumb and index fingers on the frontal, the middle finger on the maxilla and the 4th and 5th on the zygoma. Gently evaluate the clockwise or counterclockwise rotation of the circumference of the orbits, comparing right to left for directions of mobile restriction.

Alternate Technique. Use whole 2nd and 3rd finger contacts above and below the eye.

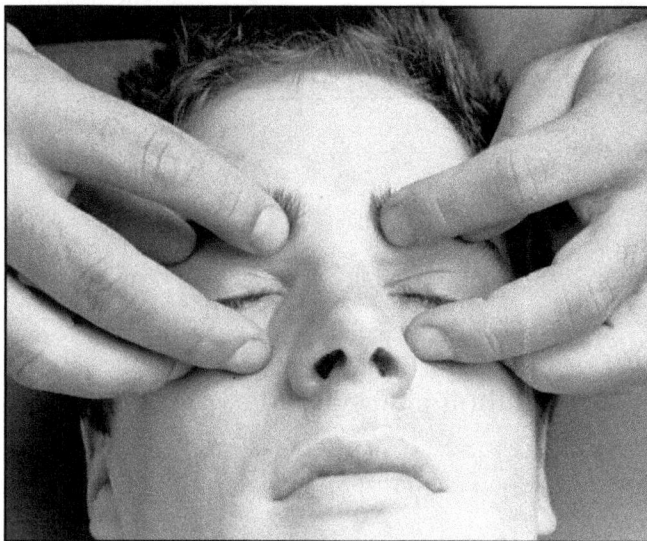

Orbit Diagnosis

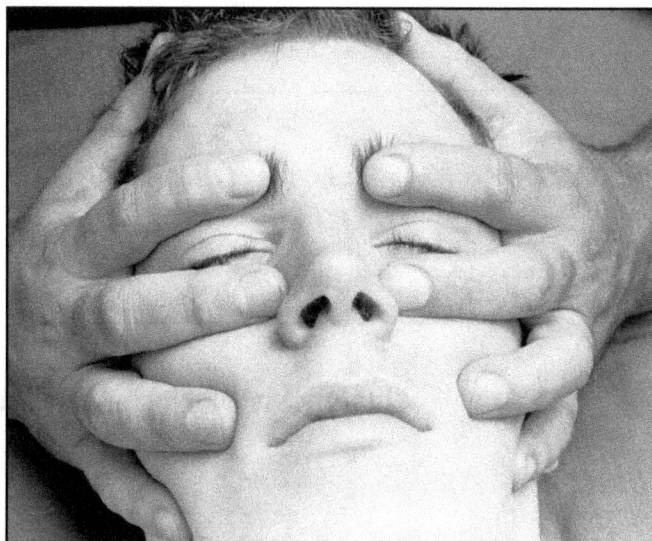

Orbit Diagnosis- Alternate Technique

Treatment. On the orbit that is restricted in one direction, introduce the direction it moves more freely and hold it there until it suddenly "softens" and assumes easy, gentle rhythmic inherent motion. The operator's free hand should simultaneously cradle the occiput on the opposite side, sending a fluid wave. Repeat on the other side.

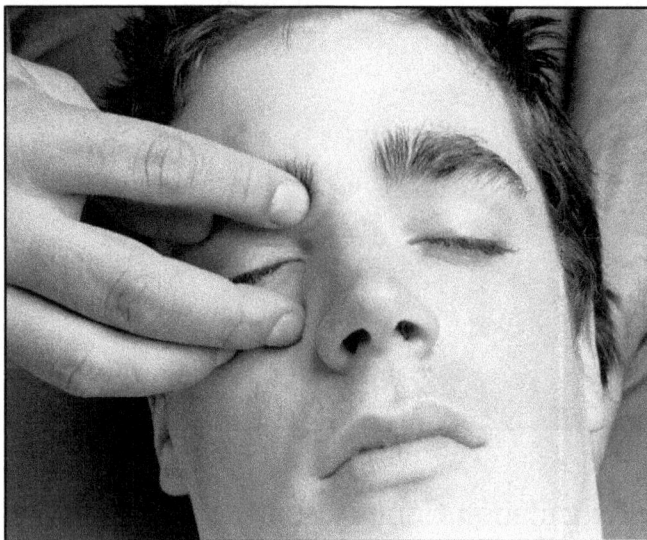

Orbit Treatment

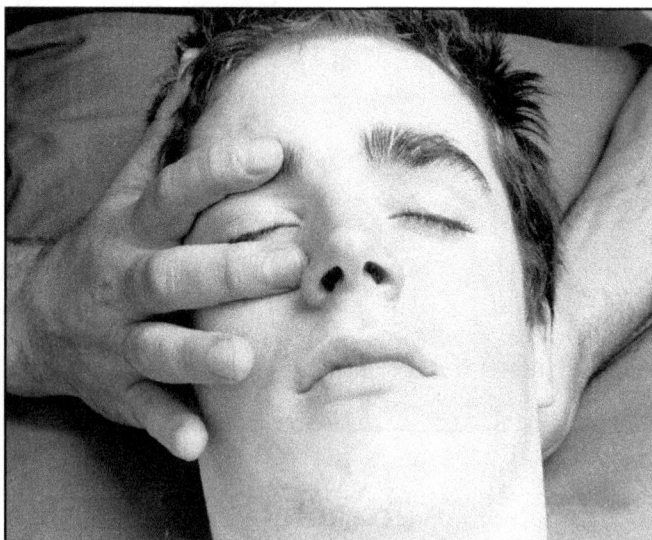

Orbit Treatment- Alternate Technique

4. The Eyeball

The eyeball is evaluated for its resilience and freedom of motion within the orbit. As it is a soft and sensitive structure, it must be handled very gently. Make sure contact lenses are out.

Diagnosis. Evaluate clockwise and counterclockwise motion of the eyeball relative to the orbit.

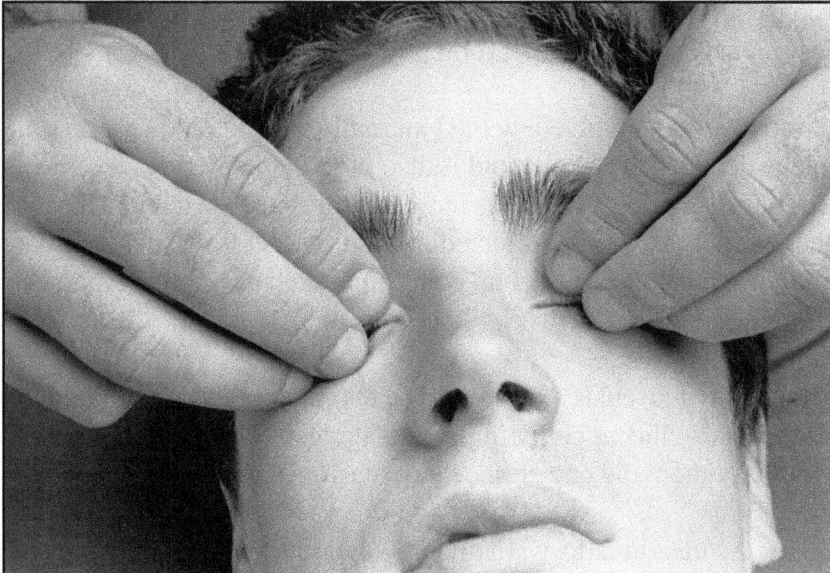

Eyeball Diagnosis

Treatment. Follow it in the direction it moves more freely, while sending a fluid wave from the opposite occiput with the other hand; hold it until there is a "softening," resistance melts, and free motion is palpated. Repeat for the other eye.

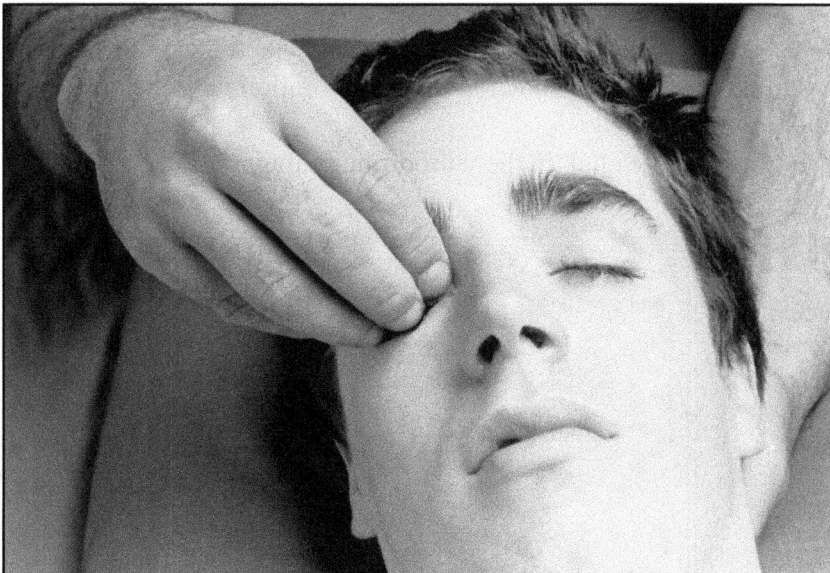

Eyeball Treatment

This series of techniques for the orbits and eyes is profoundly relaxing to the patient who has had restrictions for a long period of time. It is very helpful in the clearance of eyestrain as well as the more complex muscular imbalances, circulatory insufficiencies, and ocular hypertension.

Temporomandibular Joint Dysfunction

Normal function of any joint relates to its motion characteristics. Therefore, temporal mandibular joint dysfunction (TMJD) is strictly defined as altered motion of the TMJ. This may be associated with pain locally in the TMJ, face, jaw or head and/or distally. (e.g., cervical and costal cage regions.) TMJD may strongly influence motion disturbances in distal body regions and often plays an important role in clinical management of these problems.

The temporal bone is almost always involved, being externally rotated on the same side to which the mid line of the mandible is deviated. The sphenoid is also high on the same side (SBS torsion). The mandible slides posteriorly on this side and places increased pressure on the TMJ leading to degenerative conditions of the internal disc if not corrected in time. TMJD is usually associated with cranial dysfunction and trauma that leads to dental conditions such as bruxism, malocclusion, internal disc derangement, etc.

We must also consider the many muscular attachments to the mandible and temporal bone in order to appreciate the importance of this clinical entity in the management of many, head, neck, upper back and extremity problems (e.g., omohyoid and sternocleidomastoid).

Treatment involves pulling the mandible forward and downward (considering the relationships with the spheno and stylo mandibular ligaments) and restoring normal temporal bone motion. In more complex cases where malocclusion is from above, the maxilla and palatine arch must be considered as well.

Diagnosis of Temporomandibular Joint Dysfunction

1. Jaw deviates to the side of the externally rotated temporal bone and high sphenoid.
2. There is a palpable asymmetry of temporomandibular joint motion with the operator's fingers over the temporomandibular joint, bilaterally.
3. There is an audible and/or palpable click in the temporomandibular joint.

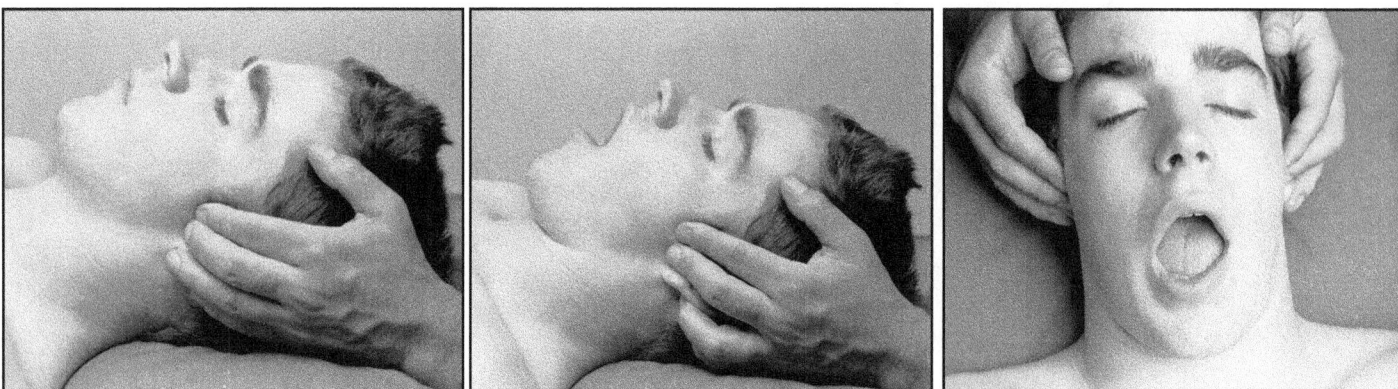

Diagnosis of Temporomandibular Joint Dysfunction

Temporomandibular Joint Treatment

1. Sphenomandibular Ligament

Place caudad thumb on occlusal surface of last lower molar teeth on opposite side of the mouth. Gently grasp greater wings of sphenoid externally with the other hand. Note the motion of the greater wing as the mandible is depressed in a caudad direction. If there is reduced resiliency of the sphenomandibular ligament the greater wing will move superiorly on the same side. If this occurs gently encourage the sphenoid toward flexion while depressing the mandible, until the tissues yield permitting free mandibular motion. If it will not release, then compress the mandible superiorly while directing the sphenoid into extension awaiting the indirect release, then proceed with the direct ligamentous release.

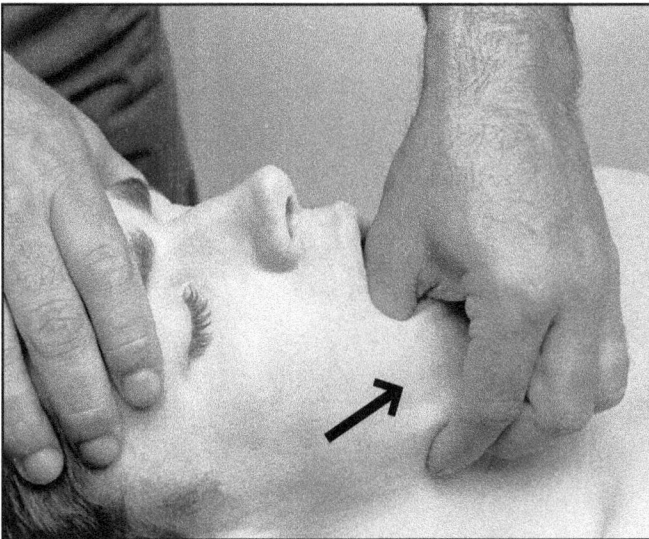

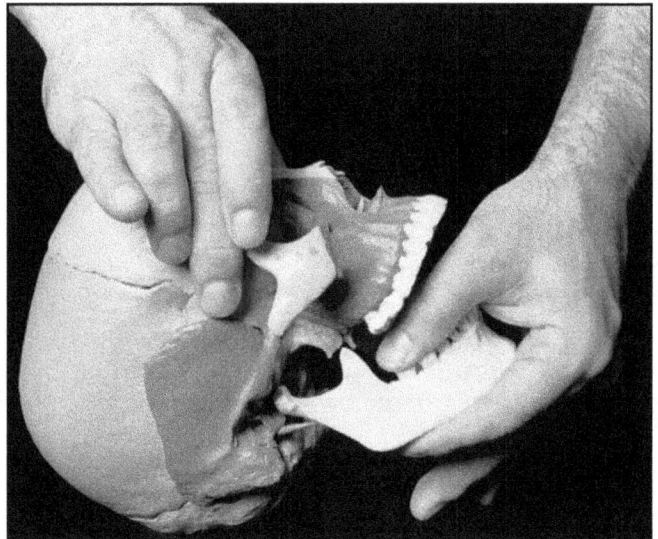

Sphenomandibular Ligament Treatment

2. Stylomandibular Ligament

With thumb on last molar tooth as above, wrap the other fingers around the angle of the mandible. Grasp the temporal with the other hand (little and ring fingers on mastoid process, middle finger in external auditory meatus, index finger and thumb on zygomatic arch). Apply gentle traction between the two hands along the direction of the stylomandibular ligament, i.e., obliquely down, medial and forward; the temporal bone will move into external rotation if there is increased tension, bring the temporal bone into internal rotation simultaneously, to directly stretch the ligament. Hold until free motion is palpable. If it will not release, then apply gentle compression of the head of the mandible into the glenoid fossa with external rotation of the temporal bone until spontaneous decompression occurs. Follow this with a direct method of release.

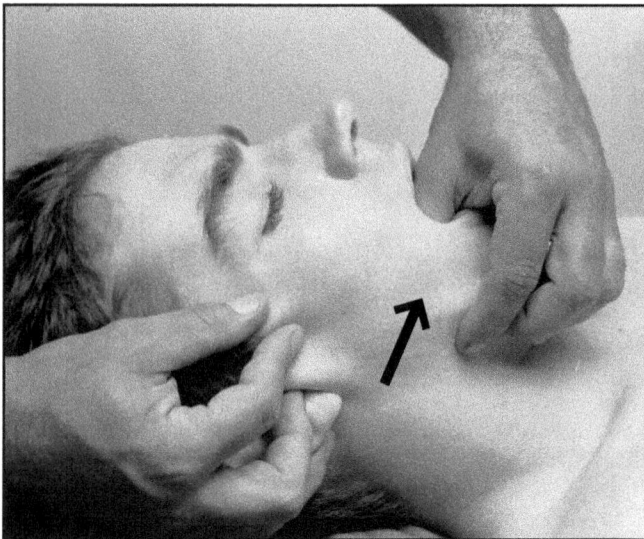

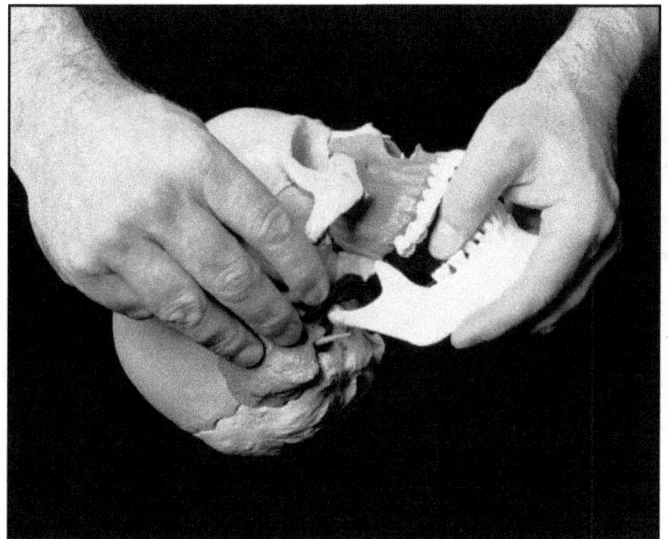

Stylomandibular Ligament Treatment

3. Capsular Elements

Sitting at the head of the supine patient, operator contacts the anterior tip of the mandible with both hands. Gently compress the mandible to one side and then the other, each for a few seconds. Feeling the resistance in these tissues, continue alternating until this resistance is decreased on the side of the temporomandibular joint dysfunction.

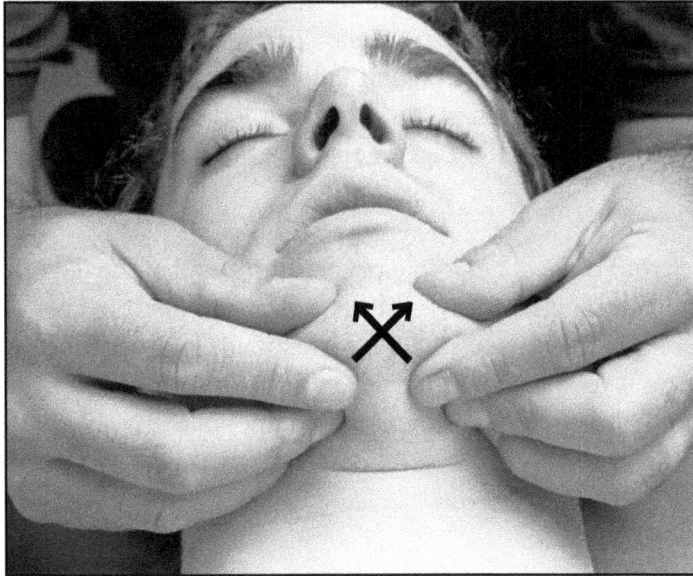

Treatment of Capsular Elements

4. Hyoid

Extensive muscular attachments from the tongue, mandible, and neck involve the hyoid bone. The hyoid is located deep in the supracrycoid region and is contacted with the thumb and the index finger of one hand on its lateral aspects. Lateral translation, rotation, and side-bending movements are introduced in their direction of ease and held until release occurs.

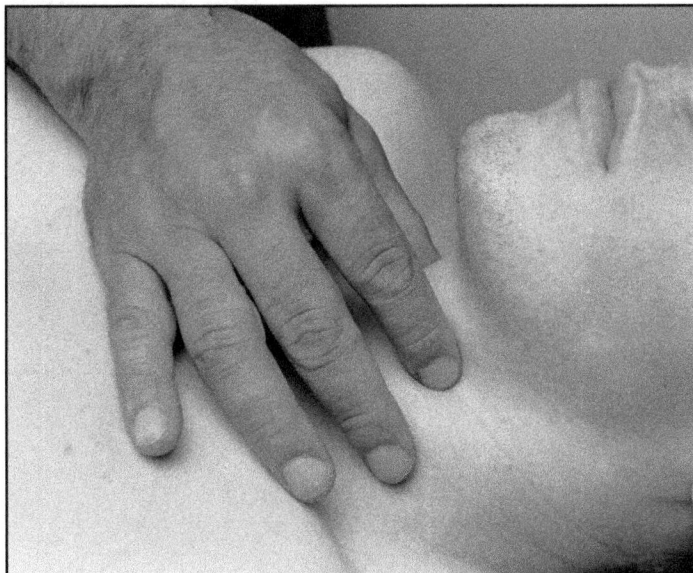

Hyoid Treatment

Geometric Axes in the Cranium

Precise geometric patterns are found within the healthy cranial mechanism as well as in the rest of the body. The axes of the orbits intersect above the posterior boundry of the sella turcica and are then projected into the contralateral posterior cranial fossa about the tentorium cerebelli and the occipital side of the occipital mastoid suture. This may be referred to as the orbital axis. The auditory (petrous) axis begins at the petrous portion of the temporal bone and intersects within the sella turcica anterior to the intersection of the orbital axis and projects into the body of the zygoma on the other side of the orbit. These diagonal axes are part of the body's normal physiologic development and function so that nerve impulses are directed contralaterally and diagonally. This occurs in both the CNS as well as the peripheral nervous system. The disturbed arrangement of the basic parts of the cranium will cause a derangement in these geometric axes and the corresponding nerve impulses of the involved structures.

The hypothesis derived from clinical anatomic observations is that the developing nerve pathways are laid down within these geometric forms. If these forms are distorted prior to the completion of the development of these nerve pathways, then a corresponding disturbance will appear in both the sensory and motor functions associated with these geometric forms. Distortion in later life may also lead to disturbance of both structural and functional components involved. (e.g. in the first two years)

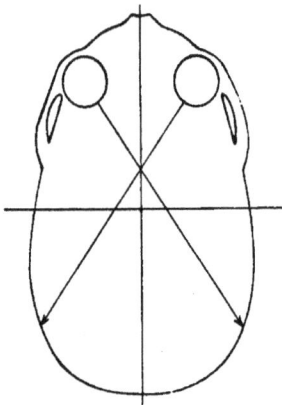

Fig. 16: Diagram showing symmetric orbital axes

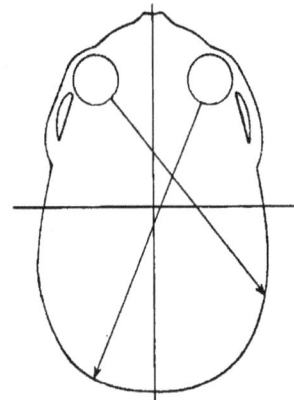

Fig. 17: Diagram showing distortion of orbital axes in right lateral sphenobasilar strain

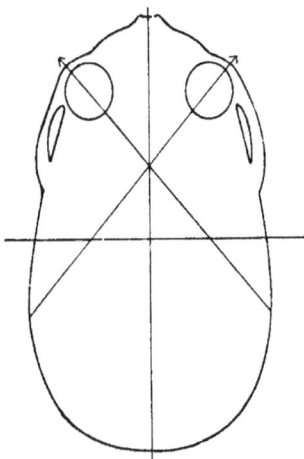

Fig. 18: Diagram showing symmetric petrous axes

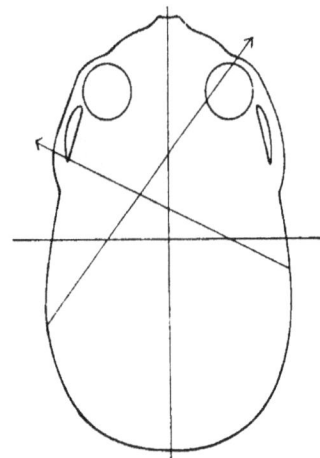

Fig. 19: Diagram showing distortion of petrous axes in right lateral sphenobasilar strain

Orbital/Auditory Axis Release of Tentorium Cerebelli

Diagnosis. Alteration in the proper diagonal axis of the orbital cranial structures can be appreciated as follows. With fingers clumped over the eyeball and the other hand resting on the opposite occipital mastoid suture, a fluid wave should be sent from the orbit to the occiput. If there is an alteration in this axis, the resulting fluid wave will be felt to fall in a place other than around the occipital mastoid suture. For example, at a more medial spot on the occiput. (Likewise for auditory axis, by placing the fingers in the external auditory meatus and sending a fluid wave to the opposite anterior zygoma where the other hand rests, the placement of the fluid wave can also be appreciated.)

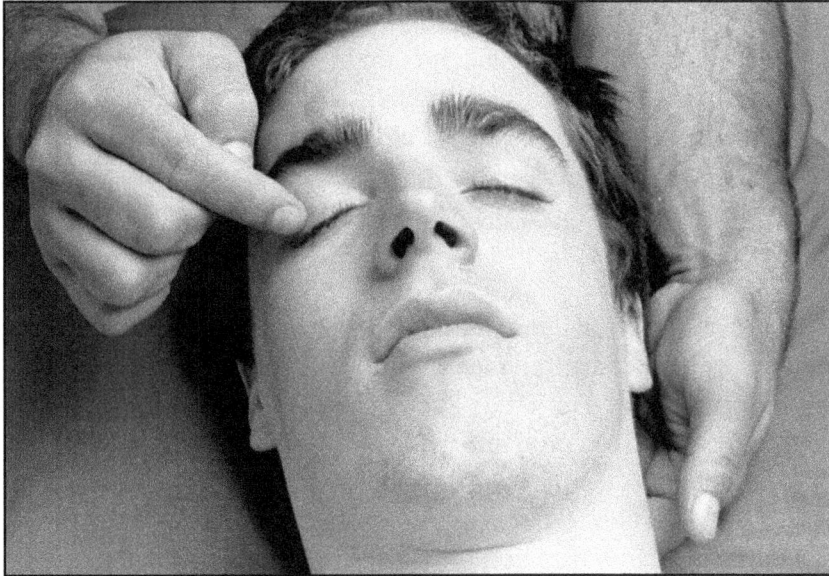

Orbital Axis Diagnosis

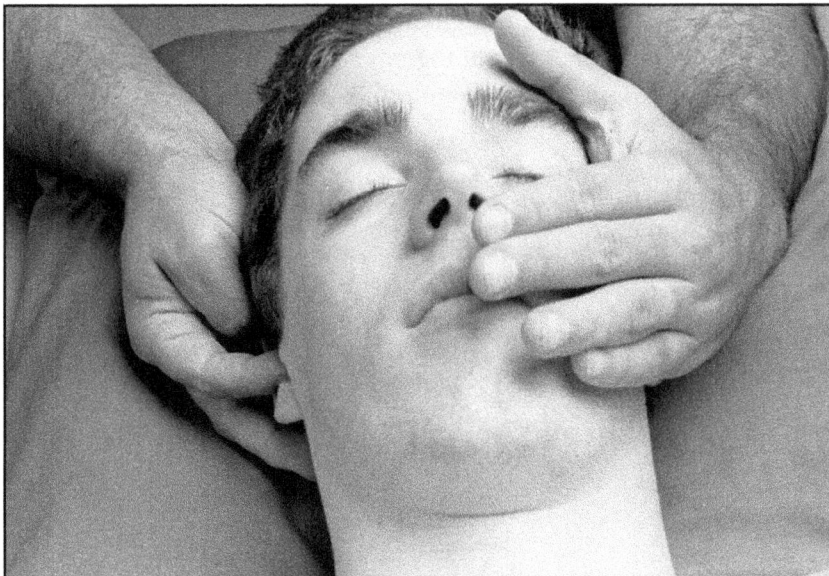

Auditory Axis Diagnosis

Treatment of this dysfunction begins with the sequence of treatment already taught for the cranial sacral approach. Oftentimes, these dysfunctions are the result of SBS strain patterns, which alter the normal geometric configuration of the cranium. The following technique will also assist in normalizing the dural strain in deep-set geometric distortions.

Phase One. The patient is supine, the operator contacting the cranium in the vault hold. The operator instructs the patient to think about turning both their eyes in one direction, to either the left or the right. After a moment, the operator instructs the patient to look to that same side they were thinking about looking to and informs the patient that they are going to be slowly turning the patient's head, in the same direction, passively. When the head arrives at the end range of that rotation, the operator instructs the patient to stop turning their eyes and to think about turning their eyes in the opposite direction. Next, the operator instructs the patient to actually look in the opposite direction and as they are doing so, informs the patient that they are going to be turning their head in that new direction again without patient effort, passively. The operator continues with this procedure going back and forth the same manner until a release is felt in the resistance to rotation palpated in the vault hold. Normally with a geometric distortion, there is a resistance felt in the tissues to the rotatory component involved.

Phase Two. When this release is felt, the operator then instructs the patient to think about turning their eyes in one direction as before, and then instructs them to actually turn their eyes in that direction. Simultaneously, the operator will turn the patient's head in the opposite direction informing the patient that they are turning their head in such a manner. So for example, the patient thinks about turning their eyes to the left and is then instructed to actually turn their eyes to the left and also are informed that they will have their head turned in the opposite direction to the right, passively, by the operator. Again when the end range of rotation is met, the patient is instructed to relax their eye directions to think once again about turning their eyes in the opposite direction and instructed to actually turn their eyes in the opposite direction and then informed that their head will be turned in the direction opposite from the direction that their eyes are now turning. This same procedure is repeated. The operator should be able to palpably perceive the resistance in the rotatory forces. This resistance will increase and then will decrease at the point when a release in the tentorium is accomplished. The resistance that is felt in the rotatory component of this technique is actually the tension that is held in the tentorium cerebelli along the diagonal axis of the orbital structures. At the end of the technique, the orbital axis should be rechecked for change.

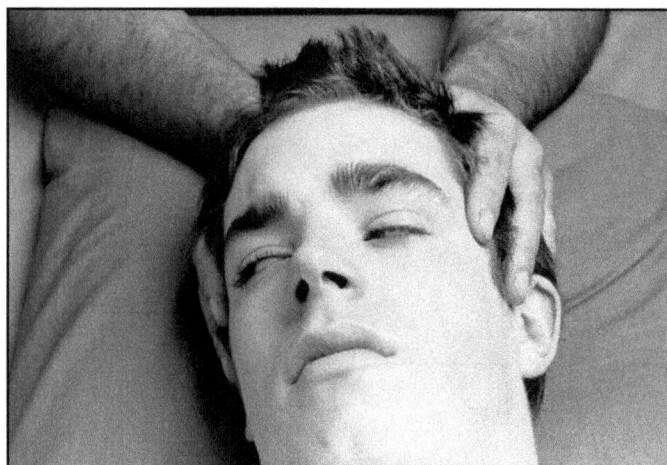 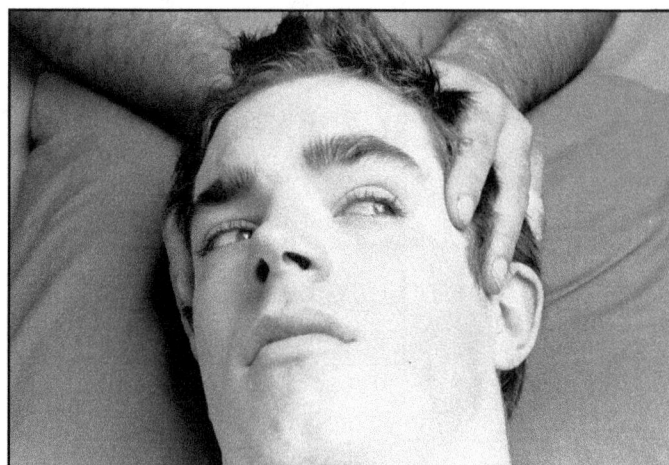

Phase One   Orbital/ Auditory Axis   Phase Two
Release Treatment

Table 7: Facial Bones
Sequence of Treatment

Assessment

Vault Hold

Frontal Lift

Cruciate Suture

Treatment

Maxilla – Palatine

Intermaxillary

Sphenopalatine

Zygoma

Vomer

Ethmoid

Frontomaxilla

Nasofrontal

Nasomaxillary

Orbit/Eye

Recheck Cruciate

Sphenopalatine Ganglia

Frontosphenoid

Sphenosquamous

Face Lift

Reassess Screening Tests

Temporomandibular Joint (if necessary)

Orbital/Auditory Axis

Venous Sinus Drainage Technique

Indications

1. At the initiation of the treatment for a hard, rigid head compressed at the sphenobasilar synchondrosis and at many peripheral sutures, this technique is invaluable for restoring inherent physiologic potency and mobility.

2. In the patient with a throbbing, devastating, severe congestive headache, especially if it is concentrated at the vertex or in the frontal and maxillary sinuses, this technique can bring profound relief as venous drainage improves.

Review the anatomy of the venous sinuses and jugular foramen, through which 94% of venous drainage occurs. The reciprocal tension membrane encloses all the venous sinuses and influences their function. Ultimately, the orbit, nasal sinuses, and contiguous areas of the face are drained through the cavernous sinus into the petrosal sinus and to the jugular foramen. The majority of intracranial structures whose blood is collected in cerebral veins drain into the sagittal sinuses or the straight sinus and are also dependent on the patency of the jugular foramen for adequate venous drainage.

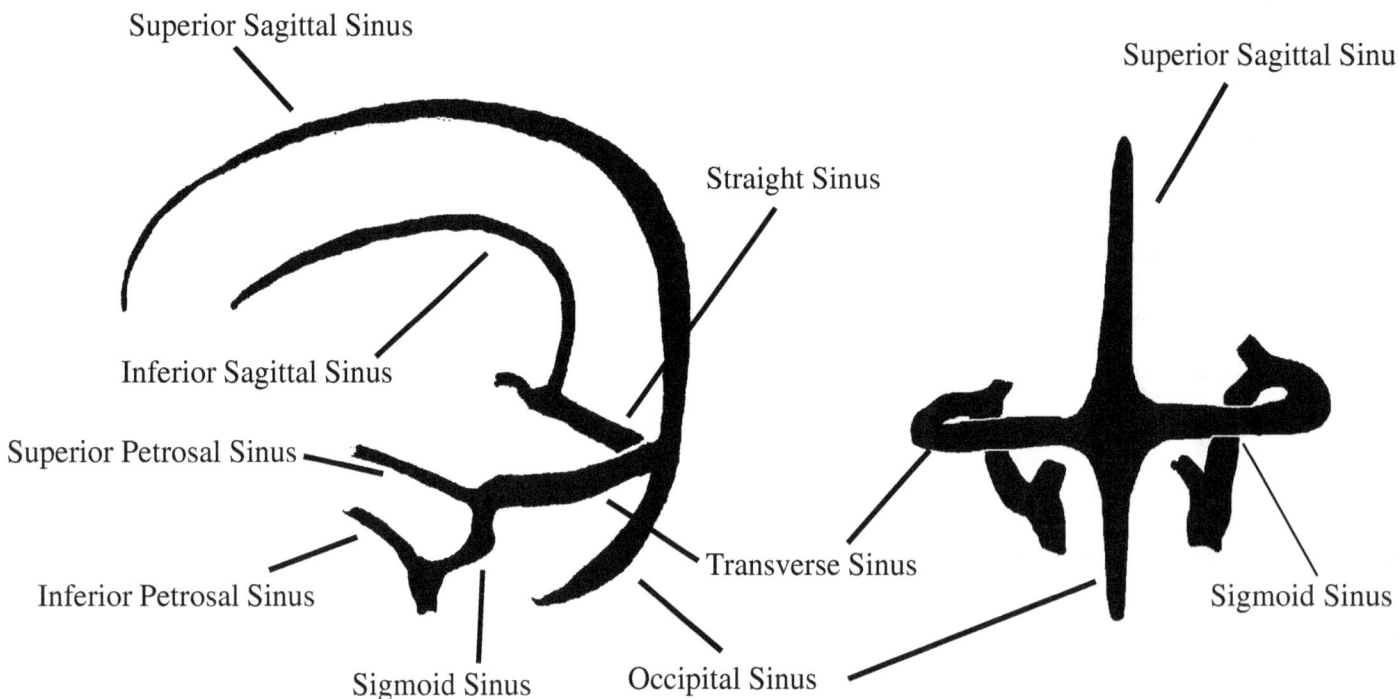

Superior Sagittal Sinus

Straight Sinus

Inferior Sagittal Sinus

Superior Petrosal Sinus

Inferior Petrosal Sinus

Sigmoid Sinus

Transverse Sinus

Occipital Sinus

Superior Sagittal Sinu

Sigmoid Sinus

Fig. 20: Dural Venous Sinuses- Lateral View   Fig. 21: Dural Venous Sinuses- PosteriorView

The operator is seated at the head of the table.
The patient is supine.

1. The Confluence of Sinuses and Occipital Sinus

The operator places his two middle fingers tip to tip with the pads of the fingers on the external occipital protuberance providing the onlt support for the patient's head. This contact is maintained until the operator senses a "softening" of the bone on his fingers and the beginning of free inherent motion. Bring fingers together along the occipital midline to release the occipital sinus. With a very gentle impulse posteriorly, the occiput is decompressed from the atlas and the condylar parts of the occiput are also released. Wait until "softening" and inherent motion are palpated.

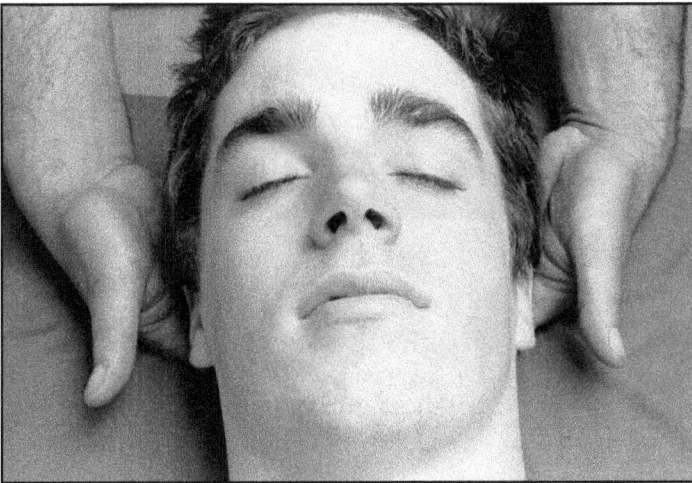

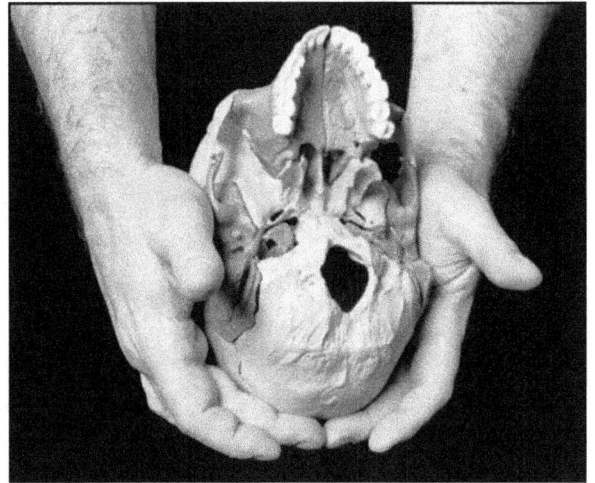

Treatment of Confluence of Sinuses and Occipital Sinus

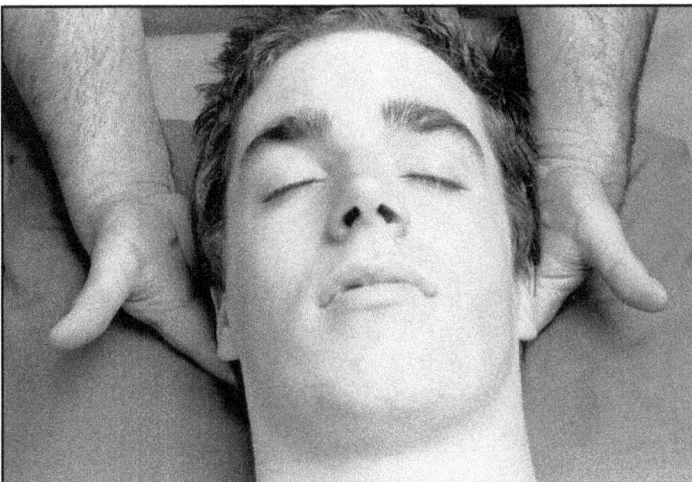

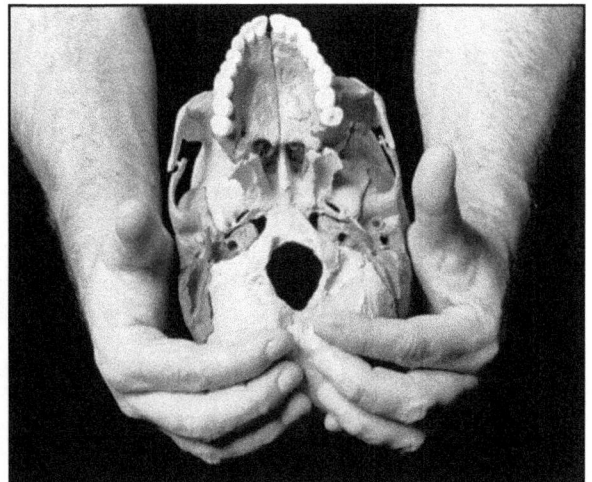

Treatment of Occipital Sinus

2. The Transverse and Straight Sinuses

Approximate the pads of the little fingers beneath the external occipital protuberance and let the pads of the other fingers support the head by contact along the superior nuchal line to the inferior lateral angle of the parietal. The head rests on the fingers and the thumbs are placed one on top of the other over the most anterior aspect of the sagittal suture at bregma. Imagine a line from the thumbs into the center of the head and visualize its intersection with the anterior end of the straight sinus. Maintain these contacts until "softening" and motion are noted.

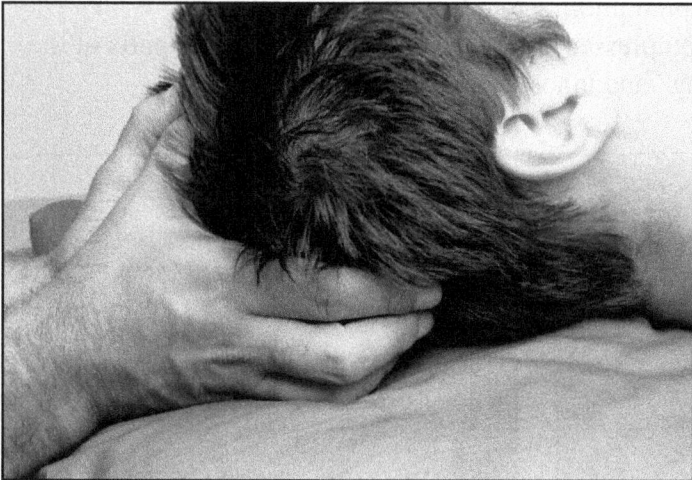

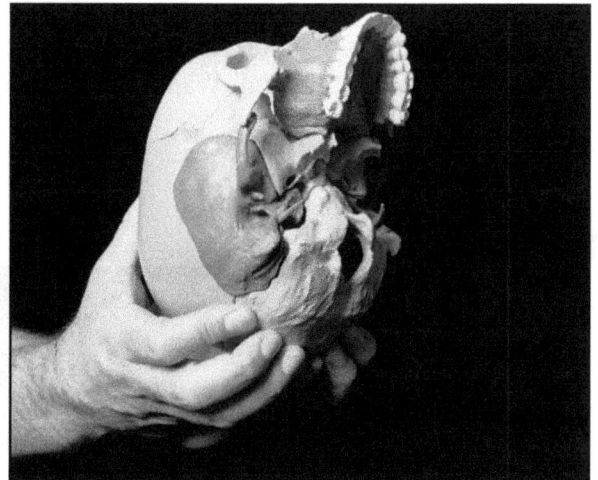

Treatment of Transverse and Straight Sinuses

3. The Superior Sagittal Sinus

Return to the external occipital protuberance as in (1). Note that inherent motion is palpable. Now address an area about an inch superior to the protuberance. With the palms of the hands facing the surface of the head, place the pad of the left thumb just to the right of the midline, and the pad of the right thumb just to the left of the mid-line. The thumbs therefore are crossed and apply a gentle separative force, the right thumb directed toward the left, and the left thumb toward the right. When "softening" and motion are palpated, move the thumbs about an inch forward and repeat the procedure. Continue step by step along the sagittal suture to the bregma (the intersection of sagittal and coronal sutures).

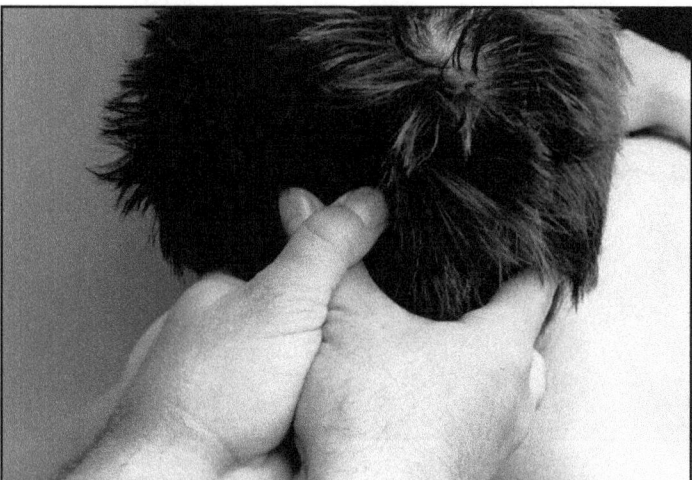

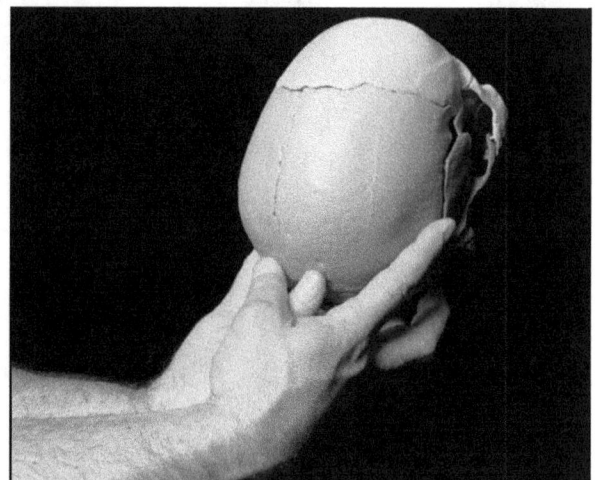

Treatment of Superior Sagittal Sinus

3. The Superior Sagittal Sinus (Continued)

To complete the anterior portion of the sinus, place the pads of the fingers on either side of the metopic suture (the midline) of the frontal i.e. the index finger just anterior to the bregma, the little finger above the nasion and the other fingers in between: the right fingers are on the right of the suture, the left fingers are on the left side. Gentle pressure with slight separation is maintained until "softening" and physiologic motion are palpated. If the frontal bone is large, two operator releases may be required, one superior and one inferior. Thumb separation is also applied to the glabella just above the frontonasal articulation until a "softening" is palpated.

In a very hard, restricted mechanism, this technique may take a long time, to reach its completion, but if every area is maintained until "softening" and motion are palpated, there will be a profound change in the whole patient with a dramatic decrease in tension throughout the body.

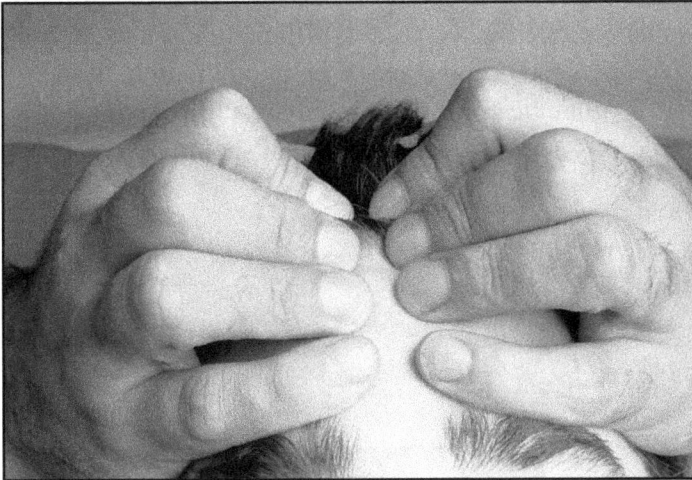

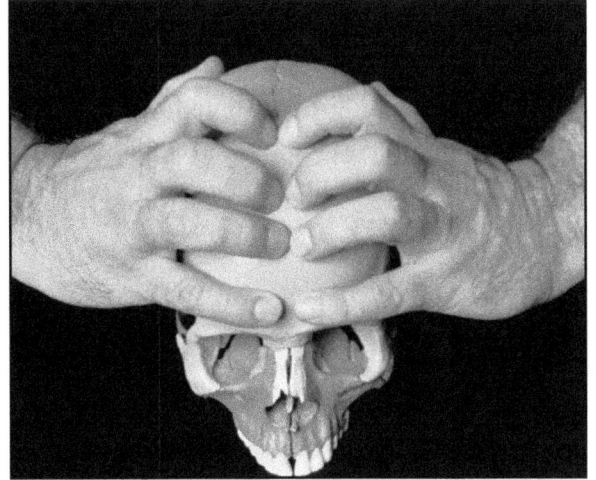

Treatment of Metopic Suture

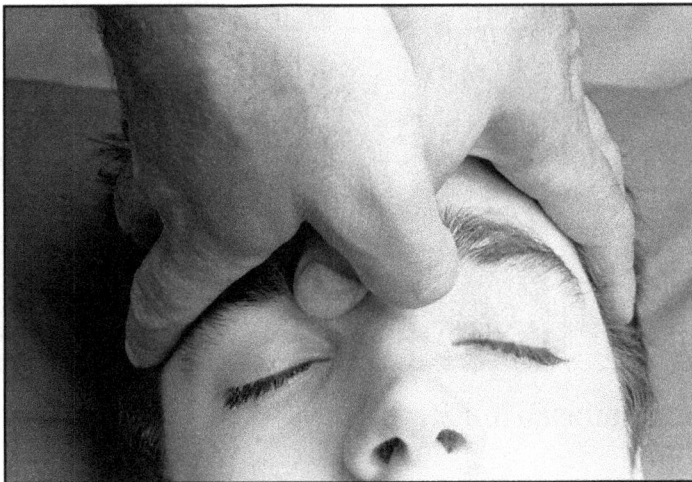

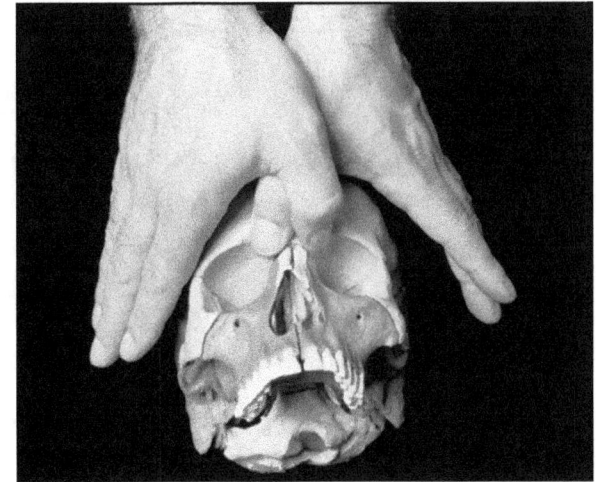

Treatment of Glabella

Summary of Venous Sinus Drainage Technique

1. *Confluence of Sinuses and Occipital sinus* Start by draining the confluence of sinuses, then the occipital sinus down to the condylar parts, opening the jugular foramen.
2. *Transverse and straight sinuses* Simultaneously with fingers lined up over the external occipital protuberance and superior nuchal line with thumbs projecting downwards through an upper contact at the bregma.
3. *Superior sagittal sinus*, including metopic suture and glabella.

Two-Operator Technique

Excercise 1: Face Lift.

This procedure is indicated in facial mechanisms that are not responsive to other approaches or in situations where the sphenoid is fixed as with intrasosseous strains. Patient is supine with one operator at the head of the patient with a firm bilateral temporal hold to stabilize the posterior elements of the cranium. The other operator stands to the patient's side, holding the left and right sides of the frontal bone in one hand and the left and right zygomae in the other hand. This operator lifts the facial bones straight up, pulling equally on the left and right sides. The second operator tells the first if temporal bone pressure is equal on both sides and, if not, to which side the first operator must increase or decrease their pressure. When the sphenoid release occurs, this will be felt as a sudden easing of the membranous tissue between the two operators' hands, and after an unwinding, tissue expansion will be appreciated by both operators. Zygomatic compression may result from this procedure due to the forces required to lift the face. Its evaluation and treatment should be carried out after completing the face lift.

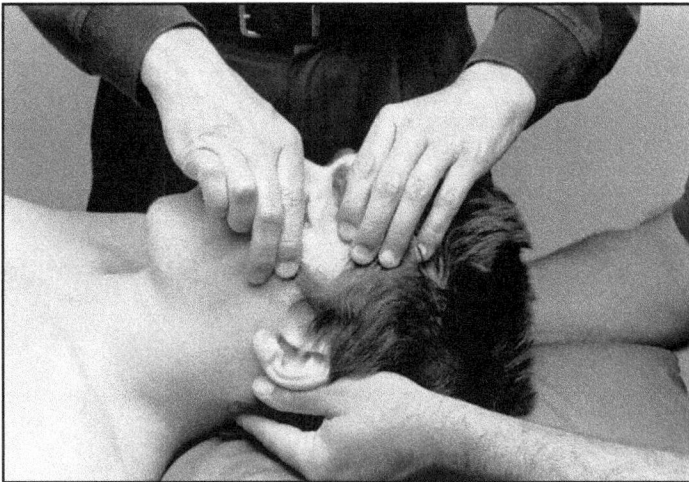

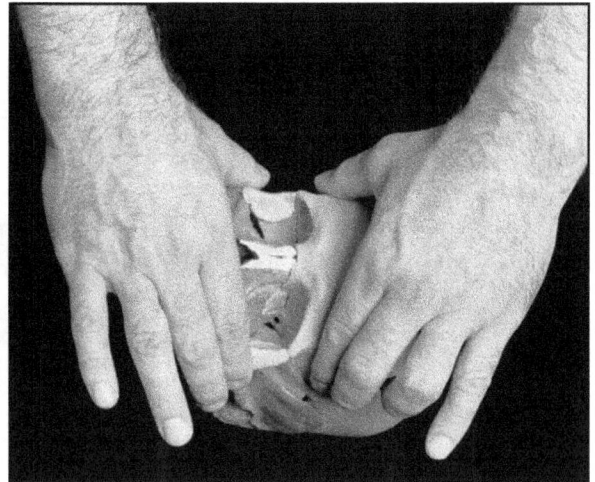

Two-Operator Face Lift

Excercise 2: Dural Stretch- Sacrooccipital Release

Operator one performs a lumbosacral decompression, while operator two performs an occipital condylar release, both with the following important modifications: (Each technique can also be performed by a single operator, independently)

Operator one: Occipital contact.

<u>Diagnosis</u>. Operator seated at the head of the supine patient. During flexion of the CRI and with the head slightly extended, gentle cephalad traction is applied to the right, left, and then midline of the occiput, noting which of these three is the most restricted or least complaint.

<u>Treatment</u>. During flexion of the CRI and with the head slightly extended, the operator places two finger pads (one on top of the other) on the occipital base where restricted traction was noted. With the topmost finger cephalad traction is introduced and held until extension of the CRI begins. The traction is partially released and reapplied with the next flexion phase of the CRI. Each subsequent flexion is met with a stronger traction force until a release is felt, in which the membranous tensions glide cephalad through what feels like a great distance. (The patient may feel this stretch into their low back.)

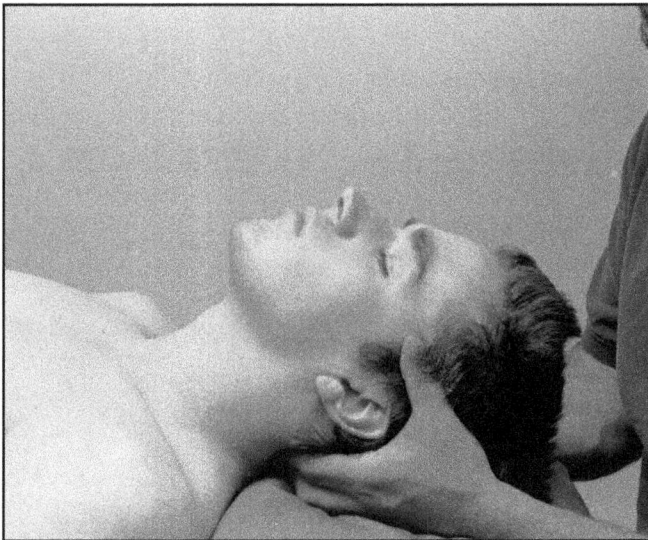

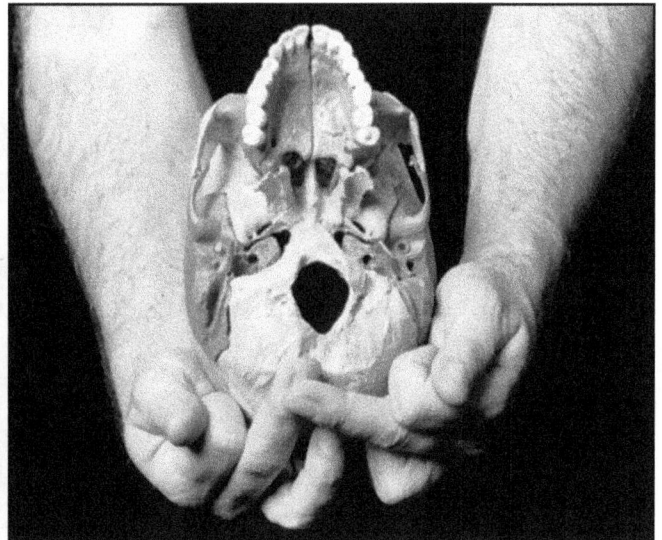

Two Operator Sacro-occipital Release: Occipital Contact

Operator two: Sacral Contact.

Diagnosis. Operator sits at the side of the supine patient with hands in position to perform a lumbosacral decompression. The finger pads are firmly contacting the sacral base bilaterally and during extension of the CRI gentle caudad traction forces are applied to the right, left, and then midline of the sacrum, noting the most restricted or least compliant of the three. Findings are compared with operator one, but they do not have to be on the same side.

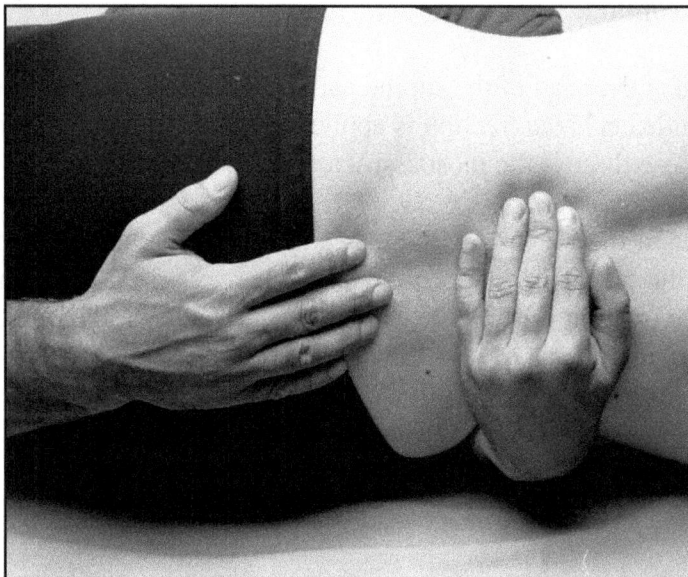

Two Operator Sacro-occipital Release: Sacral Contact Hand Positioning

Treatment. During extension phase of the CRI anterior and inferior traction is placed on the sacral aspect noted to be most restricted and held there until flexion of the CRI begins. The sacral traction is partially released and reapplied with the next extension phase of the CRI. Each subsequent extension is met with a stronger traction force until a release is felt, in which the membranous tissues glide caudad for what feels like a great distance. (The patient should feel the stretch into their upper back.). Note: Both operators must synchronize their relative traction forces at the proper time so that both operators do not apply traction force simultaneously. The operator at the head controls the timing of the procedure.

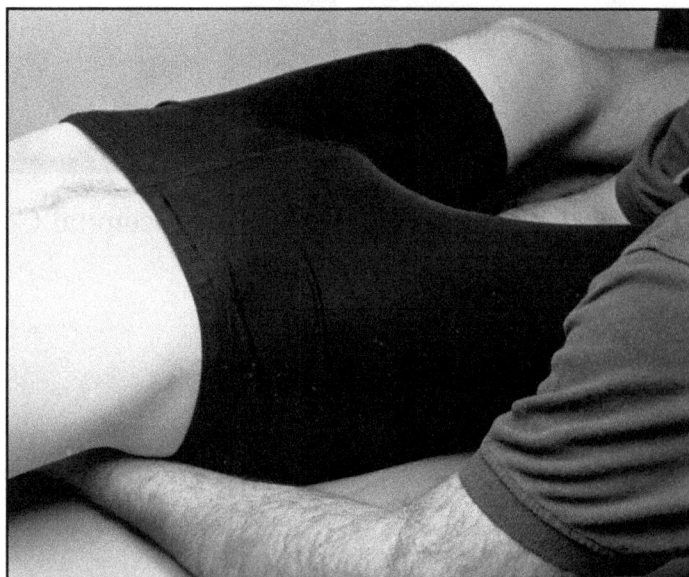

Two Operator Sacro-occipital Release: Sacral Contact Treatment Position

138

Level II Course Schedule- Day 1

8:00 am   (*0900*)   Course logistics

                                     Discussion of participants' experiences since last course

9:15 am   (*1015*)   Break

9:30 am   (*1030*)   *Table Session-* Review #1

12:00 pm   (*1300*)   Lunch

1:00 pm   (*1400*)   *Table Session-* Review #2

3:30 pm   (*1630*)   Break

3:45 pm   (*1645*)   Review, summary and questions

5:00 pm   (*1800*)   Adjourn

Level II Course Schedule- Day 2

8:00 am	*(0900)*	Questions
8:30 am	*(0930)*	*Lecture*: Embryology, Birth, Infant Anatomy
9:30 am	*(1030)*	Break
9:45 am	*(1045)*	*Lecture:* Embryology, Birth, Infant Anatomy (continued)
10:15 am	*(1115)*	*Lecture:* Pediatric Exam and Treatment
10:45 am	*(1145)*	Pediatric case study with demonstration
12:00 pm	*(1300)*	Lunch
1:00 pm	*(1400)*	Practice parameters of pediatric evaluation and treatment Questions
2:00 pm	*(1500)*	Effects of Trauma on breathing and diaphragm function
2:45 pm	*(1545)*	Break
3:00 pm	*(1600)*	*Table Session* •Shock Release •Lateral Rib Cage •Anterior Rib Cage •Sternum •Clavicle •Shoulder
4:45 pm	*(1745)*	Breathing exercises
5:00 pm	*(1800)*	Adjourn

Level II Course Schedule- Day 3

8:00 am   (*0900*)   *Table Session*
- Balancing 3-diaphragms
- Diagonal vector release

9:00 am   (*1000*)   Facial trauma, cranial nerve entrapment, anatomy review

10:00 am   (*1100*)   Break

10:15 am   (*1115*)   Demonstration of Intraoral Technique – I and II

12:00 pm   (*1300*)   Lunch

1:00 pm   (*1400*)   *Table Session*- Intraoral technique I
- Cruciate suture and four-quadrant diagnosis
- Maxilla-palatine and intermaxillary sutures
- Sphenopalatine suture, superior and inferior fixations

2:30 pm   (*1530*)   Break

2:45 pm   (*1545*)   *Table Session*- Intraoral technique II
- Zygoma
- Vomer
- Ethmoid

4:15 pm   (*1715*)   Demonstration of intraoral technique – III

5:00 pm   (*1800*)   Adjourn

Level II Course Schedule- Day 4

8:00 am	(*0900*)	*Table Session*- Intraoral technique III
		•Sphenopalatine Ganglion
		•Frontosphenoid
		•Sphenosquamous
9:00 am	(*1000*)	Orbital technique
		•Anatomy review
		•Demonstration of diagnosis and treatment technique
		Table Session
		•Nasofrontal
		•Nasomaxillary
		•Orbit
		•Eyeball
10:00 am	(*1100*)	Break
10:15 am	(*1115*)	Temporomandibular joint
		•Anatomy review
		•Demonstration of diagnosis and treatment techniques
10:45 am	(*1145*)	*Table Session*- Temporomandibular joint
		•Sphenomandibular ligament
		•Stylomandibular ligament
		•Capsular release
		•Hyoid release
12:00 pm	(*1300*)	Lunch
1:00 pm	(*1400*)	*Table Session*- Orbital Axis Release
2:30 pm	(*1530*)	Break
2:45 pm	(*1545*)	*Table Session* Venous Sinus Technique
5:00 pm	(*1800*)	Adjourn

Level II Course Schedule- Day 5

8:00 am	(*0900*)	Review
8:30 am	(*0930*)	*Table Session*- Two-Operator Technique
		•Face lift
10:00 am	(*1100*)	Break
10:15 am	(*1115*)	*Table Session*- Two-Operator Technique
		•Dural stretch
12:00 pm	(*1300*)	Lunch
1:00 pm	(*1400*)	Clinical Integration
3:00 pm	(*1600*)	Adjourn

Notes:

OSTEOPATHIC MANIPULATIVE MEDICINE APPROACHES TO THE PRIMARY RESPIRATORY MECHANISM

Level III
Harnessing the Fulcrum, Unleashing the Tide

OMM Approaches to the Primary Respiratory Mechanism

Level III
Course Objectives

Be familiar with the concepts of fluid matrix and midline fuction, tidal potency, and the related use of fulcrums.

Develop palpatory skills to appreciate reciprocal tensions within the fluid matrix.

Develop palpatory skills to harness fulcrums within the reciprocal tensions in fluid, membrane, and bone.

Develop palpatory skills to palpate tidal potencies within fluid, membrane and bone.

Be familiar with the concept and palpatory experience of the anterior dural girdle and its relations to other dural rings within the cranial vault.

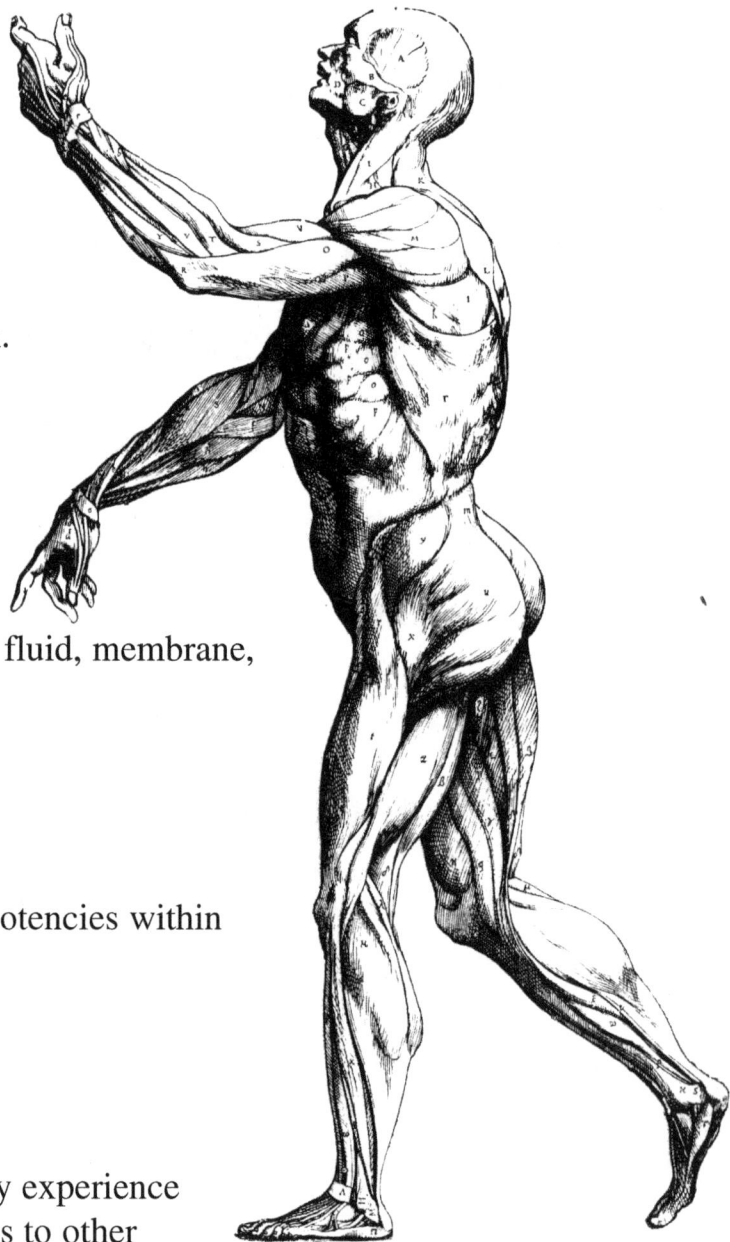

Fluid Matrix and Midline Function

The osteopathic approach stresses a dynamic relationship to the patient as a whole. Such a holistic approach emphasizes a palpatory experience of the patient's inherent healing capacity and functional equilibrium, as well as the underlying structural and motor disturbances that contribute to altered form and function.

Palpatory perceptions and responses to treatment are unique to each patient. The therapeutic summation of diagnostic perceptions and treatment responses establishes a fulcrum of dynamic balance through which health and vitality can return to the patient.

Health and vitality have their origins in the embryonic fluid matrix from which living form and function are expressed. Its expression unfolds through interactive electrochemical and electromagnetic forces within the body's living fluids, forming an intelligent matrix of life potentials and potencies. This fluid matrix organizes itself around a three-dimensional axis of fluctuating motion, establishing a functional midline as well as a blueprint for all subsequent life. Embryologic growth proceeds in relation to this midline, establishing a vital relationship to all body tissues. This ongoing midline relationship is essential for the optimal health and vitality of all living tissues throughout life.

Midline function resides at the core of our being, and interfaces with every physical, emotional, intellectual, and spiritual aspect of our lives. It is present before our central nervous system develops, and its biodynamic vitality is not a function of any one or even all the systems of our body together. Such vitality is indivisible, an intelligent self-generating matrix of originality and intention.

This original fluid matrix is called the *tide* or *tidal body*, and the biodynamic force active within this tidal body is called *potency*. Potency is the fluid drive within the tide bringing the tidal body into a vital relationship with all other bodily functions. Coiling and uncoiling of the fluid-membrane matrix constitutes the basic movements of the tidal body. The potency within this matrix is called the "breath of life" and the tidal body is its core container. Tidal movement occurs through suspended, automatically shifting fulcrums around the original midline forming a biodynamic blueprint for all subsequent growth and development. The embryologic expression of this blueprint is the neural tube through which tidal movement creates living form and function. Automatic shifting is directed by tidal potency expressing originality and intention through this midline fluid matrix. Reciprocal tension patterns are established by this tidal movement, the core of which centers at the Sutherland fulcrum just at the junction of the great vein of Galen and the straight sinus at the posterior end of the third ventricle.

As tissue relations become disturbed over time by stress and traumatic forces, these reciprocal tension patterns are altered and tidal function is disturbed. Tissue orients around a new fulcrum, and midline relations are altered from the original matrix, distorting originality and misguiding intention. Bone development and growth also become disturbed within this fluid membrane matrix. By palpating through the bone and into the membrane and the potency of the fluid matrix within, we can contact the tidal body and stimuate the breath of life.

In order to reorient tissues around their original midline and enhance the vital potency of the tidal body, functional midline anatomy must be understood. The neural tube is anchored in lamina terminalis with its superior attachment at the anterior inferior aspect of the third ventricle, its inferior attachment in the pia of the filum terminale, which attaches to the end of the coccyx. The Sutherland fulcrum began embryologically at lamina terminalis, but migrated during embryologic coiling/uncoiling to its adult position. This migration occurred in conjunction with the development of the central nervous system, establishing the automatically-shifting fulcrum, which balances the tension and movement in the whole system.

Cranial flexion and extension reflect the original embryologic movements of the neural tube in its coiling (flexion) phase and uncoiling (extension) phase. During flexion, the Sutherland fulcrum and the lamina terminalis converge along an axis that passes through the third ventricle. The pituitary and pineal move toward one another similarly. The tentorium rises anteriorly with the sphenoid and it flattens and falls posteriorly with the occiput like a bird preparing to land. The cerebral ventricles expand in the flexion phase, widening and shortening like wings, the tail of the bird rising as the tube is lifted superiorly. As uncoiling occurs in extension, the ventricles lengthen and narrow as the lamina terminalis and Sutherland fulcrum move away from each other. The tentorium moves inferiorly at its anterior attachment with the sphenoid and superiorly with the occiput. Simultaneously, the leaves of the tent become more angulated in response to the lengthening and narrowing of the ventricles and in association with the temporal bones internal rotation. This biodynamic movement of the tidal body creates a longitudinal axis or fluid drive that establishes and maintains the body's physiology and midline function.

Fig. 22: The Motility of the Neural Tube

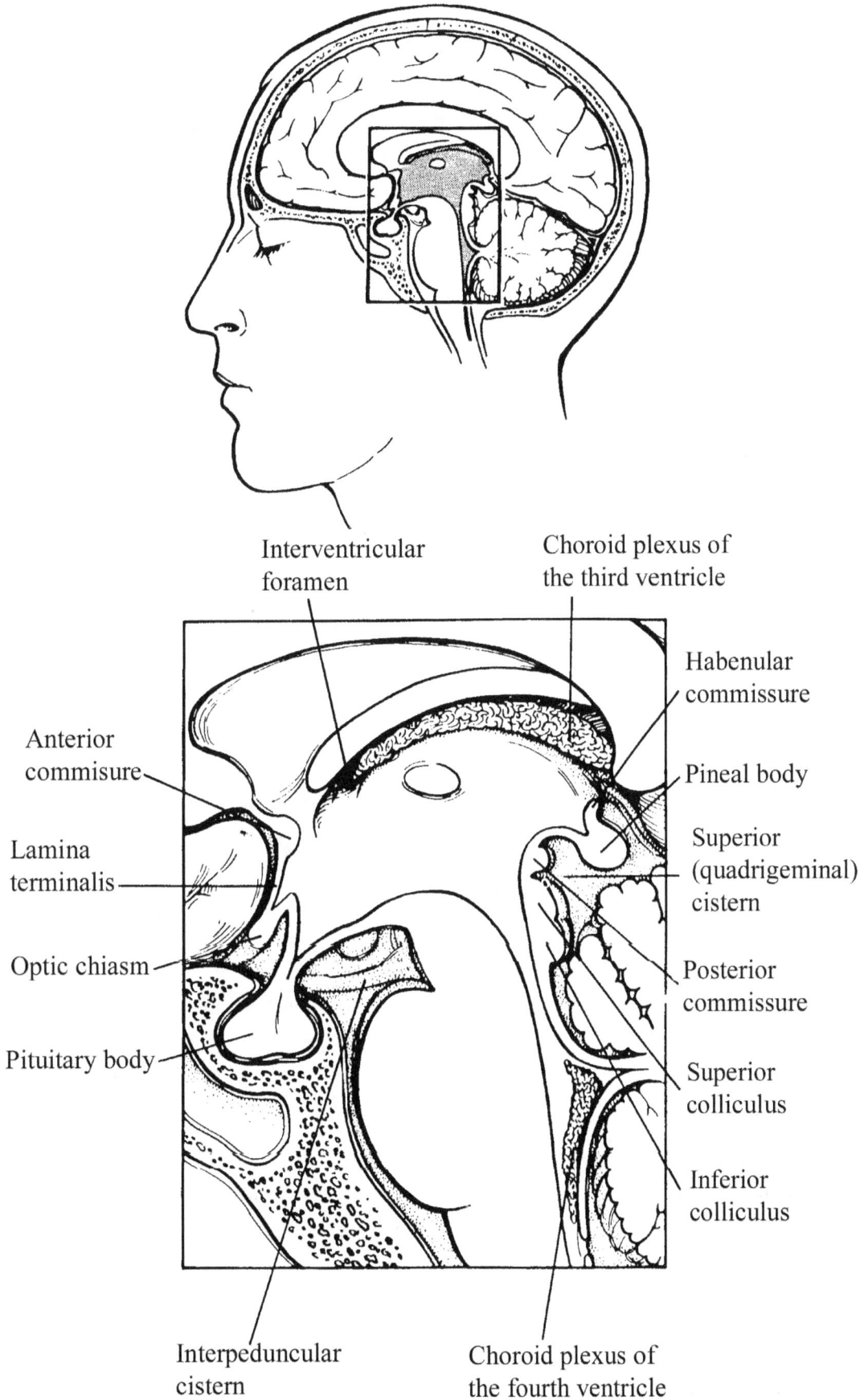

Interventricular foramen

Choroid plexus of the third ventricle

Habenular commissure

Pineal body

Anterior commisure

Superior (quadrigeminal) cistern

Lamina terminalis

Optic chiasm

Posterior commissure

Pituitary body

Superior colliculus

Inferior colliculus

Interpeduncular cistern

Choroid plexus of the fourth ventricle

(Reprinted with permission from the Sutherland Cranial Teaching Foundation)

149

Biodynamic Versus Biomechanical Approach

As physicians trained in the osteopathic concept, we recognize altered form and function, and their role in the natural history of disease and suffering. Structure and function are reciprocally related—linked together in a biomechanical continuum that interplays with all other body systems, and influences the integrity of the whole system. Improved structure enhances function; enhancing function improves structure. These are concepts that provide a mechanical basis for osteopathic problem-solving and therapeutic intervention. There is, however, a more permanent and powerful therapeutic potency than this mechanical realignment/enhancement. Such a therapeutic potency is found within the patient as a dynamic impulse of health and vitality that instills corrective vitality on contact.

Such health and vitality lives within the tidal body representing the potential for bringing health to any patient experiencing any illness. Health can then be seen as ever present within the embryonic potencies of each individual, always active and yet latent within ordinary (disturbed) physiologic function. Static patterns of motion contain reciprocal tensions around disturbed midline fulcrums. Establishing balanced tension around those fulcrums allows the inherent forces to shift, freeing the potency within to correct associated disturbances to optimal healthy function. The potency within is corrective because it contains the intelligence (blueprint) of the original midline fluid matrix. This biodynamic force is ever-present in one form or another, and always receptive to the practitioner skilled in it's palpatory perception.

Table 8: What is the difference between this biodynamic approach and the traditional biomechanical approach?

Mechanical	Biodynamic
Neutral is passive reference point or axis for motion	Midline is active
Forces are applied by operator to realign structures	Operator unleashes inherent healing forces within the patient
Diagnostic skills focus on identifying altered positional relations and their associated altered motion patterns	Diagnostic skills focus on identifying reciprocal tensions in tissue, fluid, and potency
Treatment skills focus on returning tissues to their structural and functional midline	Treatment skills focus on bringing tissues into a dynamic balance so that their inherent fluid potency can be unleashed
Removes traumatic forces in body	Stimulates corrective forces in body

Palpating the Fluid Membrane Matrix and the Breath of Life

Embryonic life begins within a highly intelligent and vital fluid matrix. Initial development proceeds along midline structures and fluid gradients that move in a longitudinal direction establishing the basic structures of the nervous system. This longitudinal axis forms a functional midline reference for all subsequent growth and development. Its structural matrix flexes and then extends in a coiling and uncoiling movement that establishes the inherent motility of the CNS present throughout life. Once the longitudinal axis is established, lateral fluctuations begin the differentiation process of all the other organ systems, which depend on this inherent longitudinal motility for their vital function.

Indications for Breath of Life Treatment:
    1) Paradoxical Motion
    2) Absent vertical rise of the sacrum
    3) SBS Compression

In this exercise, we begin to appreciate the coiling and uncoiling of the longitudinal axis as well as the vitality present within the system called the "breath of life." The patient is supine and the operator sits at the head of the table with fingers coming together in the midline of the occiput in a vertical fashion. To re-establish the longitudinal movement of the long axis, we must first initiate the flexion phase of motion, which is the axis of motion through which the coiling of the nervous system occurs. By drawing the basi-occiput in a cephalad and anterior direction, we bring it into its relative phase of cranial or SBS flexion. Our next goal is to create a neutral point within the long axis by moving into areas of tension within the dural tube (i.e., rotation and side-bending) to balance the tension in three dimensions. Traction is put into the mechanism by spreading the fingers across the midline of the occiput while simultaneously holding the position of balance as a fulcrum through which the longitudinal motion will be re-established like a doorway through which the breath of life inspires. When the inherent force of the breath of life coils, it causes a strong fluid fluctuation within the membrane matrix, palpated as a pulsating movement with both flexion and extension characteristics, but with a rate that is consistent with the slow tide occurring at a rate of approximately 1 1/2 cycles per minute. This is the frequency that the breath of life moves through the fluid membrane matrix. Both the patient and the operator will experience a profound sense of relaxation and "self."

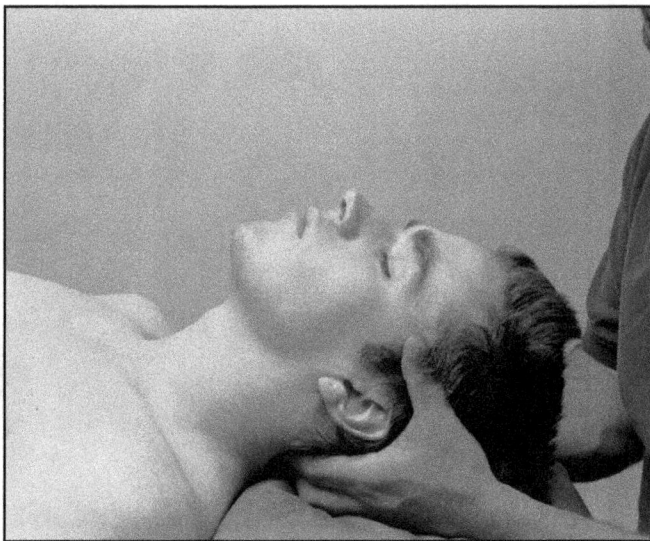

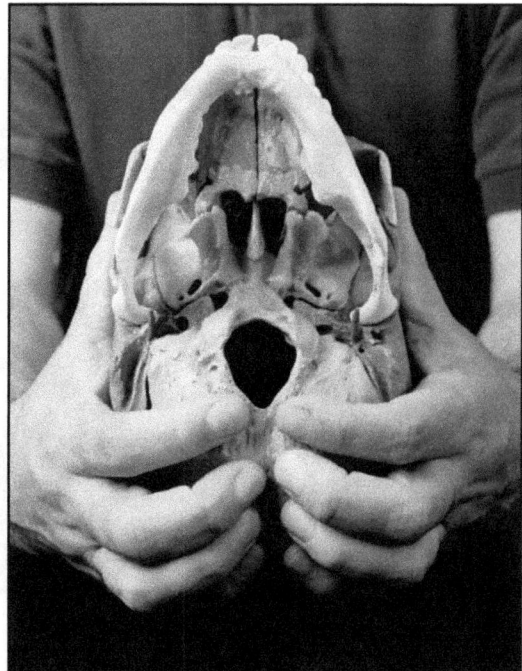

Palpating the Breath of Life- Occipital Approach

Temporal Approach

By lifting the cranial base cranialward we can also accentuate coiling/flexion movement within the CNS. This exercise is performed by pulling the zygomatic process of the temporal bones superiorly (cranially) and simultaneously bringing the mastoid processes medially (into external rotation) and posteriorly (focusing a cephalad vector through the SBS). Balance is established between temporal bones while traction is held until a lengthening is perceived along the midline axis. The rise and fall of the tentorium cerebelli can also be oberved to enhance the treatment.

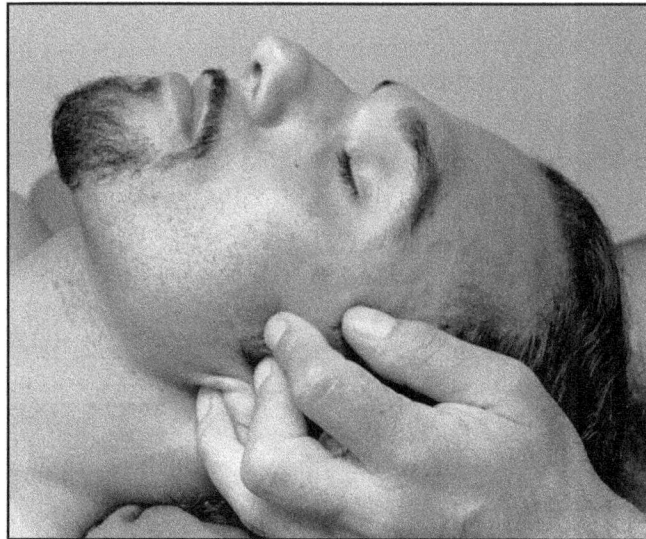

Palpating the Breath of Life- Temporal Approach

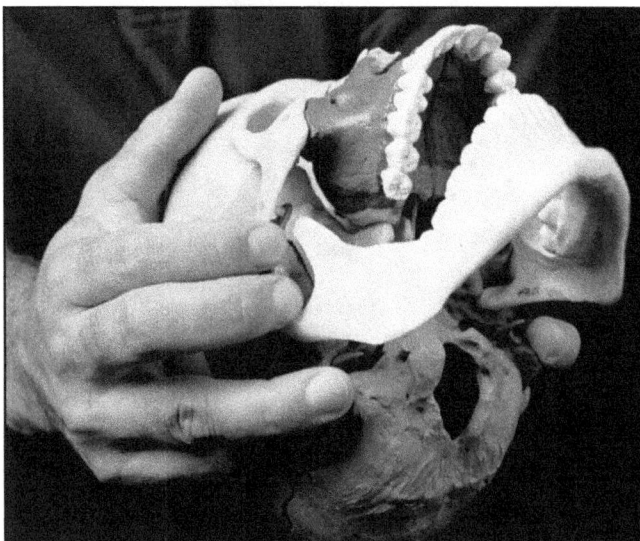

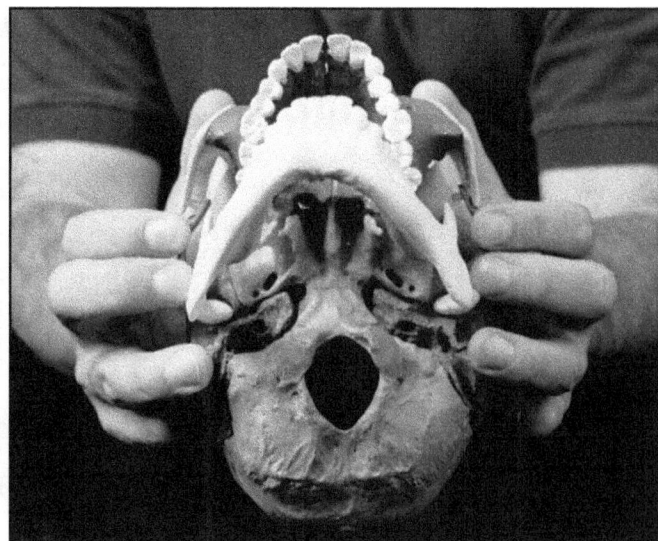

Anatomical Placement for Temporal Approach

Tidal Potency and Respiratory Function

Fluid and membranous functions of the CRI reflect tidal movemements mechanically and biodynamically. Mechanical motions exist at the periphery of the system like waves crashing on the sand. Biodynamic motions occur more centrally in association with midline function in the depths of the ocean. Perception of this deeper tidal movemement is slower and more dynamic, stimulating deeper responses in the potency of the CRI.

There are two distinct kinds of potency, one pointed and sharp, the other soft and very sweet. The very pointed, sharp form of potency can be sensed in a lateral fluctuation or by directing the tide longitudinally. This potency has a sense of direction and only operates along geometric lines related to the formation of the body, i.e., longitudinal axis. If we do not have our hands aligned properly with the intrinsic geometry of the body, then the tidal forces will not reveal their potency with much intensity. This type of potency is dependent on vectors, and to sense the proper vector we must align our hands with the forces of health hidden in the body and not focus on just the altered structure/function. As this potency becomes active, it feels electric, quick and sharp like a spark, and has an absolute ability to reorganize unhealthy patterns of health in the tissues.

The other form of potency active within the tidal body is softer and slower, like liquid moving within a liquid. It does not move with a vectorial or directional orientation, and it does not have an axis of motion, nor does it function through a fulcrum. Such potency moves through the tidal body all at once, like a carpet of warm fog filling every nook and cranny, down to the deepest core of our perceivable self. This soft potency leaves in its wake a warm wellness and fresh fullness that permeates areas of strain with the breath of life. It restores the vitality of every living cell in the body. It is a power so subtle (if you are not looking for it, you could easily miss it), and yet so powerful that it envelops and transforms us.

Tidal potency is modulated by diaphragmatic (respiratory) function. Unrestricted cardiorespiratory and circulatory mechanics fuels tidal potency by stimulating midline fluid and pressure gradients. Unrestricted respiratory movement clears the way for a wave of fluid potency to bathe body tissues from head to toe. Respiratory function is limited by areas significantly restricting the cranial rhythmic impulse, especially tissues above and below the respiratory diaphragm, and through viscerosomatic reflex disturbances. It is important to clear and optimize this respiratory function before unleashing the tide.

Potency represents what is indivisible within the body, the inherent intelligence "present" within the primary respiratory mechanism. This is the truest perception we can have of the cranial rhythmic impulse.

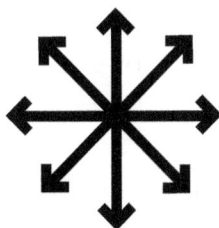

Fig. 23: Directional Potency   Fig. 24: Soft Potency

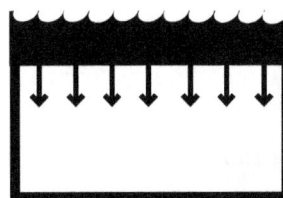

Structural and Functional Midline

We have spoken about unleashing longitudinal fluid potency in the tidal body to re-establish the body's original matrix for midline function. Stimulating tidal potency and the body's self-healing, self-regulatory intelligence accomplishes a primary objective in osteopathic manipulative management. Maintaining this functional midline in part is a self-generating phenomenon, but often requires the support of midline structures to optimize the ongoing benefits of a functioning tidal potency.

Midline structures have relationships to themselves and to each other that can facilitate proper tidal function. These relationships are enhanced by a proper postural foundation from the ground up. Gait mechanics also reinforce productive or counterproductive structural patterns that may "tip the scales" of ongoing balance between corrective (self-generating) tidal forces and traumatic (degenerative) inertial forces. Therefore, maintenance of optimal structural relations is a worthwhile endeavor, especially as it relates to midline structures of the spine, sacrum, sternum, and cranial vault.

Midline structures are all oriented around the original midline matrix of fluid potency; however, their axes of motion are altered significantly by macro- and microtraumas originating externally as well as internally. Disturbing the axis of motion causes a shift away from the original midline, altering the structural relations of the attached moving parts, as well as their inherent fluid potencies. Palpating such an altered axis of motion and following the inherent functional potencies of the attached moving parts to their relative state of balanced tension is "harnessing the fulcrum." The fulcrum has movements occurring around the x-, y-, and z-axis, and also has translatory characteristics that move along the x-, y-, and z-axis. Therefore, we label this complex phenomenon a *suspended three-dimensional automatic shifting fulcrum*. Midline structures oriented longitudinally have six directions of freedom. Treatment incorporates these six directions of freedom, balancing tensions in all six directions and then waiting for the potency within the original tidal matrix to be unleashed (unwinding may occur before potency is palpated). The fulcrum acts as a doorway through which this potency enters into the tissues and into the hands of the operator simultaneously. The potency of the tide will always respond, without fail, in due time, but does not always appear to move in a linear fashion on or around any axis of motion.

Distal midline structures should move together in concert with longitudinal tidal forces associated with the flexion and extension phases of the cranial rhythmic impulse. Synchronized sacral and sternal movements are simultaneously moving caudad in extension and cephalad in flexion, in association with shortening and lengthening of the functional midline. Likewise, occipital and sternal movements behave similarly, but in relation to the basiocciput, which, remember, moves in the opposite direction as the occipital squama under your hands.

The sacrum during flexion makes two important excursions. One is a direct vertical rise, the other a circumflexion. The vertical rise is as important to central nervous system motion as the circumflexion. Therefore, observe the vertical rise in the sacrum that precedes circumflexion.

Intraosseous Motion and Membranous Function

Intraosseous motion must be established before normal interosseous or articular motion can be accomplished. Any distortions in intraosseous structure or function will disturb the fluid membrane mechanism of that bone. This follows the classic adage *Before you can know another, you must know yourself.* Intraosseous motion within the cellular and fluid matrix of the bone is oriented to the midline and shaped to the function it supports. This function is not only longitudinal, but also has a lateral expression, particularly during the flexion phase, which is vital to the function of the central nervous system. If we observe the occipital bone closely it defies the classical description, which focuses only on its flexion activity, a midline anterior-posterior movement. However, the living occipital bone breathes. It changes shape with each primary respiratory cycle. It opens its transverse diameter internally with greater excursion in addition to the more publicized flexion action. The basic principle for treatment of an intraosseus distortion is quite simply to follow the motion and quality of the potency during flexion phase. As one exaggerates the normal motion in synchrony with the inhalation phase, internal forces within the bone collect at the fulcrum. Tensions within the potency itself can be appreciated in this manner. The fulcrum is the point to which the tidal forces are collectively bringing their influences into focus as a wave of potency that releases the disturbed axis and pattern of motion.

Remember, it is the membranes that carry the bones into their positions of flexion, extension, external rotation, or internal rotation. The bones ride within the membranous system of the human body and are guided by the reciprocal tensions of fluid, membrane and potency. There is no recoil in this system of motion. Both phases are active. During the flexion phase of the primary respiratory mechanism, the central nervous system converges upon lamina terminalis just anterior to the pituitary. It is essential that the pial attachment to the coccyx be able to move vertically toward lamina terminalis in order to allow the full coiling motion of the central nervous system to occur. During the extension phase of the primary respiratory mechanism, the central nervous system converges upon the Sutherland fulcrum. All the bones in the body are moving in concert with this reciprocal tension membrane as it automatically shifts between lamina terminalis and the Sutherland fulcrum.

Treatment Sequence for Harnessing the Fulcrum, Unleashing the Tide

1) Palpate an area of disturbed (midline) function and sense the CRI as fully as possible.

2) While sensing the CRI, the patient's tissues will inherently move, orienting about their disturbed axis to a point of balanced tension. This is the fulcrum around which the dysfunction is organized. Operator force must sustain the tissue balance around this fulcrum.

3) Balanced tension around this fulcrum stimulates (embryonic) midline relations, opening the doorway for tidal potencey to come into the patient's tissues.

4) Therapeutic effects of this tidal potency may include a variety of responses; large involuntary or chaotic movements, "unwinding", melting, jolting, twitching, trembling or wavelike movements, repositioning of body parts, or audible sounds of movement. Simultaneously, the patient may experience memories, visualizations (e.g. of color), emotions, feelings of warmth, softness, electricity, cold, nausea, dizziness, vertigo, sleepiness, profound relaxation or hypnagogic states.

5) At the moment tidal potencey is fully expressed in the patient's tissues, a still point will be appreciated. In this moment there is stillness and balanced tension without any operator effort.

6) The primary phases of flexion and extension of the CRI will follow the still point. This may be perceived as a gentle, slow swelling or expansion of the patient's tissues between the operator's hands. Generally the rate is slower and the amplitude greater than when the treatment began.

The wise physician knows what is happening in the patient by being aware of what is happening here in the moment. This is more potent than wandering off into various theories or making complex interpretations of the situation at hand.

Stillness, clarity and consciousness are more immediate than any number of expeditions into the distant lands of one's mind. Such expeditions, however stimulating, distract both the physician and the patient from what is actually happening.

By staying present and aware of what is happening, the physician can do less, yet achieve more.

adapted from Lao Tzu's Tao Te Ching

Sacral Evaluation and Treatment

1. <u>Sacral Apex</u>: With the patient supine, the operator sits at the patient's side and contacts the paracoccygeal tissues between their index and middle fingers. Gentle but firm contact is made with the sacrococcygeal region and a passive listening introduced to monitor the longitudinal function of the sacrum as it rises (coils) and falls (uncoils). In the flexion phase, the terminal fibers of the pia are pulled cephalad, causing a vertical rise of the sacral apex. To restore this normal longitudinal movement of the sacrum, it is necessary to observe inherent sacral motion with the intention of following it to a position of balanced reciprocal tension. This can occur in either the flexion or extension phase of the CRI. This intention must also include contacting the fulcrum through which the potency held within can be released. The operator's other hand contacts the paraspinal tissues of the lower lumbar spine to assist in locating the fulcrum, following inherent motions to the stillpoint and waiting. Continued observation on the part of the operator should begin to appreciate the stimulation of the potency within the longitudinal axis of the sacrum.

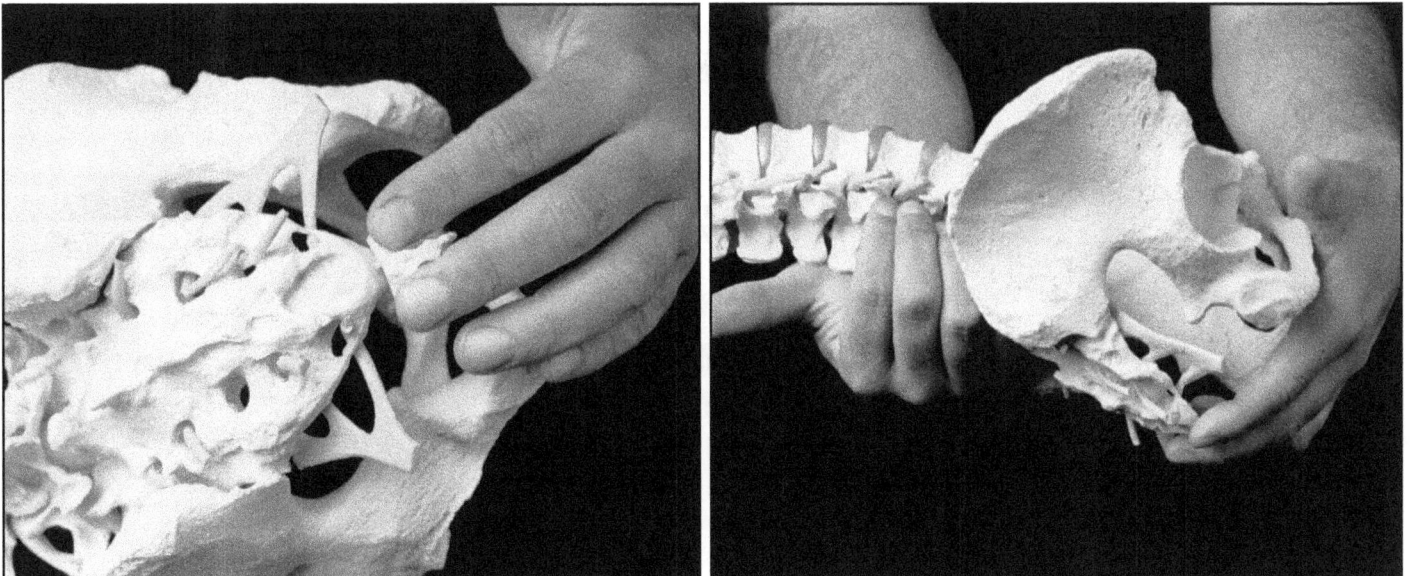

Sacral Apex Treatment

2. Intraosseous Sacral Dysfunction: Intraosseous dysfunction can be appreciated by a sense of heaviness or lack of organization within the functional characteristics of the sacrum. Such a sacrum structurally feels rigid and "bony." With the same hand contact as in #1, the operator's lumbar contact moves down to a sacral contact at about the level of S1. Again, the operator observes the direction of forces locked within the intraosseous structure, following the reciprocal tensions to their balanced point around a dynamic fulcrum, through which potency can return to the intraosseous structures. Though the mechanism is followed through both flexion and extension movements the balanced fulcrum of the flexion phase in particular should be exaggerated. This assists with unlocking tensions within the fluid membrane matrix that disturb lateral fluid fluctuation during flexion. This is repeated at multiple levels of the sacrum, S2, S3.

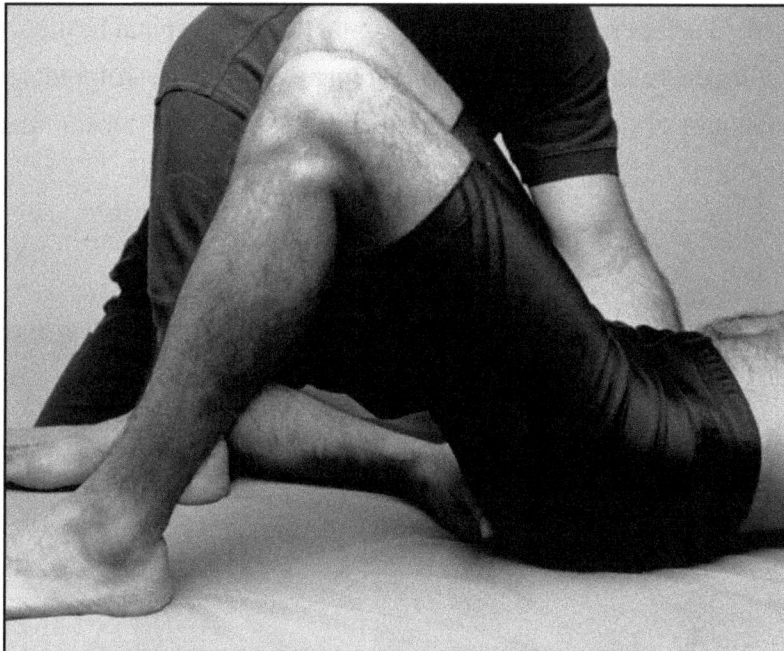

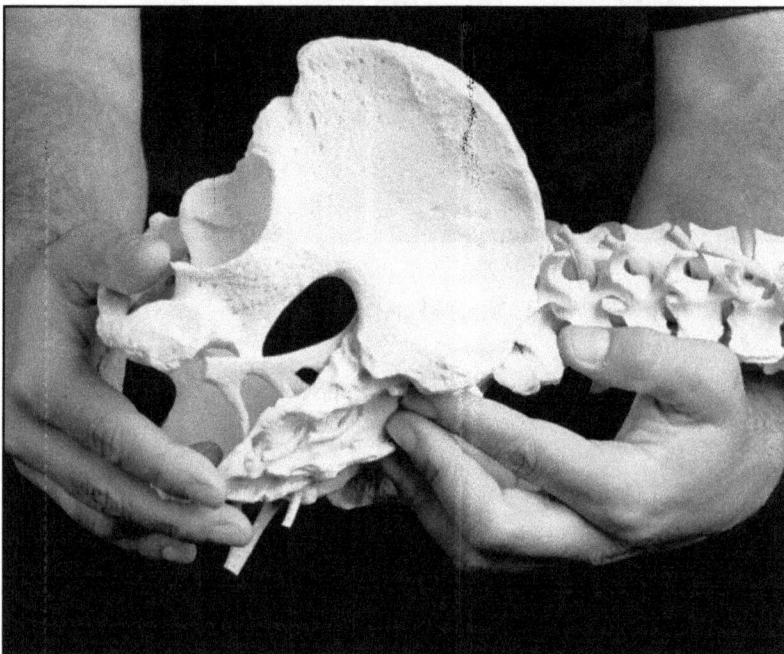

Treatment of Intraosseus Sacral Dysfunction

3. Thoracolumbar Junction: While still contacting the sacrococcygeal area, the operator contacts an area of spinal restriction in the thoracolumbar spine with the other hand. Sacral movements are used to balance points of tension in the spine and a fulcrum established between the two points. Midline finger or paraspinal hand contact can be used to accentuate balanced tension at the spinal point of focus. Release of tidal potency through the spinal midline will be felt at both points of contact.

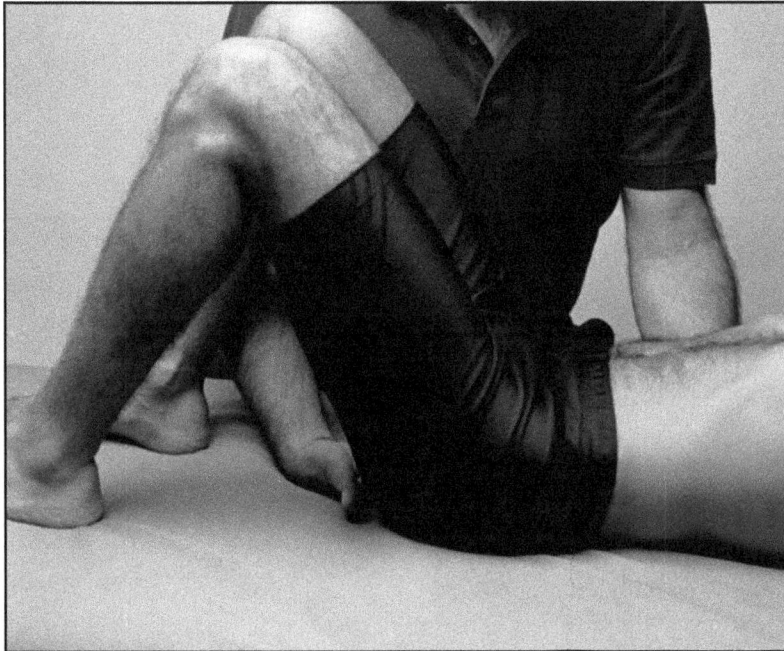

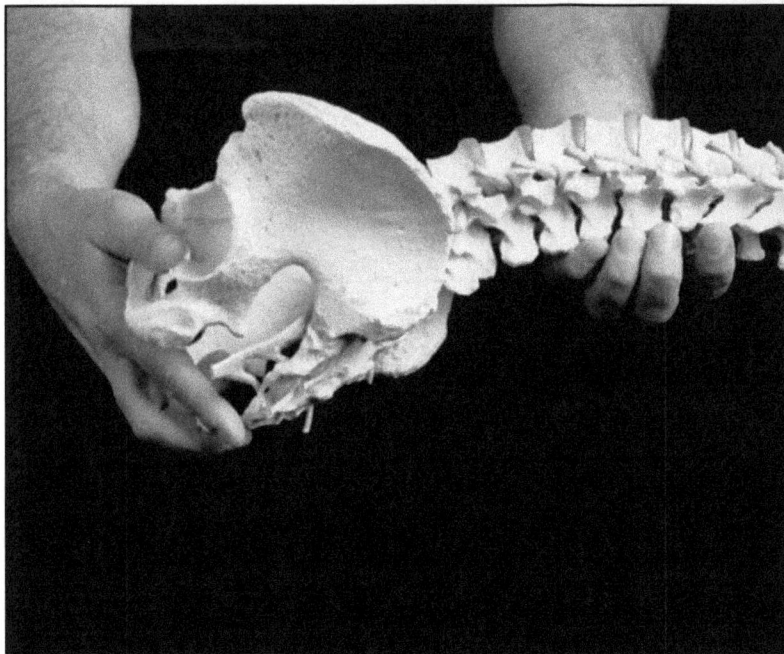

Treatment of Thoracolumbar Junction

4. <u>Sacrosternal Axis</u>: With the same sacrococcygeal hand-hold, the operator moves their other hand to a contact point of tension on the patient's sternum. This tension may be felt to be located in the upper, middle, or lower aspect of the sternum. Again, the operator passively listens for synchronized movements of the sternum and sacrum as they move together, caudad in the uncoiling, or extension phase and cephalad in the coiling, or flexion phase. The operator continues to follow these inherent movements, exaggerating the directions that are free, until potency comes into the tissue and full synchronized motion is restored. The sacrosternal axis is a vital midline fulcrum that coordinates upper and lower body functions.

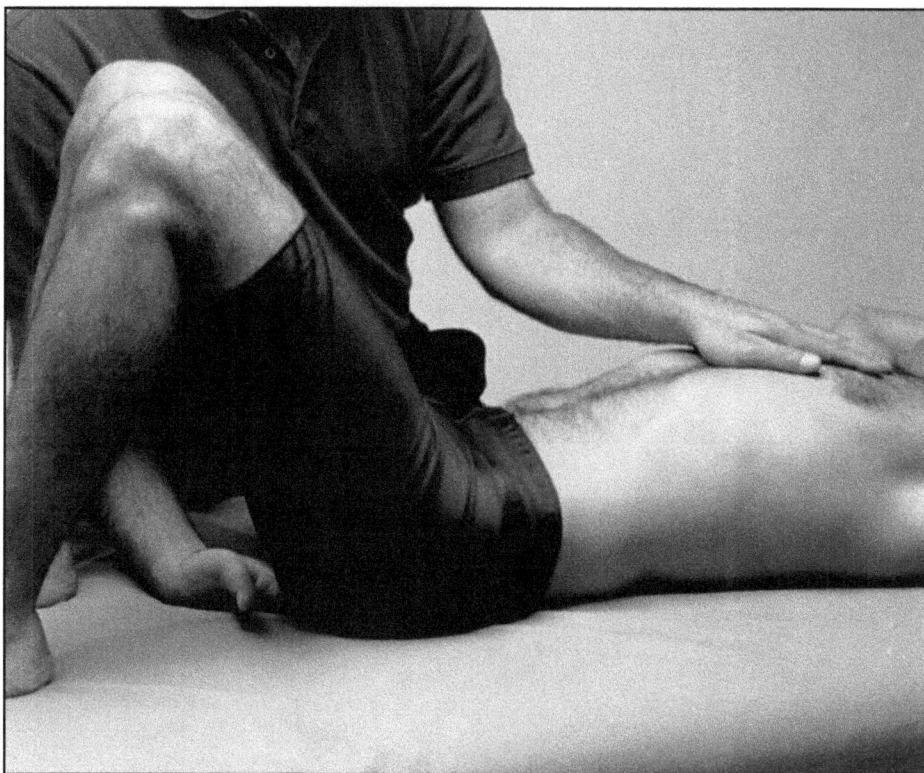

Sacrosternal Axis Treatment

Occipital Evaluation and Treatment

1. <u>Occipitocervical/Thoracic Junctions</u>: The functional midline axis coordinates regional motion patterns that can be easily appreciated by contacting a point of functional stress within one part of the body and balancing it with an important midline structure, either the occiput or the sacrum. In this exercise, we find an area of the cervicothoracic spine that is restricted and observe its inherent function with respect to the mechanics of the occipitocervical region. The inferior occiput is contacted with fingers along the vertical midline. The head can be followed toward directions that balance the tensions felt in the thoracic region including flexion/extension, sidebending and rotation. The operator sits at the head of the table creating a fulcrum between their hands around which the reciprocal tensions of these two regions are brought into balance, a stillpoint is appreciated, and the potency of the tide follows as the thoracic tension is dissipated.

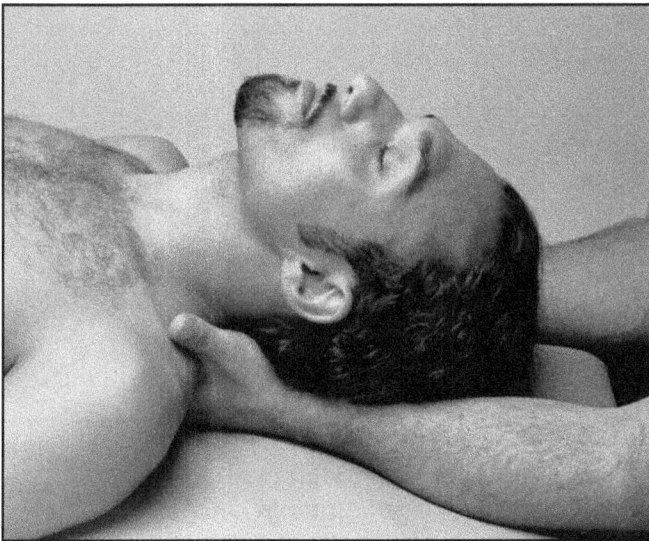

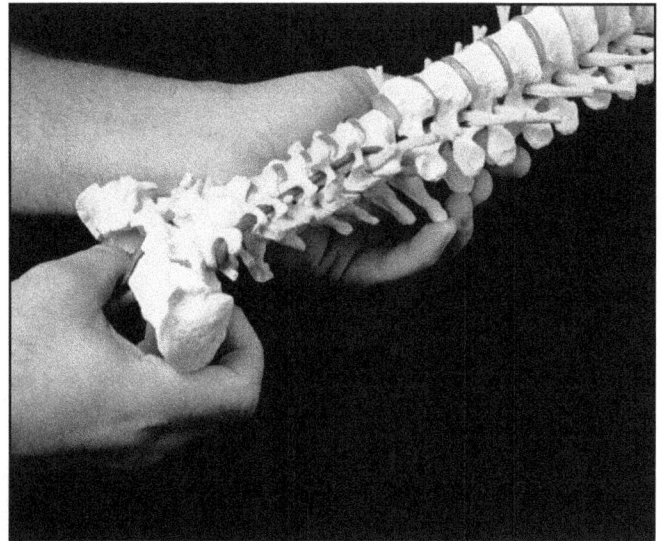

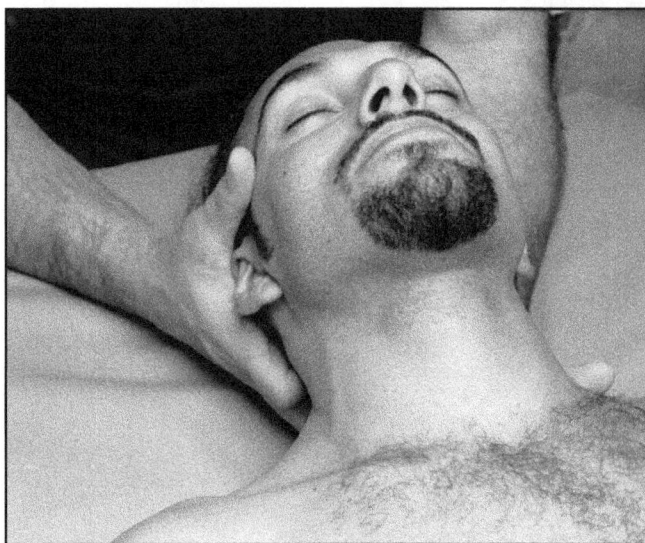

Treatment of the Occipitocervical/Thoracic Junction

2. Occipitoatlantal Junction: The operator sits at the head of the table contacting the midline of the occiput inferior to the inion and extending all the way to the first cervical segment. Intraosseous strain is particularly appreciated during this technique as the operator follows the normal flexion and extension movements and additionally focuses on sidebending and rotational movements away from the midline. The operator balances reciprocal tensions within the occiput by compressing toward or distracting away from the midline and following anteriorly or posteriorly in order to achieve balanced tension around the longitudinal axis or fulcrum. As the potency rises, lateral occipital fluctuation will be enhanced. The atlas is monitored for balanced responses throughout the procedure, and positioned to enhance fulcrum alignment (positions include more or less anterior translation, flexion/extension, rotation, and sidebending).

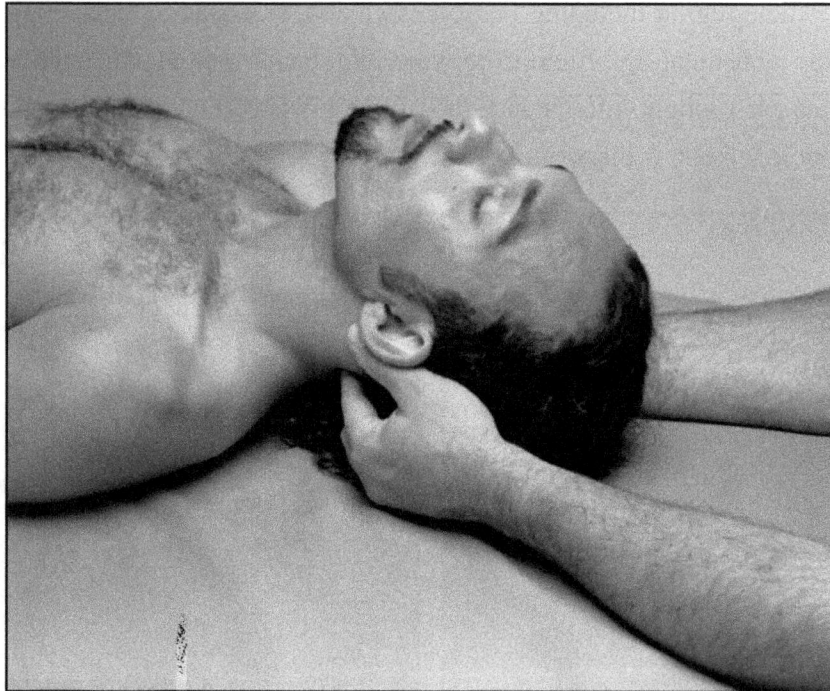

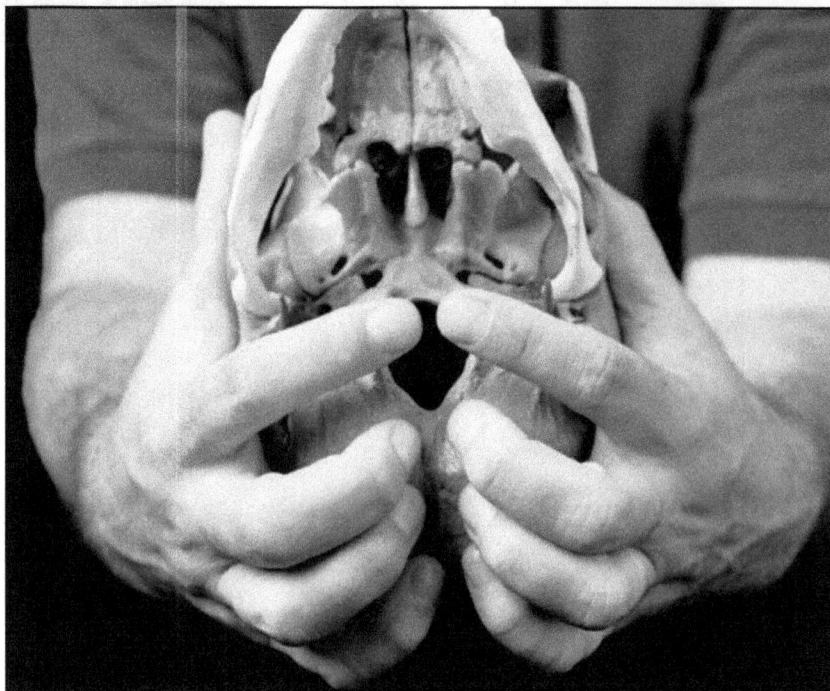

Treatment of the Occipitoatlantal Junction

3. Occipitosternal Axis: With one hand maintaining contact on the occipital midline, the other hand contacts the sternum and appreciates the respective coiling (rise) and uncoiling (fall) of both hands. (The sternum rises with the SBS as the occipital squama falls) The operator gently exaggerates the direction that moves more freely while simultaneously following movements of fluid and membranous strains within each bone. A balanced fulcrum is held until full excursion and potency is restored in both directions.

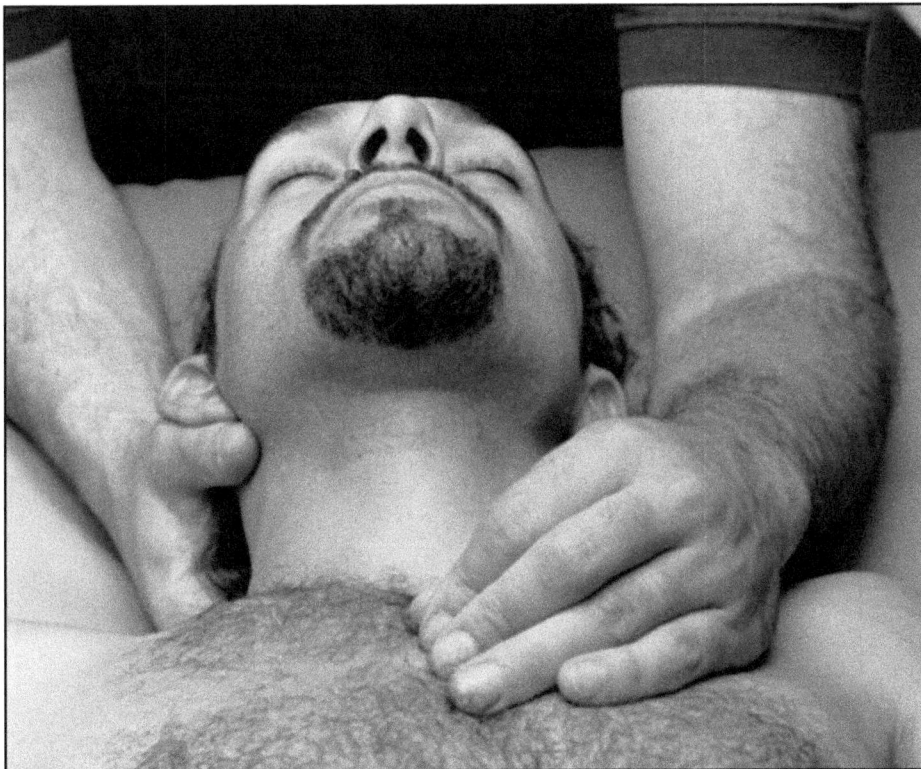

Treatment of the Occipitosternal Axis

Cranial Vault Evaluation and Treatment

1. <u>Inion/SBS</u>: The potency locked within the SBS mechanism can be unleashed along both a longitudinal and AP axis simultaneously because they are both part of the same coiled axis. Midline contact along the vertical rise of the occiput at inion is established with two hands in the midline. Gentle tension is applied toward or away from the midline in the direction of fluid membrane ease. The thumbs of both hands then contact the greater wings of the sphenoid anteriorly. The inion is a point that has a direct fluid potency relationship to the Sutherland fulcrum, and as such taps the central-most reciprocal tensions in the tidal body. This relationship includes the confluence of sinuses; transverse, occipital, straight, and superior saggital. Additionally, the coiling and uncoiling function of the third ventricle can be appreciated and the shifting fulcrum from lamina terminalis to the Sutherland fulcrum. With this focus to the fluid potency, the occiput and sphenoid are brought into dynamic balance using all available SBS motions, laying down a fulcrum, awaiting the stillpoint and subsequent deep tidal stimulation of the potency. This will often result in a soft potency being unleashed. Modulation of sphenoid fluid membrane tension can be directed toward greater balance through ocular movements.

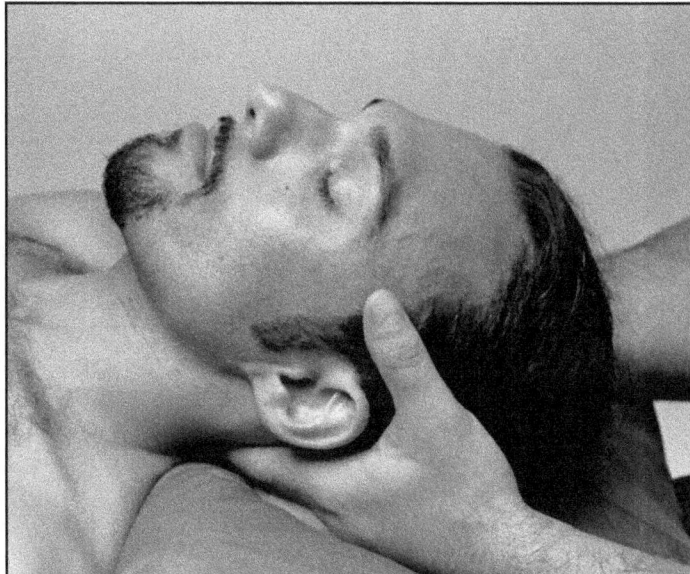

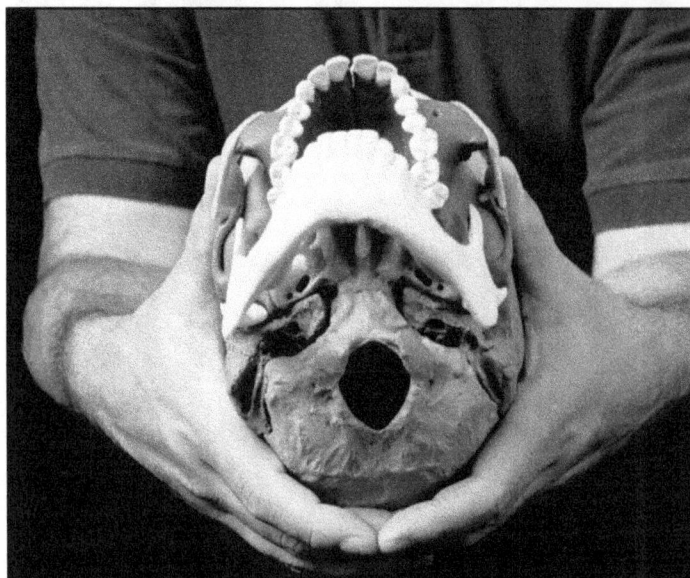

Inion/SBS Treatment

2. Bregma/Frontoparietal: The Sutherland fulcrum projects a fluid potency to the superior-most point of the cranial vertex known as bregma. With the thumbs focused on this point, the two hands spread out and contact the parietal bone just below the parietal boss in much the same manner as we have instructed previously with the parietal lift. Parietal tensions are appreciated and a midline point of balance established by following compressive or distraction forces through the parietal bones, as well as side-bending and rotation forces, in order to harness the fulcrum and unleash the tide.

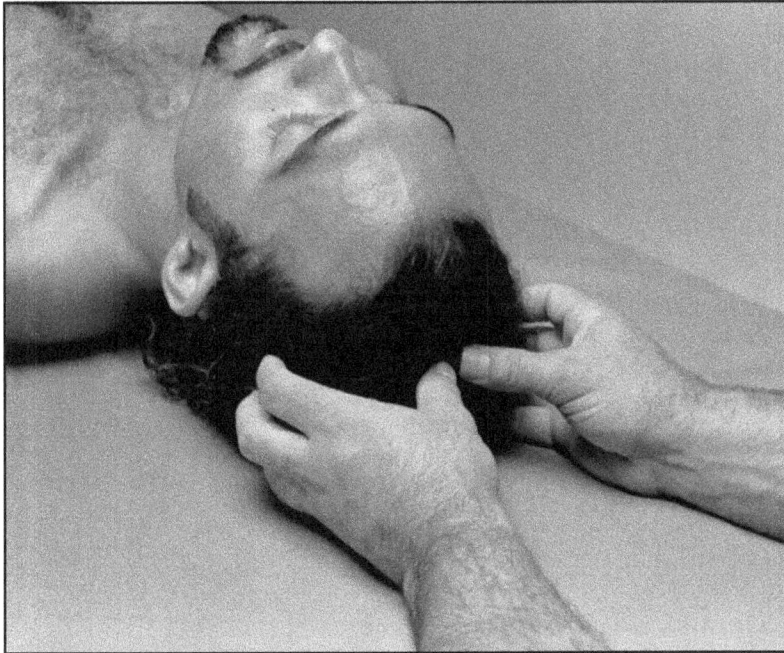

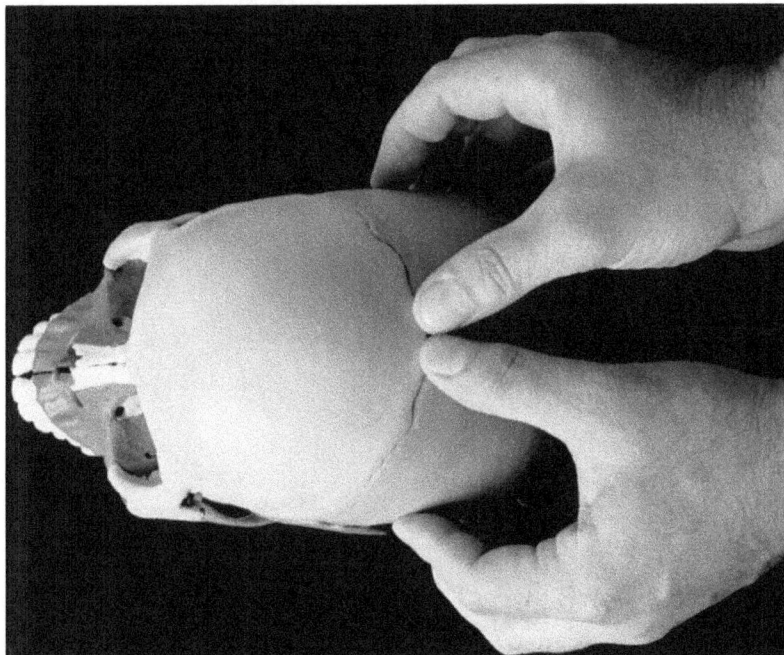

Bregma Treatment

AP Axis Evaluation and Treatment

1. Bregma-Inion Axis: Bregma and inion are connected by the fulcrum established by the inclination of the straight sinus during flexion. Fluid potency can be appreciated between these points of the tidal body as an expansion and contraction of the fluid potencies within. Gentle contact is made using one or two fingers, laying down a fluid fulcrum between these two points. Dynamic stimulation of the fulcrum will ensue with automatic shifting and eventual restoration of biodynamic function along this fulcrum.

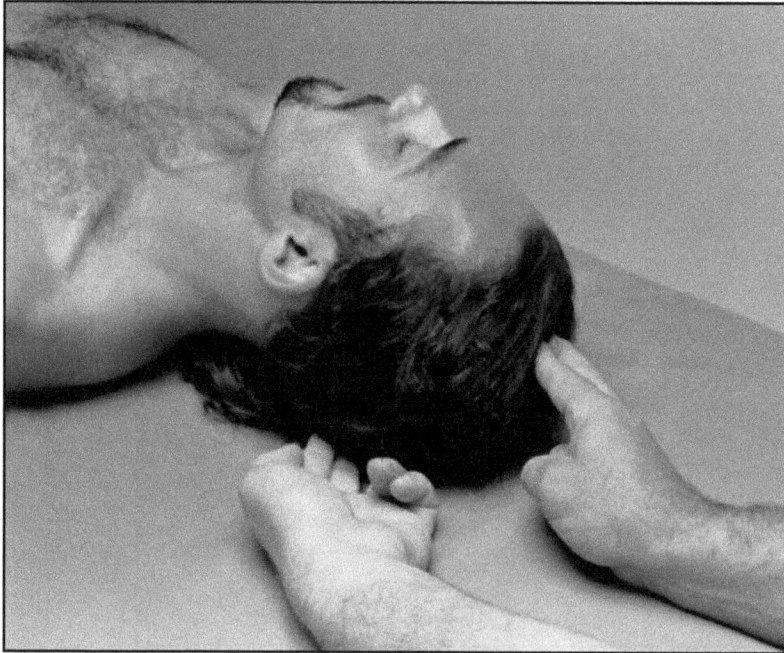

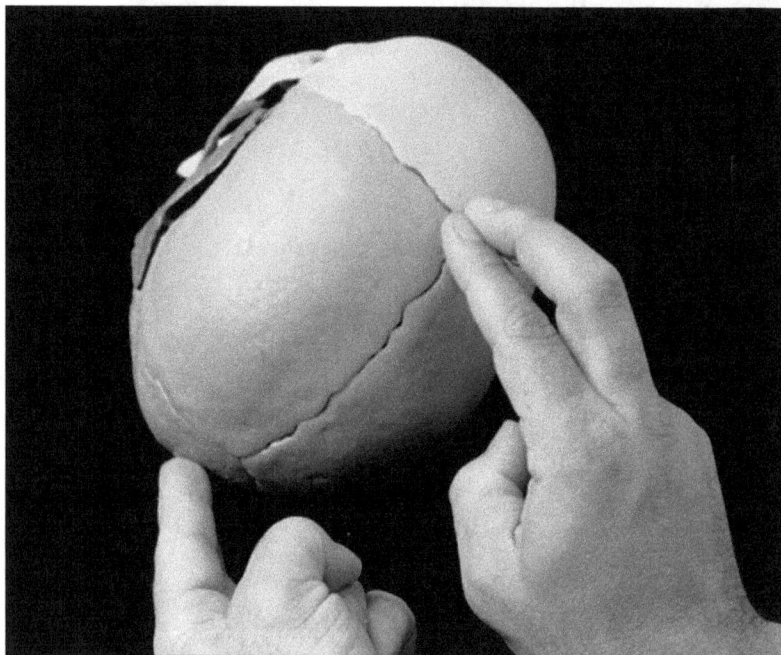

Treatment of the Bregma-Inion Axis

2. Nasion-Inion Axis: Similarly, contact is made with these two points, which transects the cranial base, waiting patiently for a similar response in the active components of this dynamic midline function.

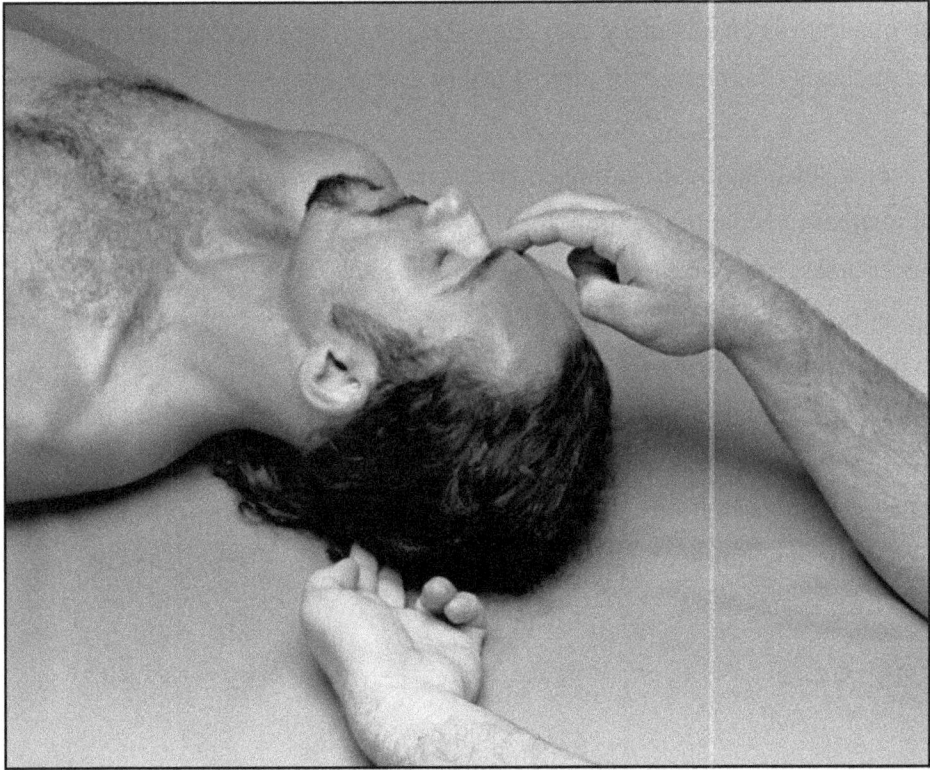

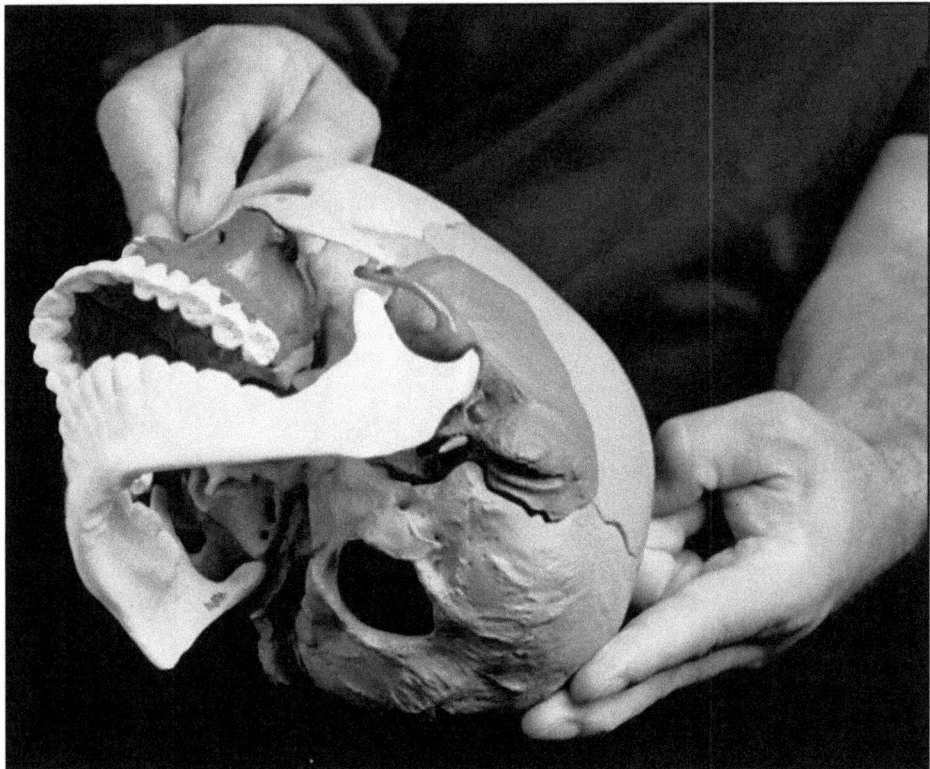

Treatment of the Nasion-Inion Axis

Four Quadrant Diagnosis and Treatment

Diagnosis. Pterion and asterion are the anterior and posterior listening posts for cranial vault diagnosis. Monitoring flexion and extension movements of the CRI and observing for any motion disturbances in each quadrant is an advanced palpation skill. As a screening exam to localize cranial dysfunctions, four quadrant diagnosis is of utmost utility.

Treatment. Once identified, these findings help to assess important changes in CRI mobility to measure treatment response. Most of the time, resolution will occur with the treatment sequence detailed in the previous courses; however, treatment can be focused to the pterion or asterion itself. A fluid wave from the opposite side can be directed into the restriction using a v-spread, but this is often insufficient to overcome the strong forces that frequently accumulate at these conversion points. Using the coronal or lambdoidal sutures, we can introduce forces from both sides into the suture. Treatment can be modified with superior/inferior shear and compression forces in the direction the tissues move most easily. Unwinding may occur, and increasing therapeutic forces can be applied as the release occurs. Gentle separation of tissues between the thumbs can be palpated as the potency arrives.

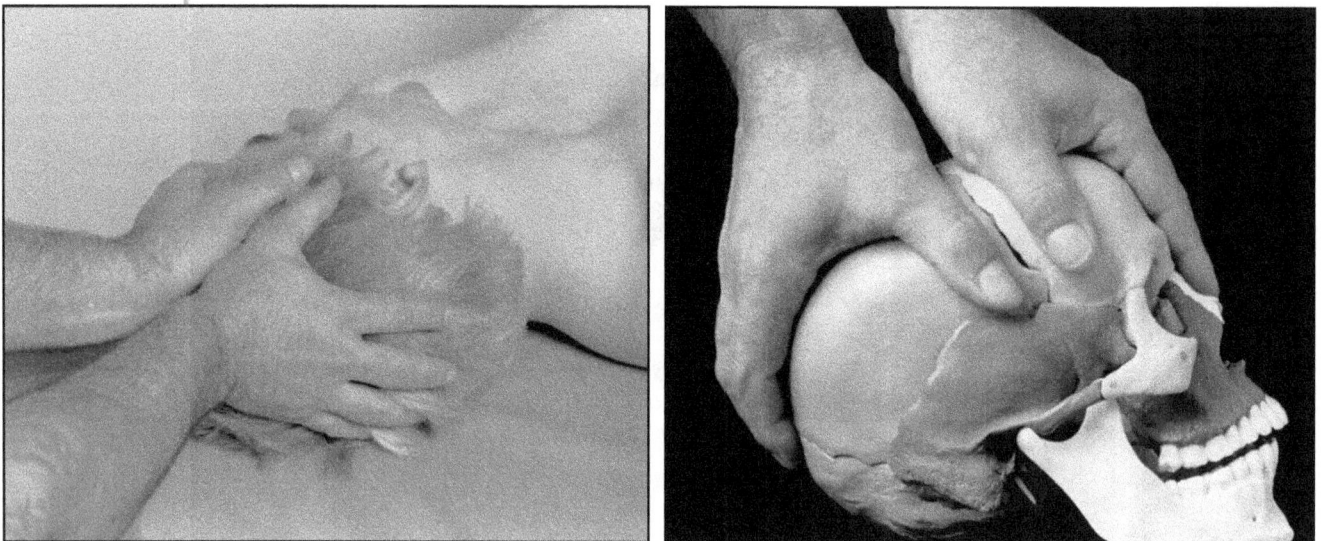

Pterion Treatment

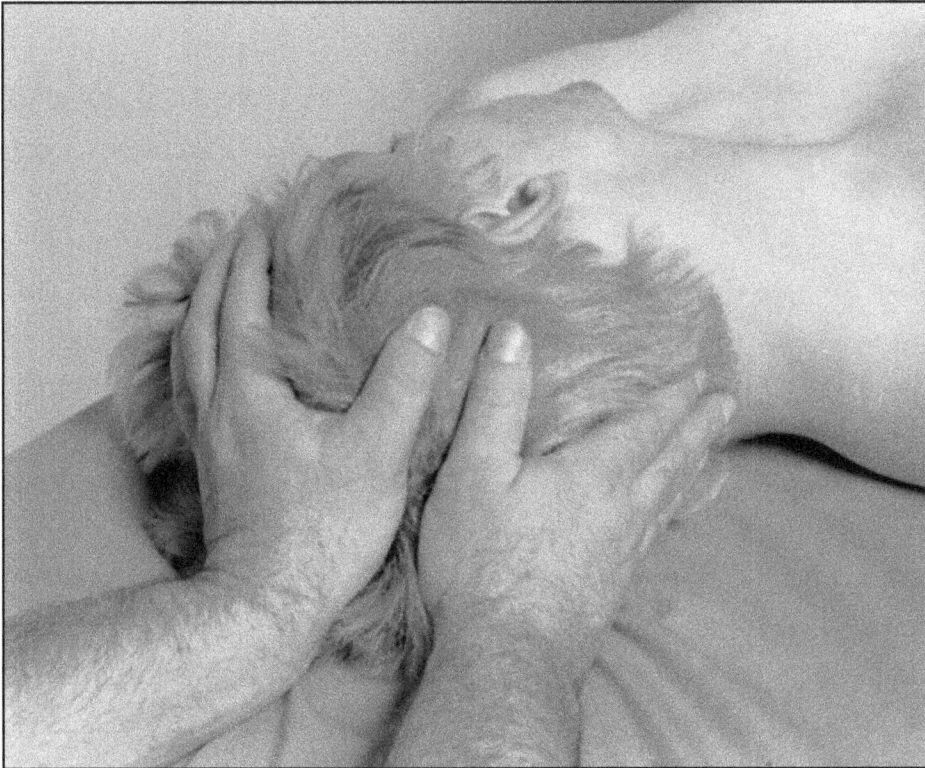

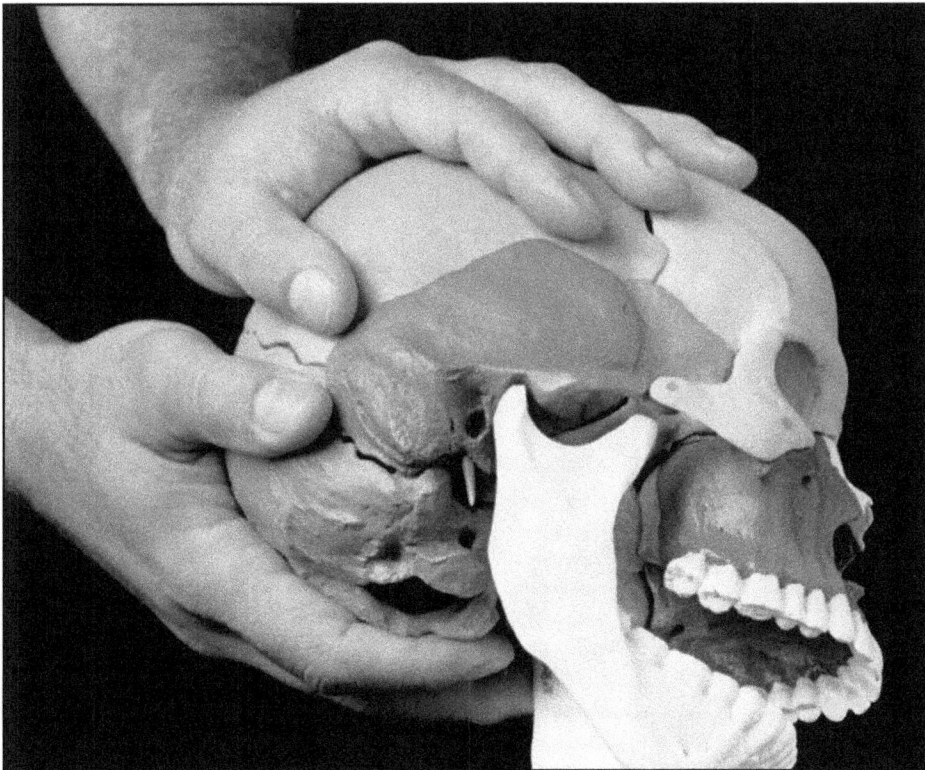

Asterion Treatment

Venous Sinus Dural Technique

Purpose: This technique takes the basic handholds taught in the venous sinus technique and extends their effects into the dural tissues surrounding the venous sinus and deep into the cranial membranous structure.

With the **transverse venous sinus** hold along the superior nuchal line, the examiner should project his sensory awareness through the sinus and into the actual dural tension of both sides of the *tentorium cerebelli.* You must imagine the tent rising into the cranial vault and coming to a point at the Sutherland fulcrum. A normally functioning tent will have equal tension throughout the entire periphery of its attachment to the transverse sinus, as well as rise and fall with the normal flexion and extension phases of the CRI. Any asymmetry in this pulling sensation coming from deep within the cranium or a restriction in the rising and falling action of the tent should alert the examiner to a dural restriction. The examiner is applying an indirect technique by bringing the parts that are loose or normal and bringing them into the tight parts of the membrane, so the examiner takes the occipital contact of the tent and moves into the sensation of where the tightness is coming from. Care should be taken to avoid temporal bone contact which may compress the occipitomastoid suture.This point is held as a point of balanced membranous tension, and a still point should be appreciated, followed by a return of normal symmetry of the rising and falling of the dura. There may be some unwinding as the stillpoint is approached.

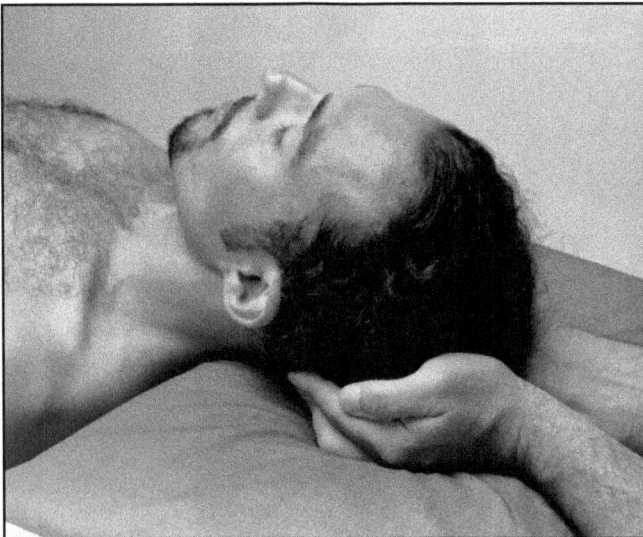

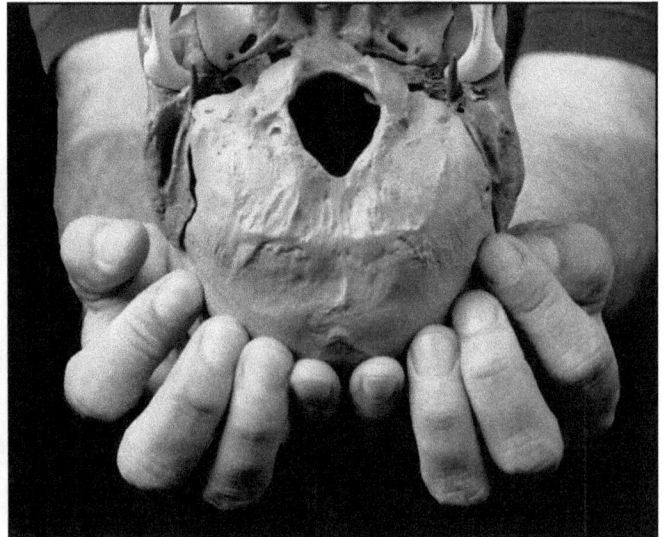

Transverse Venous Sinus Treatment

The **occipital sinus** is approached from it's midline attachment to the transverse venous sinus. The fingers of both hands come together along the vertical midline of the entire occipital sinus. This is a point of entry into the *falx cerebelli* and the posterior cranial fossa. The operators fingers move into areas of tension projecting awareness through the sinus into the falx itself until a release is appreciated and a stillpoint occurs.

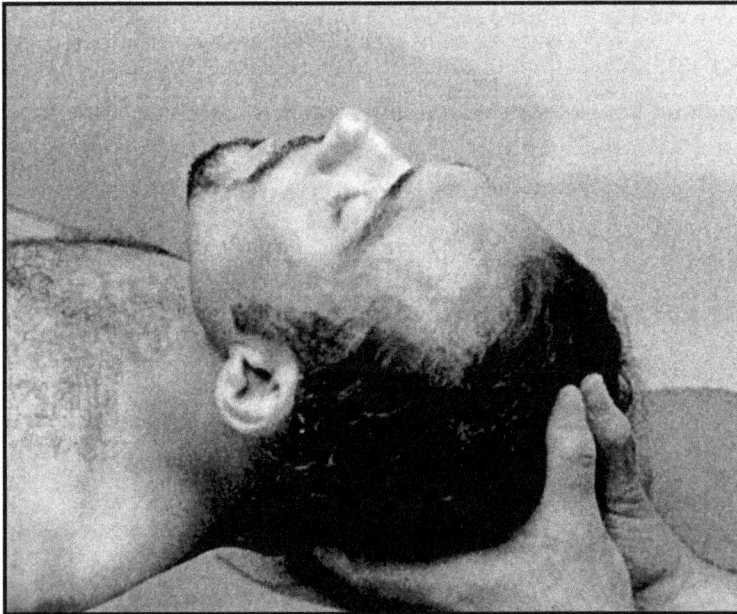

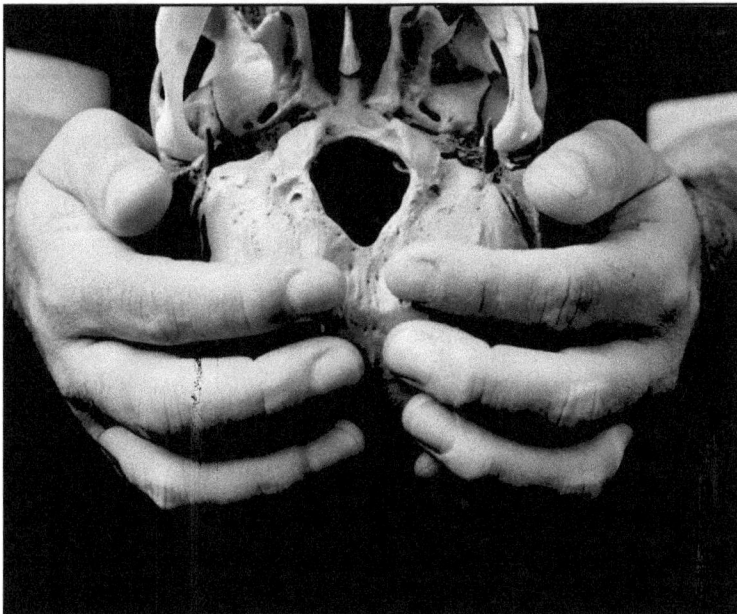

Occipital Sinus Treatment

The **straight sinus** can be approached in a similar fashion. Remember that the straight sinus is oriented diagonally up towards bregma. You want to hold the external occipital protuberance with two fingers and bregma with two thumbs trying to balance the head up on your fingers. The fulcrum of the entire reciprocal tension membrane should be appreciated through the tips of your fingers and thumbs and into the cranium to the *Sutherland fulcrum* creating a fluid fulcrum. Again, the examiner is attempting to find a point of balanced membranous tension by moving from areas of looseness into or towards the area where the tension seems to be the tightest. As the membrane unwinds, the point of balance may shift; be certain to have a good contact on the patient's head as it goes through this unwinding process. Fluid potency will rise and expand between the points of contact.

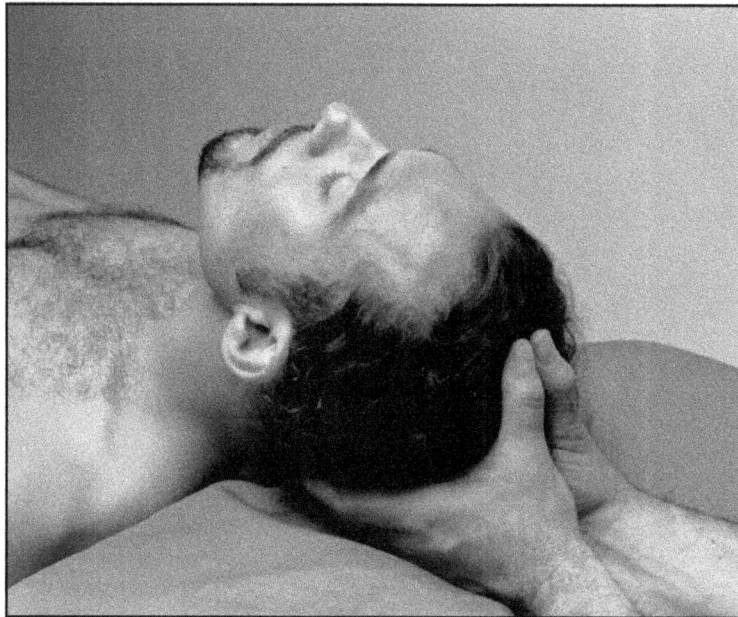

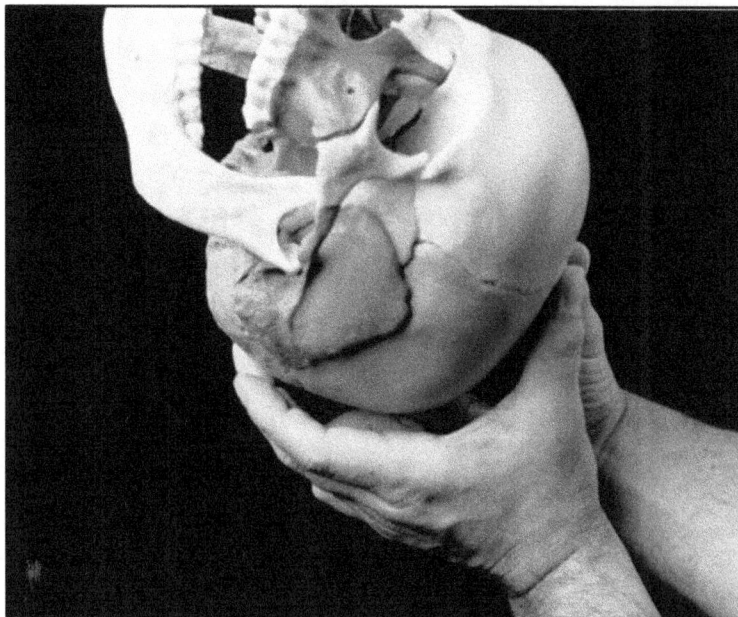

Straight Sinus Treatment

The **superior sagittal sinus** and sagittal suture can be used as an entry point to the *falx cerebri*. Using the same spreading technique with the thumbs that we used in the venous sinus technique, the release can be appreciated deeper into the dural membranous space down to the inferior sagittal sinus. Again, at each point of contact the tensions in the dura may go through an unwinding process and then come to a still point and then resume their normal rising and falling or expanding and contracting motion.

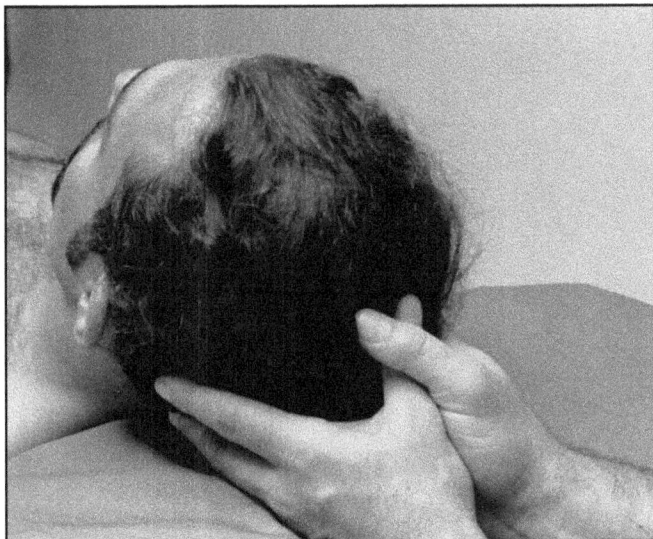

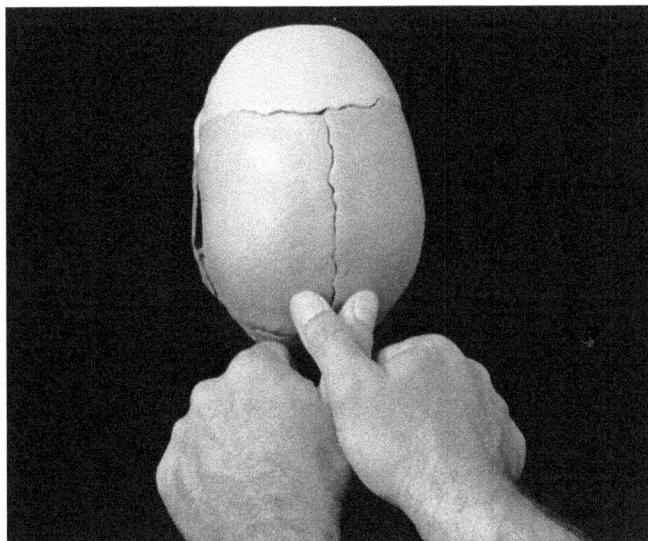

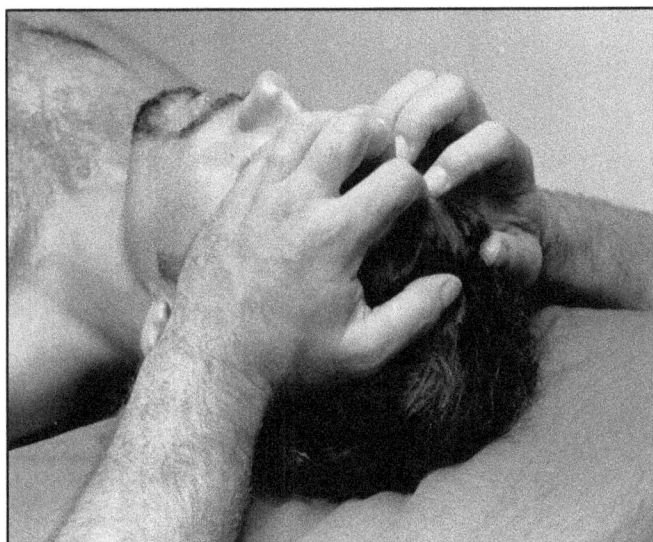

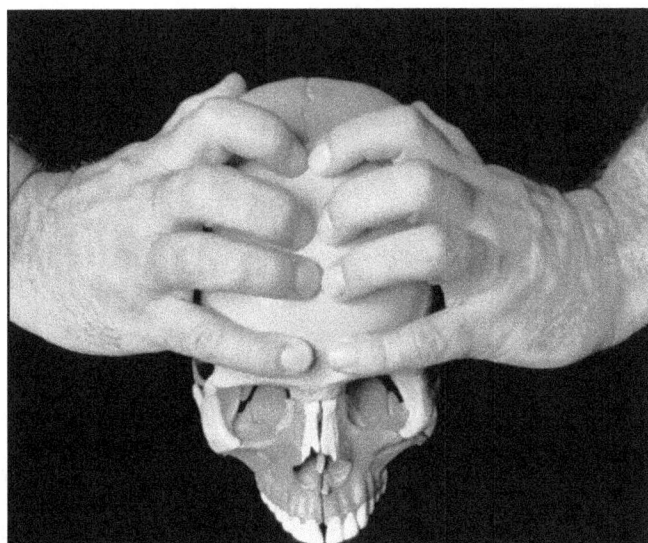

Superior Sagittal Sinus Treatment

Dural Ring Balancing

The **<u>anterior dural girdle</u>** has attachments that connect it to the top of the head along the coronal suture to bregma, down to the greater wings of the sphenoid. Its fluid membranous function is considerable, especially with respect to its functional relations to anterior cranial structures including the sphenoid and temporal bones, orbital elements and associated anterior cranial nerves. The anterior dural girdle can be best contacted with the operator sitting just to the side of the patient's head, their hand shaped as a hoop, overlying the coronal suture in its entirety. The operator's other hand makes contact with various other membranous rings, bringing the relationship between the two contact points into balance around a fulcrum that stimulates tidal potency.

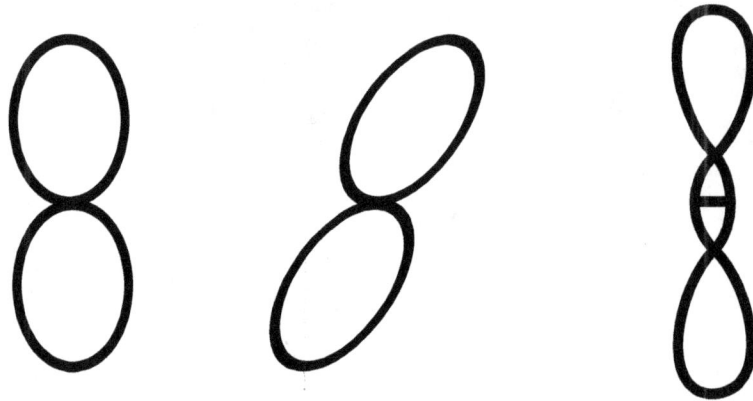

<u>Fig. 25</u>: Depictions of Dural Ring Imbalances

<u>Exercise-</u> Two handed contact with hoop in vault hold focuses operator's attention on this dynamic membranous structure

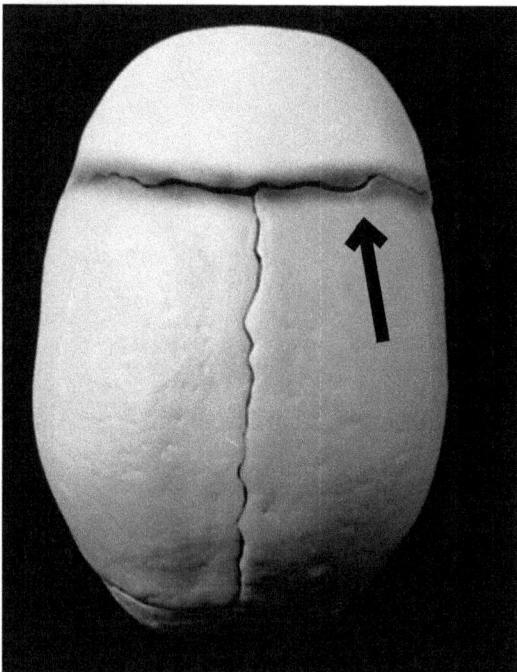

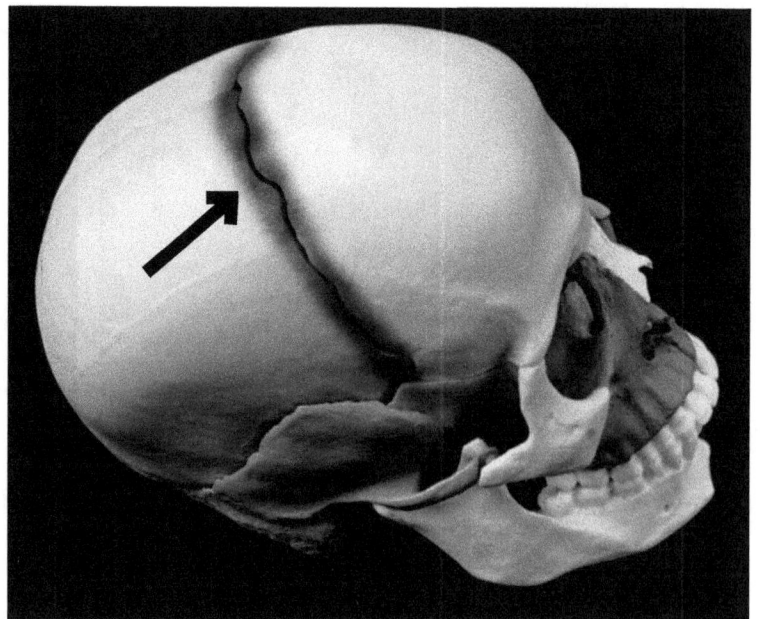

Darkened Regions Indicate Location of Anterior Dural Girdle

1. The first contact is through the **<u>mandibular rami</u>**, a moment should be taken to feel through the bony anatomy into the fluid and membrane matrix. Translatory, rotational, and compressive forces are followed to their point of balanced tension around the gyroscopic fulcrum between the membranous rings of the mandible and anterior dural girdle. The operator's hands should feel connected around an eliptically shaped fluid potency, eventually palpating an expansion as the release occurs.

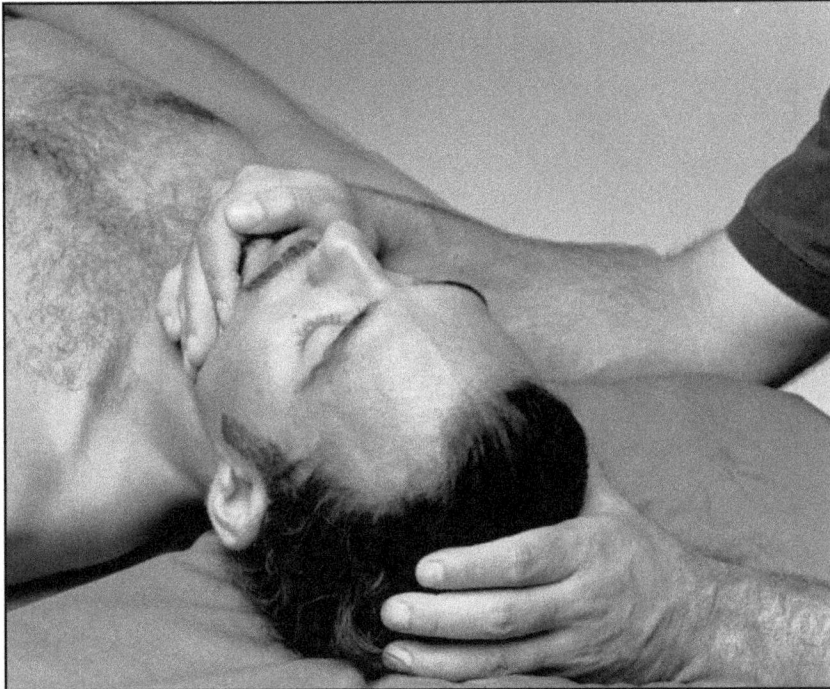

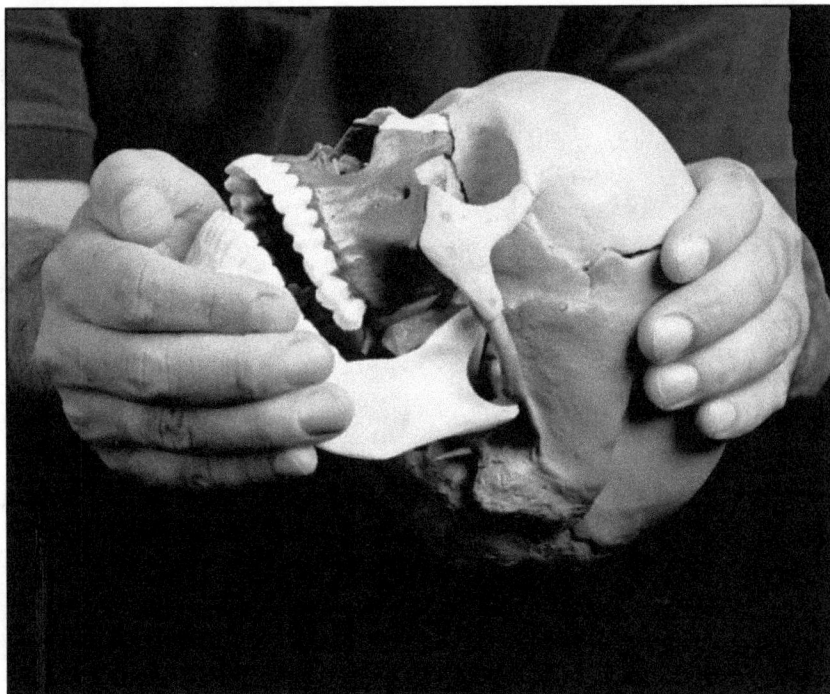

Treatment of Mandibular Rami

2. The **maxillary arches** are appreciated using intraoral contact with bilateral maxillae by performing an intermaxillary spread. The operator stands so that exessive supination of the forearm can be avoided. If the patient's hard palate is too narrow, contact can be made on the inferior aspect of the upper teeth or by single finger pad contact on the cruciate suture. Tensions within the maxillary arches are followed through anterior/posterior and superior/inferior shear, rotation and compression/distraction movements. Reciprocal tensions between these dural rings are appreciated and balanced through a dynamic fulcrum, which again stimulates tidal potency. Upon release, external rotation of maxilla bones will accompany expansion between hoops.

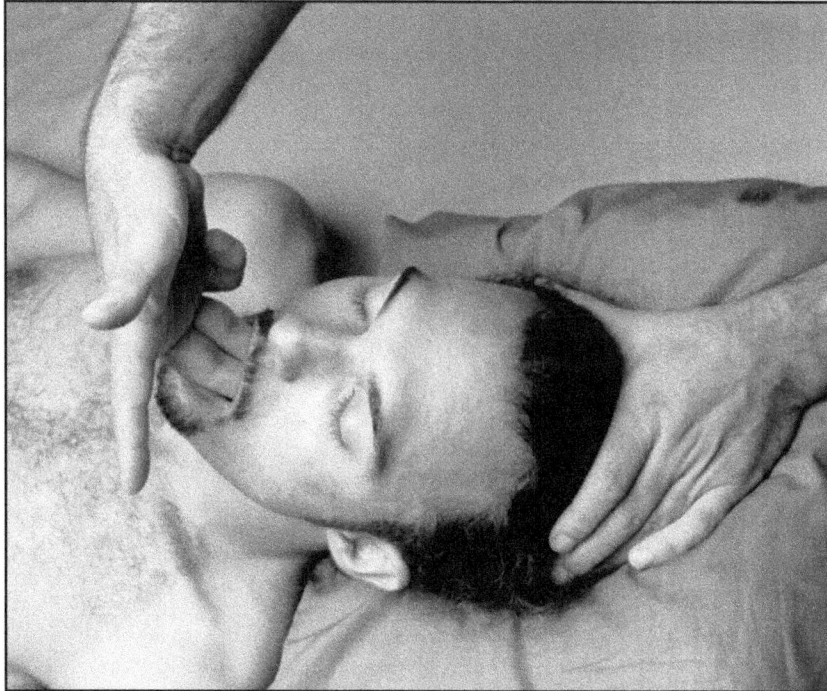

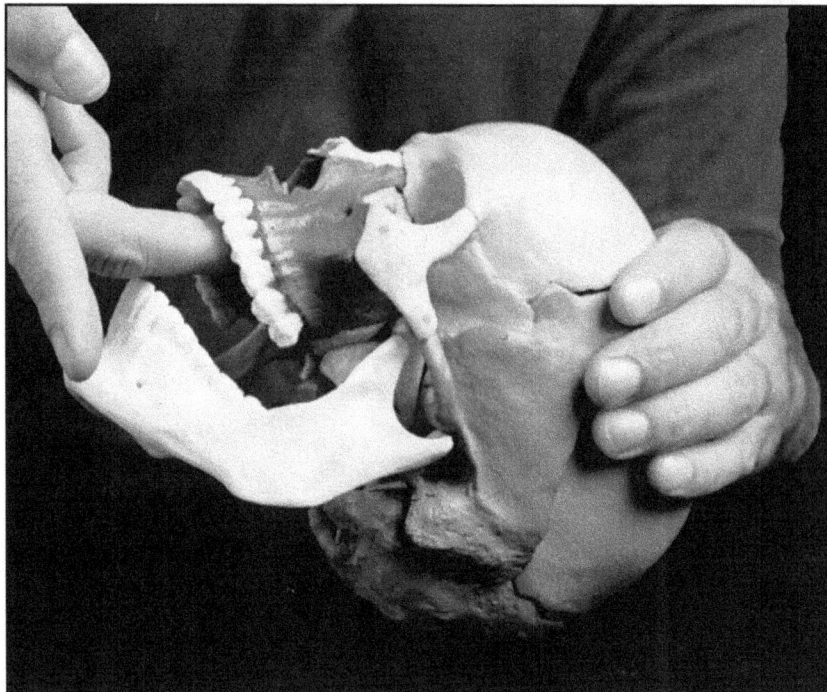

Treatment of Maxillary Arches

3. Tentorium Cerebelli: The operator's second hand forms a hoop-like structure around the posterior aspect of the cranial vault overlying the transverse sinus and inion. Care should be taken to avoid compression of the occipitomastoid suture. Reciprocal tensions are assessed in multiple planes of motion, introducing dynamic balance so that the fulcrum can be harnessed and the tidal potency unleashed.

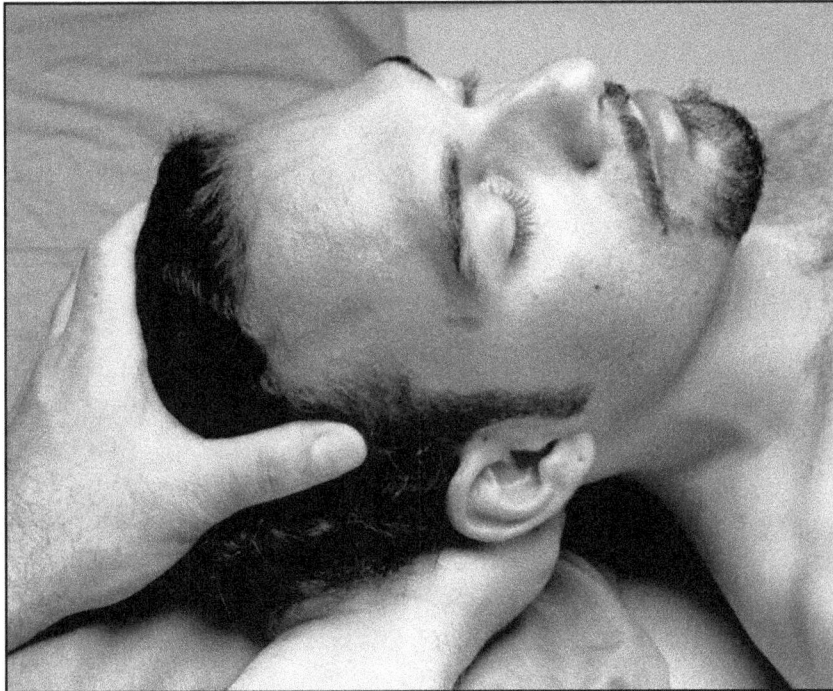

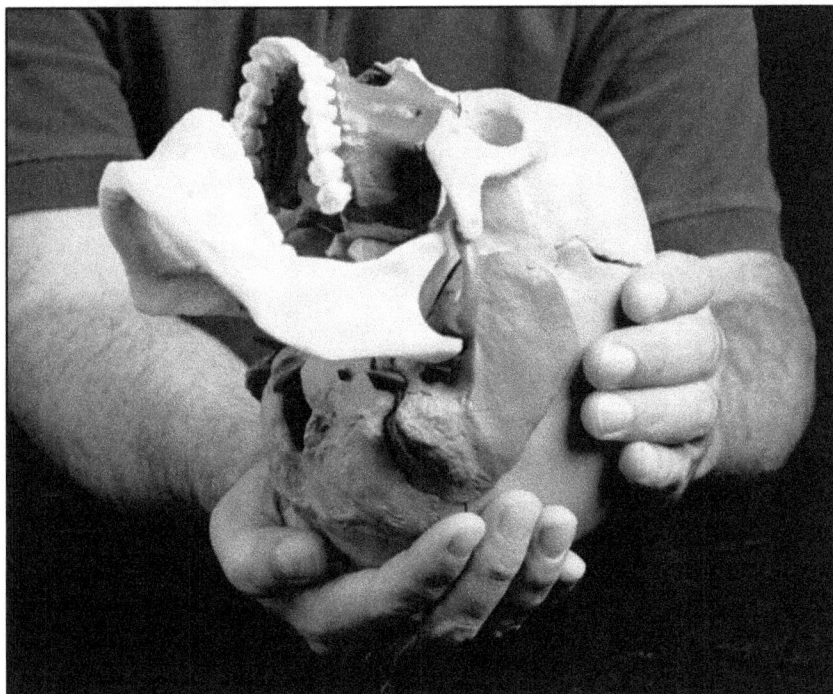

Treatment of Tentorium Cerebelli

4. Sphenoid: The operator's hand comes to rest bilaterally over the greater wings of the sphenoid, with dynamic tension being perceived between the sphenoid and the anterior dural girdle until a dynamic fulcrum can be appreciated, and again tidal potency restored. Ocular and SBS movements can be used to modulate releasing response (lateral and vertical strains, sidebending, torsion and compression/distraction).

Alternate treatment: With both hands together over bregma and both index fingers over greater wings, a fluid wave can be sent from bregma into the body of the sphenoid. Wait for lateral fluctuations of the CRI to be felt in index fingers. This technique is helpful for treating intraosseous sphenoid problems. (See page 165, Bregma/Frontoparietal technique, for similar hand positioning)

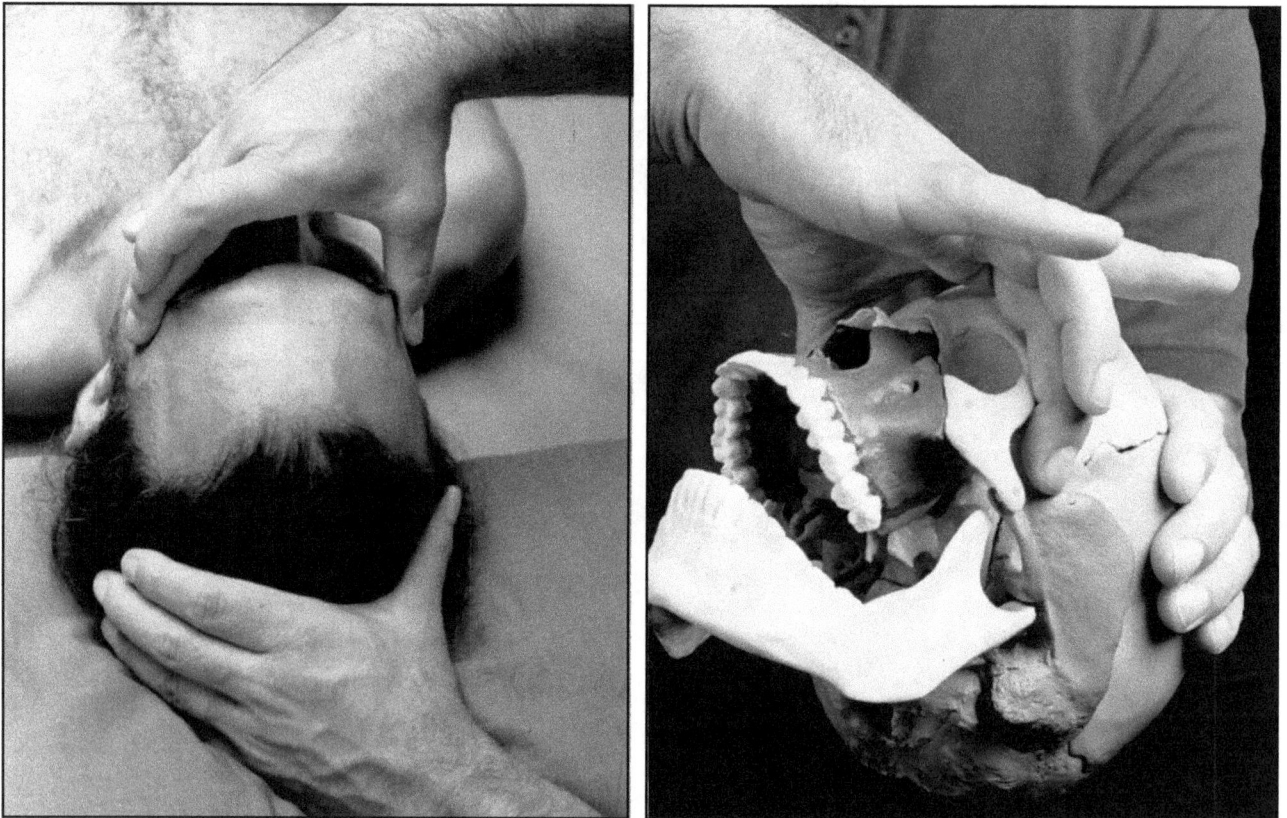

Treatment of the Sphenoid

Two-Operator Technique

1. Dural Tube Release: This can be accomplished with profound results using very basic approaches already discussed in this course. One operator sits at the head of the supine patient using a midline occipital hold balancing inion and the SBS, while the other operator sits at the side of the patient, contacting the sacrococcygeal area and lumbosacral spine as instructed previously. Both operators assess the dural tube tension and mobility, and follow the reciprocal tensions simultaneously to a point of balance about a fulcrum, awaiting the stimulation of the tidal potency.

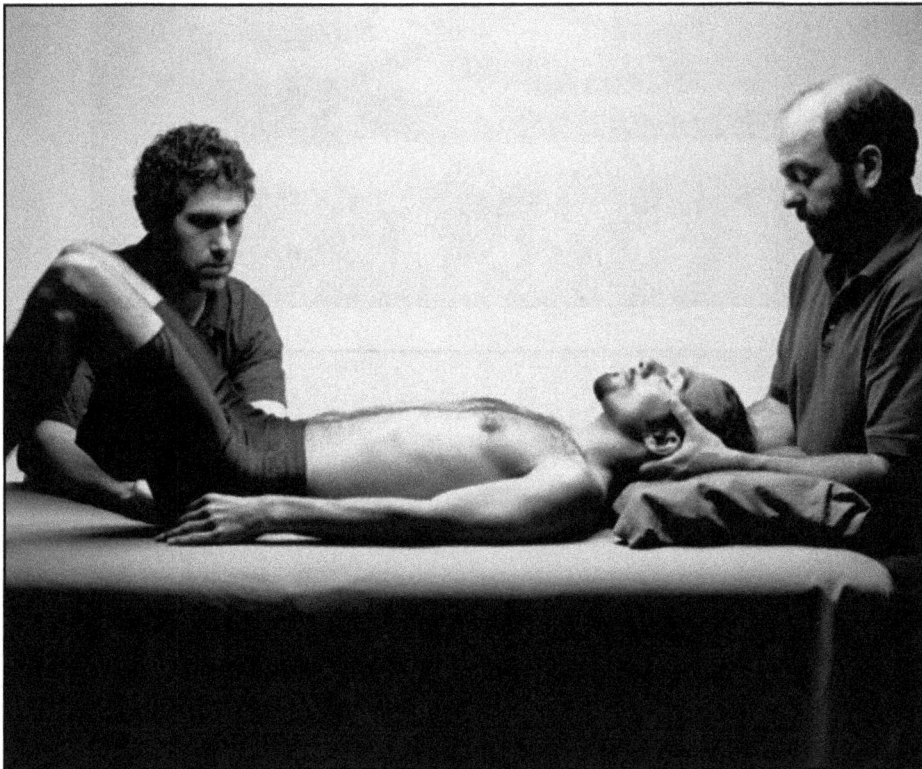

Dural Tube Release

2. Occipital-Sternal-Sacral Release: The two operators maintain one-hand contact on either end of the dural tube, while the other hand contacts the sternum. Both operators simultaneously assess for synchronized movements between their two hands, exaggerating the directions that move more easily until a balanced midline excursion and intensity is palpated.

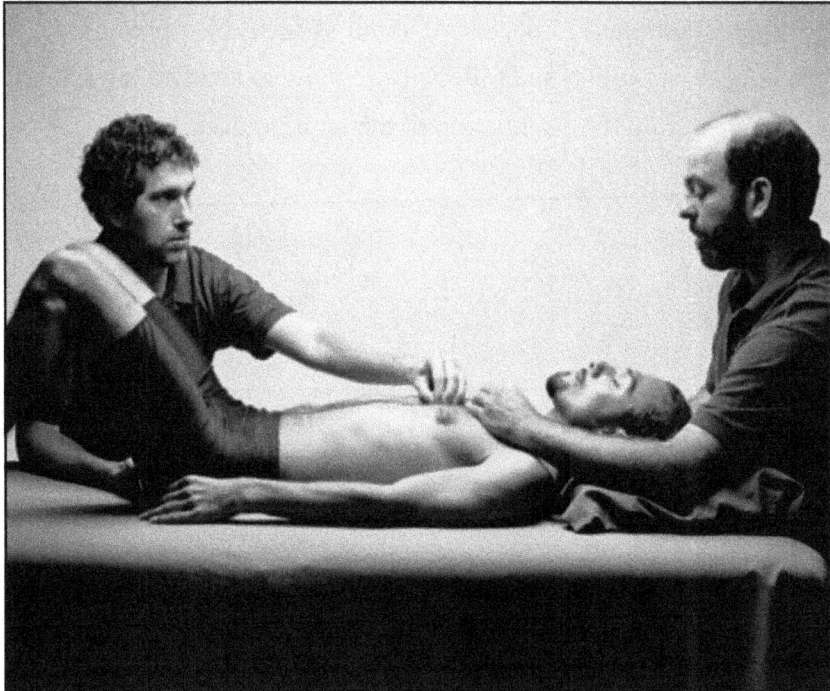

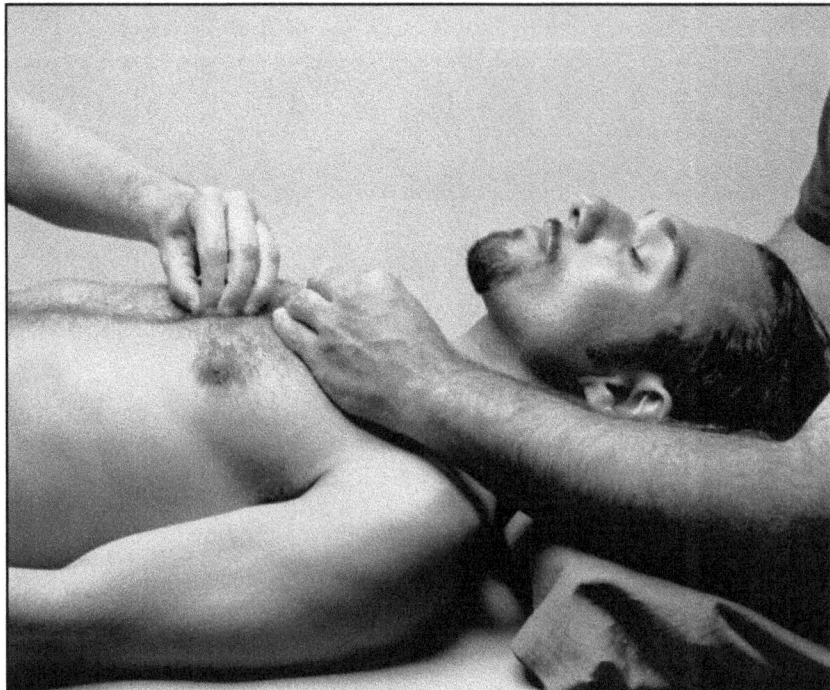

Occipital-Sternal-Sacral Release

Level III Course Schedule- Day 1

8:00 am	(*0900*)	Course Objectives
8:30 am	(*0930*)	*Table Session-* Facial Bone Review and Update
9:45 am	(*1045*)	Break
10:00 am	(*1100*)	*Table Session-* Facial Bone Review and Update, continued
11:15 am	(*1215*)	Diaphragm / Costal Cage Review
11:45 am	(*1245*)	Lunch
1:00 pm	(*1400*)	Cranialfascial Screening Exam Review
2:00 pm	(*1500*)	Fluid Matrix and Midline Function

- Embryology
- Tidal Body and CNS behavior
- The biomechanical versus biodynamic approach

2:45 pm	(*1545*)	Break
3:00 pm	(*1600*)	Fluid Matrix and the Breath of Life

- Paradoxical motion

4:00 pm	(*1700*)	*Table Session-* Functional Midline

Unleashing longitudinal tidal function
- Occipital approach
- Temporal bone approach

5:00 pm	(*1800*)	Adjourn

Level III Course Schedule- Day 2

8:00 am   (*0900*)   Participant Responses

8:30 am   (*0930*)   Laying Down the Fulcrum
- Tidal Potency and respiratory function
- *Table Session-* Fulcrums: Finding the area of primary restriction using the cranial rhythmic impulse

9:15 am   (*1015*)   Structural versus Functional Midline
- Longitudinal fulcrums and pendular function
- Intraosseous motion and membranous function

9:45 am   (*1045*)   Break

10:00 am   (*1100*)   *Table Session-* Sacral Evaluation and Treatment
- Sacral apex
- Intraosseous sacral dysfunction
- Thoracolumbar junction
- Sacrosternal axis

11:45 am   (*1245*)   Lunch

1:00 pm   (*1400*)   *Table Session (Continued)-* Sacral Evaluation and Treatment

2:00 pm   (*1500*)   *Table Session-* Occipital Evaluation and Treatment
- Occipitocervical/thoracic junctions
- Occipitoatlantal junction
- Occipitosternal axis

2:45 pm   (*1545*)   Break

3:00 pm   (*1600*)   *Table Session-* Cranial Vault Evaluation and Treatment
- Inion/SBS
- Bregma/Frontoparietals

4:00 pm   (*1700*)   *Table Session-* AP Axis
- Bregma-Inion
- Nasion-Inion

5:00 pm   (*1800*)   Adjourn

Level III Course Schedule- Day 3

8:00 am	(*0900*)	Questions and Answers
9:00 am	(*1000*)	*Table Session*- Four Quadrant Diagnosis and Treatment
9:45 am	(*1045*)	Break
10:00 am	(*1100*)	*Table Session (continued)*- Four Quadrant Diagnosis and Treatment
10:30 am	(*1130*)	*Table Session*- Venous Sinus Dural Release
11:45 am	(*1245*)	Lunch

1:00 pm   (*1400*)   *Table Session*- Dural Ring Balancing
Anterior dural girdle relations
- Mandibular rami
- Maxillary arches
- Tentorium cerebelli
- Sphenoid

2:45 pm   (*1545*)   Break

3:00 pm   (*1600*)   *Table Session*- Palpatory Exercises
Two-operator techniques
- Dural tube release
- Occipitosternal-Sacral release

5:00 pm   (*1800*)   Adjourn

Notes:

SFIMMS SERIES IN NEUROMUSCULOSKELETAL MEDICINE

OSTEOPATHIC MANIPULATIVE MEDICINE APPROACHES TO THE PRIMARY RESPIRATORY MECHANISM

Level IV
Osteopathic Approach to Infants and Children

OMM Approaches to the Primary Respiratory Mechanism

Level IV
Course Objectives

Introduce concepts of osteopathic embryology and embryonic intelligence.

Introduce concepts and treatment approaches for fetal and infant stimulation.

Demonstrate and practice maternal treatment approaches before and after delivery.

Introduce the osteopathic view of birth mechanics and functional anatomy of the infant.

Review and demonstrate principles of newborn examination and treatment.

Introduce the osteopathic approach to perinatal health promotion with emphasis on brain function and Neurologic organization.

Introduce treatment approaches for overlapping sutures with articular and membranous approaches.

Introduce assessment and treatment approaches for movement re-patterning.

Introduce the osteopathic view of pediatric health and illness with selected health topics including introducing the idea of osteopathic pediatric ecology.

Participate in pediatric clinical case evaluation and treatment clinics.

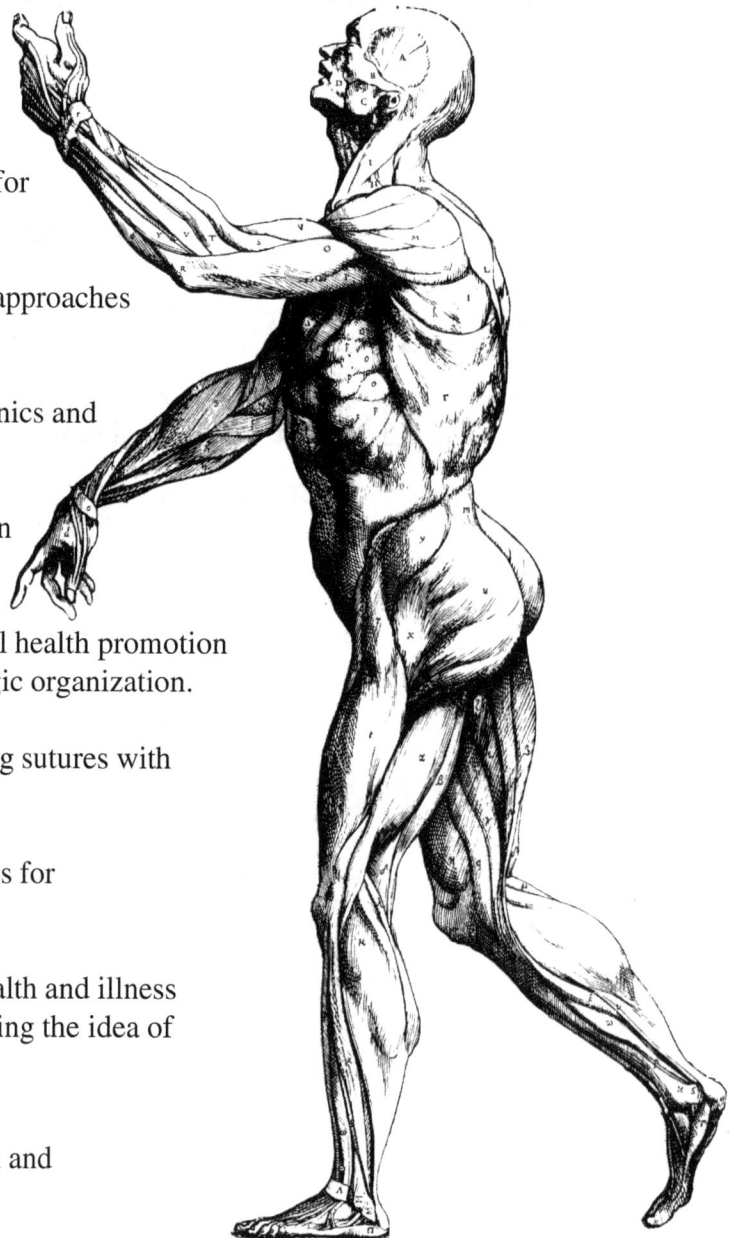

Embryonic Intelligence:
It's Design and Function

What is intelligence?

Intelligence is the fundamental (perceptual) force of life with a self-generating, self-sustaining motile function, originating from conception. Its expression is given form through the electromagnetic fluid membrane matrix of the embryo before any development of the central nervous system. Such intelligence has awareness as it fluctuates between motile phases of fluid expansion and contraction. This awareness is driven by the ebb and flow of its own motile function and midline potency. Midline potency functions as a "fluid drive," giving direction and serving as a reference point for the animating forces of life. Axes of motion are all oriented around this midline potency, which acts as a fulcrum for all subsequent growth and development. The midline fluid matrix contains the blueprint for intelligence to function physiologically for a lifetime.

Intelligence functions optimally when experiencing a full and free movement between its polar opposites (ebb and flow); between sleeping and waking, inhalation and exhalation, introversion and extroversion, giving and receiving, creation and destruction, fullness and emptiness ... Fixation of movement limits self awareness and self expression and is often the result of unresolved (traumatic) forces within the fluid membrane matrix. Even neurosensory experiences within the womb may transmit psychic conflicts into the electromagnetic field of intelligent awareness.

Intelligent awareness of this type is sensitive in particular to maternal influences, both within and outside of the womb. Mobile relations, chemical and nutritional factors, as well as sensory stimulation, are all contributing to the development and evolution of embryonic intelligence and fetal development. Maternal host factors are inextricably linked to this process and exert significant influences on intelligence. Even certain emotional factors such as the mother's attitude at the moment of conception her relationship to her mother and to the child's father have a profound impact on embryonic intelligence, its self awareness, self expression and, ultimately, its development and evolution.

Embryonic intelligence is active and evolving through fetal, infant, childhood, adolescence and adult stages of development. Within this intelligence is the blueprint or matrix of life that enables healthy vital function. Therefore, after birth, intelligence continues to act as a mobile perceptual function through self awareness, self expression and evolution. This intelligence seeks to know itself through meaningful interactions with the outside world in order to develop greater self awareness, greater self expression and, ultimately, contribute to its own evolution. While fixation on the self leads to narcissism, movement of perceptual function between the self and the outer world leads to creative and cooperative endeavors which most reflect intelligent purpose. We cannot know the intelligent design of ourselves without coming into direct contact with that intelligence in others.

Clinical Implications of Embryonic Intelligence

When we treat patients the intention behind our treatment is always perceived by the patient and will always direct the outcome of the treatment. We can focus on many things when we treat patients. Often we think of ourselves as the mechanic or the plumber trying to realign the parts or release their blockages. We can be quite active or quite passive. We can observe and, of course, we can manipulate. What we are trying to get at here is something quite different, however, and has to do with contacting embryonic intelligence within ourselves as well as within our patients. To do this we must go beyond being therapeutic agents. Beyond being observers. And beyond being anything separate at all. We must actually disintegrate ourselves, becoming nothing but a fulcrum of pure midline function, intelligent potency around which the patient's intelligent potency can reorganize and revitalize itself. This also requires that we understand the embryonic relations that connect us in a fluid membrane matrix and make us all one intelligent potency.

Beginners acquire new theories and techniques until their minds are cluttered with options. Advanced students forget their many options. They allow the theories and techniques that they have learned to recede into the background.

Learn to unclutter your mind. Learn to simplify your work.

As you rely less and less on knowing just what to do, your work will become more direct and more powerful. You will discover that the quality of your consciousness is more potent than any technique or theory or interpretation.

Learn how fruitful the blocked patient suddenly becomes when you give up trying to do just the right thing.

adapted from Lao Tzu's Tao Te Ching

In osteopathic medicine this intelligent potency is called the "tidal body". The "tidal body" is a pregenetic, embryonic body that persists throughout life in an electromagnetic ebb and flow of fluid membrane potency. It is considered pure potency untainted by the events of life or by time. It is pure health or vitality which cannot become ill. By contacting this "tidal body" we stimulate the intelligent life-force that we all share and witness its expression and evolution. Every human being has their own intelligent design and purpose that they are here to become aware of, express and evolve. Our job in treating the patient is to facilitate the patient's intelligent potency in coming into a state of self awareness in order to realize and express that design and purpose.

"The art of healing is to bring the soul into contact with the body and bring alive the purpose for which that soul is living."

Robert C. Fulford, D.O.

Maternal and Fetal Relationships

Though the developing fetus is protected from the outside world by its fluid-filled, maternal container, the container itself becomes the fetus' outside world. Relationships between the fetus and the mother have structural and functional components that greatly influence its growth and development. The position of the fetus in an anterior, posterior, breach, or transverse lie, as well as the changing maternal posture, reflects potential structural tensions between the mother and fetus. Associated movements of both fetal and maternal structures create the opportunity for strain and dysfunction during the prenatal period. Assessment of the relative structural relationship between mother and fetus may indicate osteopathic treatment to enhance mobility and its associated fluid and membranous function.

Neurochemical continuity between the mother and fetus are greatly influenced by nutritional intake, neurosensory activity and certain emotional states. Since the fetus shares the same blood supply as the mother, many chemical compounds pass from the mother to the fetus. This means in a state of high anxiety the mother's adrenalin response is shared by the developing fetus. Conversely, the endorphin responses of loving and pleasurable experiences are also shared by the fetus. Neurosensory stimulation of both the mother and growing fetus are helpful in stimulating optimal growth and development through better chemistry. Sensory fetal stimulation may include visual patterns of lightness and darkness, speech patterns, musical sounds and vibrations, tactile kinesthetic experiences, as well as vestibular stimulation from respiratory, circulatory and maternal rocking and swaying movements. Fetal stimulation is a combination of all the above sensory experiences and has been shown to positively influence fetal growth as well as maternal fetal bonding.

Osteopathic Manipulative Treatment
of the Pregnant Mother

Osteopathic manipulative treatment of the pregnant mother focuses on the vitality of her primary and secondary respiratory mechanisms which, of course, are supporting the fluid functions of both the mother and fetus. Both the Cranial Rhythmic Impulse and diaphragm functions are assessed and treated osteopathically.

Fetal Release

The relation of the fetus to the maternal pelvis interfaces with the uterus and its attachments, (i.e. uterosacral ligaments) as well as affecting the thoracolumbar spine via the anterior weight shift.

With the mother's on all fours, the operator can approach the abdomen from the side with both hands supporting the structures within. Gentle compression is applied and torsional forces followed and held in the directions of ease to release tensions within the abdomen and between the mother and fetus. Unwinding may occur and fluid potency stimulated. Caution should be exercised in cases of observed vaginal bleeding or placenta previa.

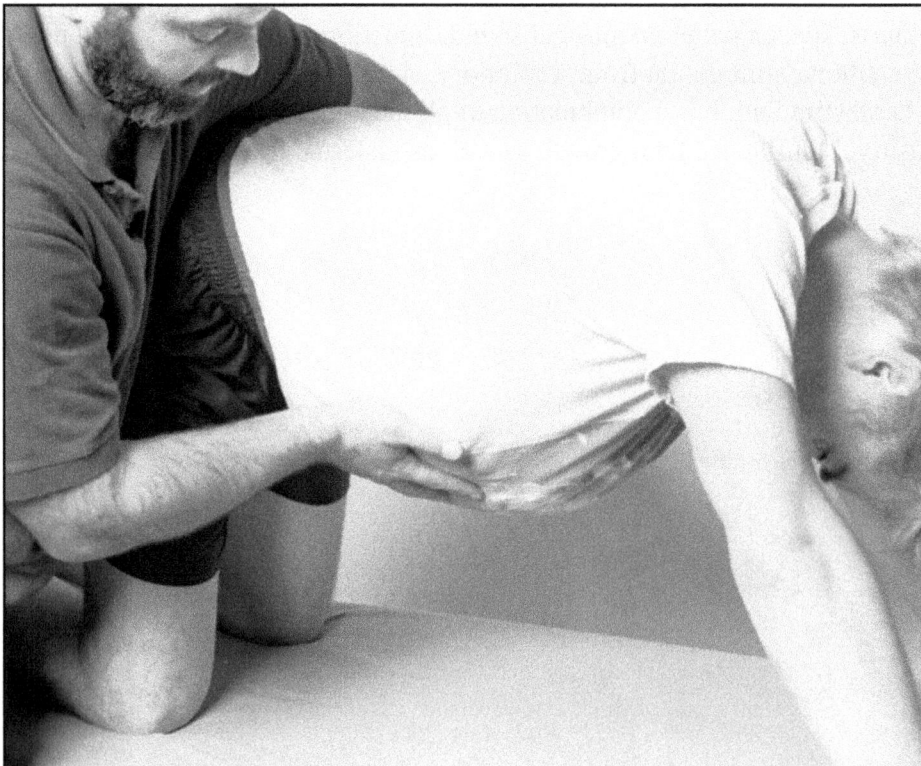

Fetal Release

Thoracolumbar/Lumbosacral Junction Release

With mother in the left side-lying position the operator sits behind with one hand contacting the thoracolumbar junction and the other over the sacrum. Directions of ease between the two hands are introduced (compression/distraction, rotation, translation, inhalation/exhalation) and tissue responses monitored to decrease tissue tension and bring about greater functional balance.

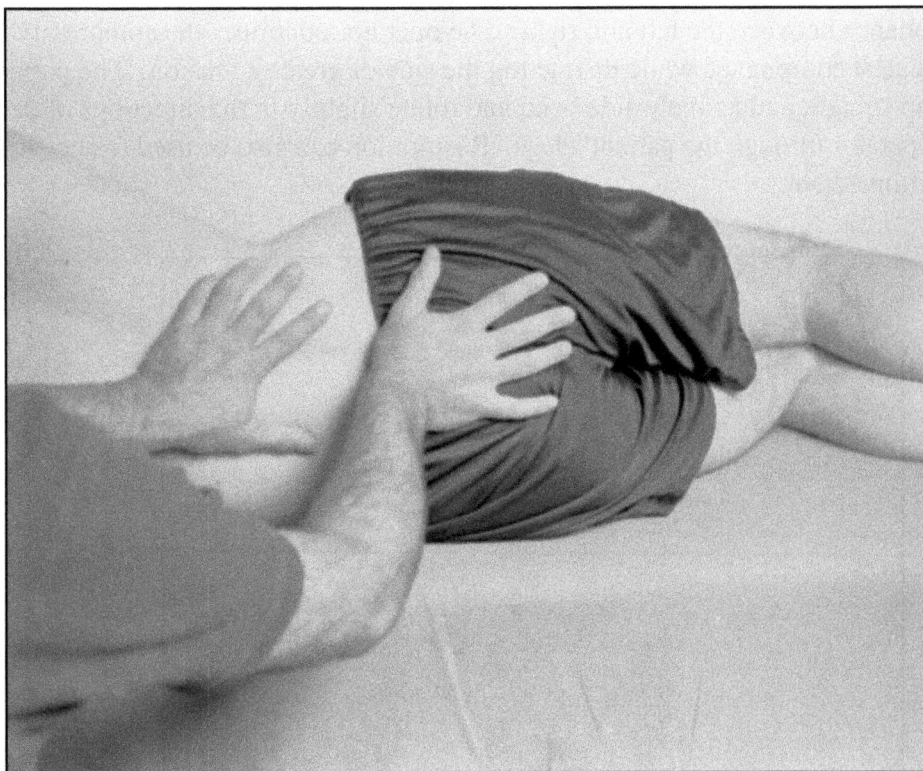

Thoracolumbar/Lumbosacral Junction Release

Seated Hip Release

The relationship between hips and lumbar spine is a central concern due to the increasing lumbar lordosis in the later months of pregnancy and the associated increase in thoracolumbar tension. Weight bearing mechanics can be assessed and directions of ease applied to help restore functional relations between these important structures.

With the patient seated, the operator sits in front of the patient with hands on the patient's knees. A gentle compressive force is applied directly into the acetabulum through the patient's legs comparing the relative compliance between the left and right. The operator continues the compressive force into the hip of greatest compliance while distracting the side of greatest tension. The patient is then instructed to sit up straight and actively side bend and rotate slightly in the directions of ease as palpated by the operator through the patient's legs. Respiration can also be used to accentuate the release, which is immediate.

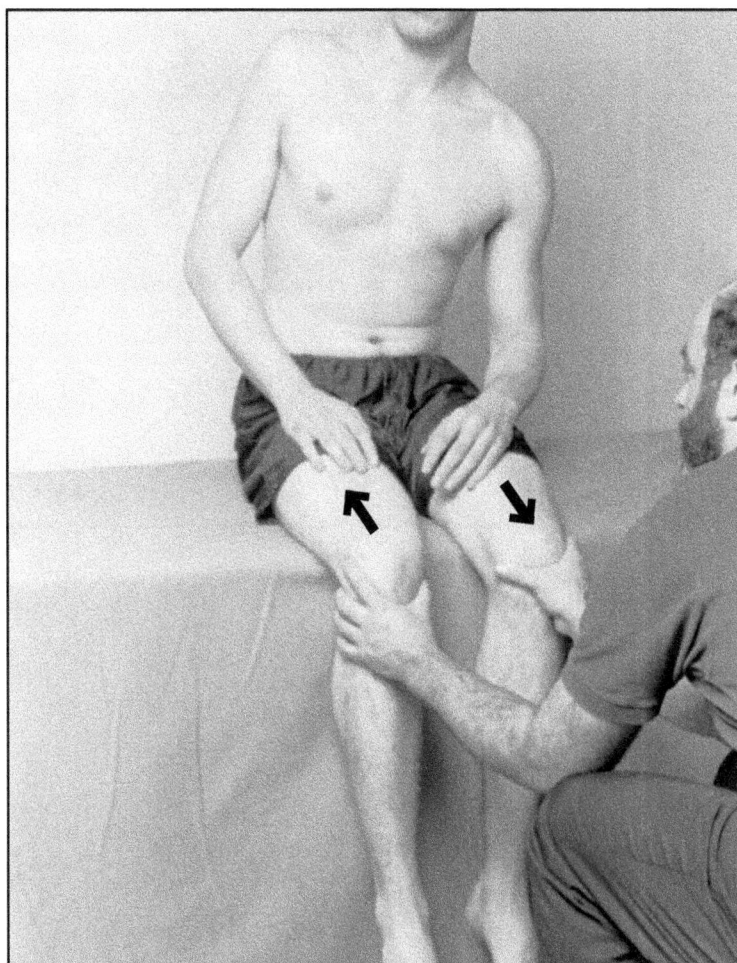

Seated Hip Release

Osteopathic Manipulative Treatment
of the Postpartum Mother

Osteopathic manipulative treatment of the postpartum mother should also focus on the vitality of the primary and secondary respiratory mechanisms of the Cranial Rhythmic Impulse and diaphragm. An area of central concern is the sacrum as it is often traumatized by a long labor or a posterior head presentation (back labor). Often this will carry the sacrum into an excessively anterior position due to the pressure of the baby's head on the sacral base. This condition may be related to the position of the patient held in stirrups in the lithotomy position. Traction applied by forceps to the head of the infant during delivery, without adequately following the natural curve of the pelvis which has an anterior concavity, can strain the base of the maternal sacrum anteriorly and inferiorly while the ilia are maintained in a posterior position by the fixed flexion of the hips in the stirrups. Treatment can be accomplished positioning the sacrum against the barrier in a relatively posterior position while using the Cranial Rhythmic Impulse and respiratory mechanisms to assist in moving the sacrum further into its normal position, more posteriorly.

The patient is seated with legs over the side of the table. The operator is seated in front of the patient. The operator introduces hand contact on the anterior ilium, introducing movement in a posterior, inferior and medial direction, bringing the sacral base posterior. The patient flexes slightly and rests her forearms on the operator's shoulders while fully exhaling. As the patient follows with an inhalation, the operator follows the sacral base posteriorly and holds it during the next exhalation and continued forward bending of the patient. When the operator feels the sacrum has made as much posterior progress as it can, he instructs the patient to exhale and hold the breath as long as they can. When they can no longer hold their breath, the patient is instructed to take a deep inhalation while at the same time lifting the head and shoulders but maintaining lumbar flexion. This will allow the patient to take a deeper inhalation thereby assisting the posterior movement of the sacrum.

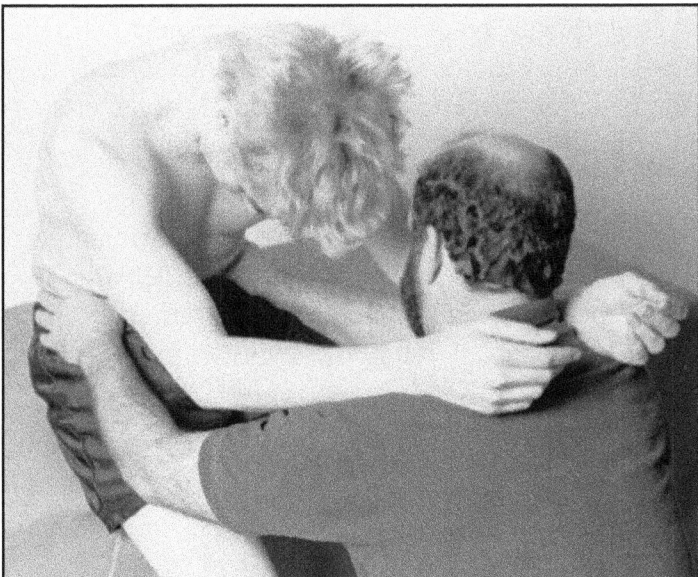

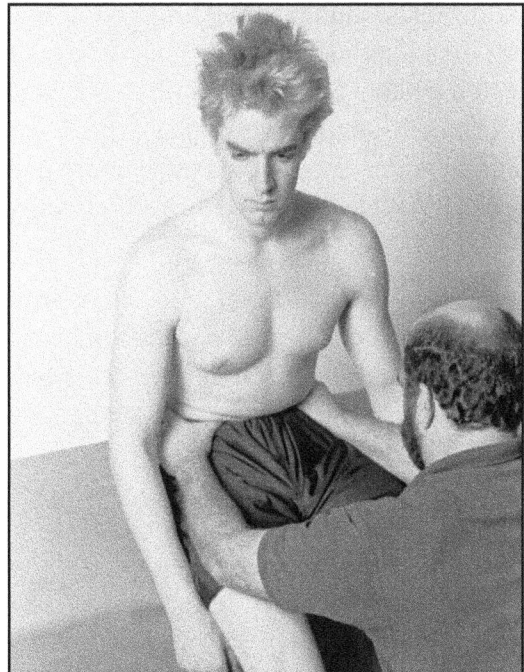

Postpartum Treatment

Perinatal Health Promotion

General health considerations essential to optimal development would include proper maternal intake of fluids, sleep and proper nutrition. For the infant the best form of nutrition is breast milk, which promotes bonding and attachment and stimulates a cascade of neurochemicals that promote optimal physiology. For example, G.I. absorption is enhanced in breast feeding babies. Additionally, the physiologic process of suckling promotes fluid fluctuation throughout the infant's body. Food sensitivities to substances within mother's milk are very common and are normally associated with rashes in the perioral and perianal regions, as well as other places on the infant's body. Colic can also frequently be managed by proper management of the mother's diet. Frequent substances that create sensitivities include wheat, dairy, alcohol, caffeine, cruciferous vegetables, and citrus. Additionally, states of stress and anxiety experienced by the mother are often transmitted from the breast to the baby.

Touching promotes wellness of both the mother and child through neurochemical stimulation of substances such as oxytocin and endorphins. Oxytocin has also been shown to be involved in stimulating maternal behavior, i.e., care of the young, bonding between mother and child, states of satiety, increased pain thresholds, sedation and decreased anxiety. Oxytocin is, of course, stimulated in response to suckling, but also is associated with touch, light pressure and warmth.

Infant stimulation and exploration help to modulate neurosensory, motor, cognitive, and psychosocial development. Signs of stimulation include dilation of the pupils, a quiet alert and inactive state of attention, reduced heart rate, reduced respiratory rate and reduced suckling rates. The infant's head will often turn toward the stimulation for 4-10 seconds. The infant's fingers and toes will stretch out to the stimulus. Infant stimulation is assisted by sitting upright or swaddling. Signs of over stimulation of the infant include brow tension, eyes that gaze away or droop down, and hands that are clasped together. Sensory experiences enhance physical growth and development and promote attachment. Motor and vestibular experiences promote sensory motor development. Olfactory stimulation often serves as an attachment marker for the infant to recognize their mother's or father's presence. Visual stimulation is most effective with high contrast items such as black and white.

For premature infants stimulation can be irritating or soothing. Positioning will often provide stimulation of either a positive or negative nature. Frequent quiet time and day/night cycling are beneficial to the premature infant. Often premature infants are hospitalized and the above stimulations or removal of irritating stimulation is essential to creating a suitable environment.

Table 9: Brain Growth Time Chart

10 to 18 weeks gestation - Phase 1	Number of brain cells is set.
20 weeks gestation to 2 years of age - Phase 2	Normal proliferation, migration and differentiation occur. Axonal growth and synapse formation follows.
20 weeks gestation to 4 years of age	Nerve fiber myelination occurs at a rapid rate and slows down after 4 years of age.
8 months gestation - 3 years of age	Brain undergoes an extra growth spurt doubling in weight. At birth the infant's brain is 25% of its adult brain weight. At 6 months of age the brain has obtained 50% of its adult brain weight. At one year of age the weight is 70% of its adult weight, and at 3 years of age it is 90%.

Table10: Infant Brain Function

Senses	Capacities Infant Experiences	Suggested Stimulators
Vision	At birth the baby looks at the edge of figures for contrast, can discriminate color, fixates for 4-10 seconds on an object up to about 13 inches away, tracks objects to the right and left of their body, identifies mother in 4 days, and perceives 3 dimensions. At 2 weeks of age the infant can perceive approaching objects and move their head away to prevent collision and can reach for an object within visual field. At 4 weeks the infant can track objects 15 inches away. At 8 weeks the infant can differentiate facial distortion from normal continence and begins to look at the center of objects. At 12 weeks accommodation is good, convergence for object 15 inches away is good.	•Human faces •Geometric shapes •Items with contrast •Bulls eye dots and checkerboards •Three dimensional objects •Animated objects and mobiles
Hearing	Can hear and discriminate loudness, tone and pitch. Can localize sounds. Can tune out monotonous sound and recognizes their name within one month of birth.	•Mother's and father's voices. •Speaking, singing and humming. •Music. •Classical pieces such as Bach, Brahms and Beethoven. •Instruments such as a violin and xylophone. •Imitating the baby's sounds. •Repeating phrases frequently. •Sound of a heartbeat. •Bells and chimes.

Senses	Capacities/ Infant Experiences	Suggested Stimulators
Touching	Can perceive touch. Myelination proceeds in a cephalocaudal direction, therefore, tactile experiences perceived in this direction as well.	• Skin to skin • Cuddling • Stroking • Massage • Introduction of different textures • Warm and cool water • Touching should be encouraged during breast feeding.
Taste	Can taste bitter, sweet, sour and salty characteristics. Mostly differentiates between sweet and sour though.	• Breast milk • Diluted sweet juices • Thumb sucking and pacifiers for saliva stimulation.
Smell	Sense of smell is very developed at birth, can distinguish mother's breast milk from all others and recognizes parents' body odors. Can distinguish sweet odor from noxious odor.	• Breast milk • Body odor through skin and clothes • Cooking odors • Sweet smells
Vestibular	Can respond to movement after fifth month of pregnancy. Senses changes in position at birth. Develops preferences for sleeping positions in first two months of life.	• Sitting upright with hips, knees and feet flexed. • Lying on tummy which encourages neck extension. • Rocking. • Riding in vibrating environments like a car. • Stroller time. • Swinging time. • Push side to side. • Stopping fall in each direction • Heel swing upside down. • 20 second side to side, up and back, alternating feet. • Spinning in a swivel chair.

Table 11: Functional Brain Stages

<u>Spinal cord and medulla oblongata</u> - Rapid development of functions pre-birth to 1 mo.

    Reflexes and life-preserving functions (breathing, sucking, etc.).

    Injuries to spinal cord or medulla usually produce severe disability and need for life-support.

<u>Pons</u> - Rapid development of functions pre-birth to 2.5 months; many functions "switch on" at 1 mo.

    Life-protecting functions (responses to threatening events).

    Some possible signs of pons dysfunction:

        Poor horizontal eye movements

        Convergent strabismus (eye deviates inward)

        Diminished vital sensation (Pain is perceived but there is little or no urgency about stopping it.)

    Some psychological/lifestyle correlates of pons dysfunction:

        Belief that the universe is basically hostile or indifferent.

        Isolation, alienation.

        Perception that survival is threatened when it isn't.

<u>Midbrain</u> (includes many subcortical brain structures) - 2.5 to 9 months.

    Sensory: Appreciating the meaning of stimuli

    Motor: Goal-directed activities

    Regulation of: Many somatic processes, cortical arousal, incoming sensory information, outgoing motor impulses

    Communication and coordination among various areas of the cortex

    Some possible signs of midbrain dysfunction:

        Diminished vital sensation

        Poor vertical eye movements

        Divergent strabismus (eye deviates outward)

        Flat affect, toneless voice, poverty of gestures

        Easily distracted (can't filter out irrelevant stimuli)

        Poor rapid alternating movements

        Hyperactivity

    Some psychological/lifestyle correlates of midbrain dysfunction:

        Disorganization (perpetually messy desk), or rigidly organized

        Overreacts to events, trouble coping, "stressed out"

        Trouble setting goals and reaching them

        Lack of balance in lifestyle

        Indecisive, can't prioritize

        "Scatter-brained"

<u>Cortex</u> - 7 months up. Many stages of cortical development.

    One hemisphere should be dominant for language and take the lead in certain other skilled activities. The other has its own areas of specialization.

    Some possible signs of cortical dysfunction:

        Learning disabilities

        Motor skills significantly worse on one side of body

        Developmental apraxias ("Never could learn to ride a bike...swim...draw...etc.")

        Speech problems (can't put things into words, stuttering, etc.)

        "Misfiled memories" (trouble retrieving info. from memory)

    Some psychological/lifestyle correlates of cortical dysfunction:

        Confused, "can't think straight", can't "see the whole picture"

        Can't apply different rules of behavior to different situations.

Table 12: Developmenttal Checklist
(Modified Denver)

AGE

Age	Question		
1 month	Can he raise his head from the surface while in prone position?	YES	NO
	Does he regard your face while you are in his direct line of vision?	YES	NO
2 months	Does he smile and coo?	YES	NO
3 months	Does he follow a moving object?	YES	NO
	Does he reach for things?	YES	NO
4 months	Will he hold a rattle and shake it?	YES	NO
	Does he laugh aloud?	YES	NO
5 months	Can he reach for and pick up objects with one hand?	YES	NO
6 months	Can he turn over?	YES	NO
	Will he sit with a little support (with one hand)?	YES	NO
	Can he transfer an object from one hand to another?	YES	NO
7 months	Can he sit by himself for 10 seconds?	YES	NO
8 months	Can he sit steadily for about five minutes?	YES	NO
9 months	Can he say "mama" or "dada?"	YES	NO
10 months	Can he pull himself up at the side of his crib or playpen?	YES	NO
11 months	Can he cruise around his playpen or crib, or walk holding onto furniture?	YES	NO
12 months	Can he wave bye-bye?	YES	NO
	Can he walk with one hand held?	YES	NO
	Can he say two words besides "dada" or "mama?"	YES	NO
15 months	Can he walk by himself?	YES	NO
	Can he indicate his wants by pointing and grunting?	YES	NO
18 months	Can he build a tower of three blocks?	YES	NO
	Does he know 10 words?	YES	NO
24 months	Can he run?	YES	NO
	Can he walk up and down stairs holding rail?	YES	NO
	Can he express himself (occasionally) in a three-word sentence?	YES	NO
2½ years	Can he jump with both feet off the ground?	YES	NO
	Can he build a tower of six blocks?	YES	NO
	Can he point to parts of his body on command?	YES	NO
3 years	Can he follow two commands involving "on," "under," or "behind?"	YES	NO
	Can he build a tower of nine blocks?	YES	NO
	Does he know his first and last names?	YES	NO
	Can he copy a circle?	YES	NO
4 years	Can he hop?	YES	NO
	Can he copy a cross?	YES	NO
	Does he use adjectives to describe pictures?	YES	NO
5 years	Can he follow three commands?	YES	NO
	Can he copy a square?	YES	NO
	Can he skip?	YES	NO

(Adjust for prematurity by subtracting the time of prematurity from the age of the child; e.g., a two-month-old infant who was one month premature should be evaluated as a month-old infant).

Table 13: Development of Neurological Organization (Brain Function) in Children Without Significant Brain Injuries

Brain Stage	Time Frame	Visual Competence	Auditory Competence	Tactile Competence	Mobility	Language	Manual Competence
VII Sophisticated Cortex	Superior 36 Mon. / Average 72 Mon. / Slow 108 Mon.	Reading words using a dominant eye consistent with the dominant hemisphere.	Understanding of complete vocabulary and proper sentences with proper ear.	Tactile identification of objects using a hand consistent with hemispheric dominance.	Using a leg in a skilled role which is consistent with the dominant hemisphere.	Complete vocabulary and proper sentence structure.	Using a hand to write which is consistent with the dominant hemisphere.
VI Primitive Cortex	Superior 22 Mon. / Average 36 Mon. / Slow 70 Mon.	Identification of visual symbols and letters within experience.	Understanding of 2000 words and simple sentences.	Description of objects by tactile means.	Walking and running in complete cross pattern	2000 words of language and short sentences.	Bimanual function with one hand in a dominant role.
V Early Cortex	Superior 13 Mon. / Average 18 Mon. / Slow 36 Mon.	Differentiation of similar but unlike simple visual symbols.	Understanding of 10 to 25 words and two word couplets.	Tactile differentiation of similar but unlike objects.	Walking with arms freed from the primary balance role	10 to 25 words of language and two word couplets.	Cortical opposition bilaterally and simultaneously.
IV Initial Cortex	Superior 8 Mon. / Average 12 Mon. / Slow 22 Mon.	Convergence of vision resulting in simple depth perception.	Understanding of two words of speech.	Tactile understanding of the third dimension in objects which appear to be flat.	Walking with arms used in a primary balance role most frequently at or above shoulder height.	Two words of speech used spontaneously and meaningfully.	Cortical opposition in either hand.
III Midbrain	Superior 4 Mon. / Average 7 Mon. / Slow 12 Mon.	Appreciation of detail within a configuration.	Appreciation of meaningful sounds.	Appreciation of gnostic sensation.	Creeping on hands and knees, culminating in cross pattern creeping.	Creation of meaningful sounds.	Prehensile grasp.
II Pons	Superior 1 Mon. / Average 2.5 Mon. / Slow 4 Mon.	Outline perception.	Vital response to threatening sounds.	Perception of vital sensation.	Crawling in the prone position culminating in cross pattern crawling.	Vital crying in response to threats to life.	Vital release.
I Medulla and Cord	Superior Birth to .5 / Average Birth to 1.0 / Slow	Light reflex.	Startle reflex.	Babinski reflex.	Movement of arms and legs without bodily movement.	Birth cry and crying.	Grasp reflex.

Neurological Organization and Patterning

Learning problems begin to be observed in the child's verbal and reading skills at 3-6 years of age. Often learning problems are related to disturbances caused by birth trauma or other developmental delays occurring in early infant and childhood development. Observing for patterns of movement are helpful in assessing possible developmental problems.

Stages of movement begin with supine symmetrical purposeless movements after birth and develop into prone flat crawling movements with the abdomen in contact with the floor. Crawling patterns proceed from homologous (worm like) to homolateral (ipsilateral arm and leg movements together) and cross (opposite movements of arms and legs). (See Figure 26.)

Next stage of movement involves creeping in which the child is on hands and knees. Creeping stage is perceived from homologous to homolateral to cross pattern as well. (See Figure 27.)

Creeping seems to trigger a variety of developmental milestones that babies reach between the ages of 6 and 9 months. Some of the changes brought about by creeping are the development of the ability to understand relationships between objects, the development of a perception of object constancy and the development of depth perception. The process of creeping provides a state of eye-hand coordination, vestibular processing, improvement of balance and equilibrium, spatial awareness, tactile input, kinesthetic awareness and social maturation. Children who have not completed this important developmental stage of movement often are lacking in other areas of motor and cognitive development. Studies also show that children who use walkers often by-pass the crawling stage, retarding development of certain cognitive skills such as reading.

A Learning Problem Indication Index (LPII) has been developed to screen for possible learning disorders of this type. Score 1 point for each positive answer.

Perinatal History
Prematurity
Prolonged Labor
Difficult Delivery
Cyanosis
Blood Incompatibility
Adoption

History of Developmental Abnormalities
Creeping Late or Abnormal
Walking Late
Tip Toe Walking Prolonged
Speech Late or Abnormal
Ambidexterity after the Age of 7 Years

Interpretation of Score

One or two - suspicious
Three - deserves more study
Four or more - further study mandatory.

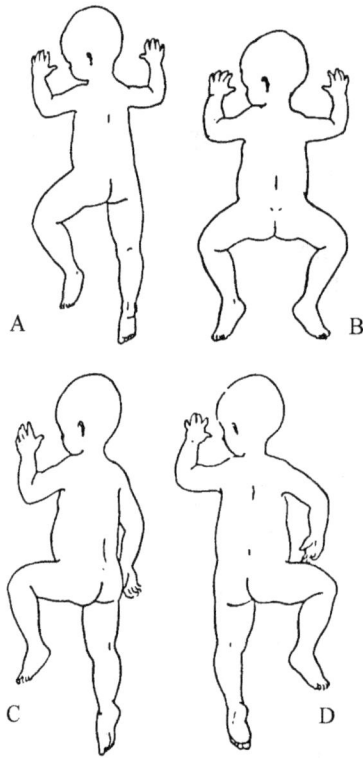

Fig. 26: Crawling Patterns: (A) Without pattern, (B) Homologous pattern, (C) Homolateral pattern, (D) Cross pattern

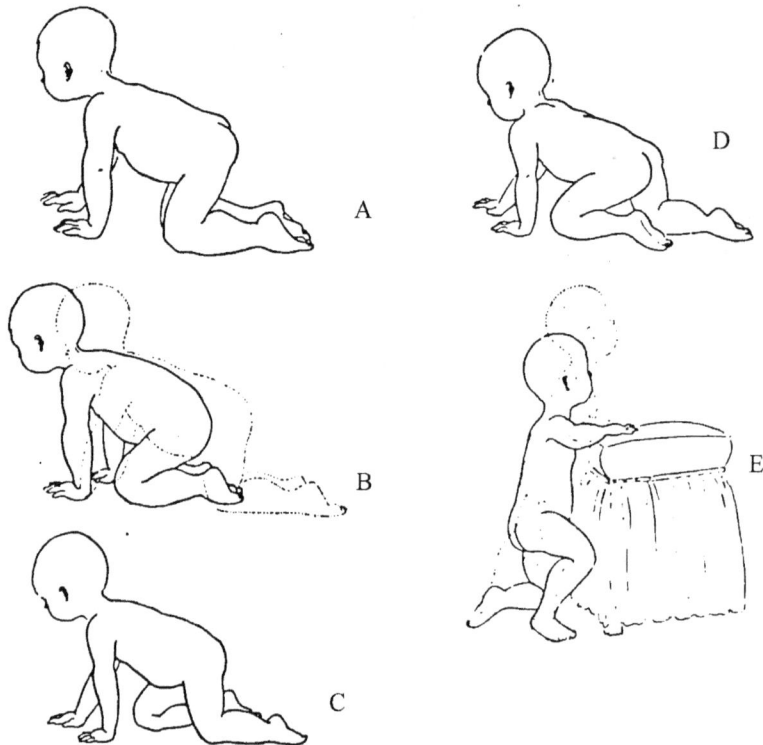

Fig. 27: Creeping Patterns: (A) Without pattern, (B) Homologous pattern, (C) Homolateral pattern, (D) Cross pattern, (E) Rising from creeping to cruise

Interventions to Enhance Sensory and Motor Integration
in Relation to Movement Patterning
Adapted from Doman and Delacato

Movement repatterning is performed after first treating osteopathically so as to optimize overall neuromusculoskeletal function. Repatterning helps to re-educate movement and coordination functions which have become neurologically impaired.

Assessment for movement dsturbance begins by observing the patient performing the most advanced patterns first (cross pattern creep, homolateral creep, crosspattern crawl, homolateral crawl), forwards and backwards.

Treatment using four man teams recreate the homolateral and cross patterns of movement, beginning with the most advanced pattern that can be performed without problem and then proceeding to the next level, which is disturbed. The patient is passive and relaxed while the 4 man team induces the movement pattern. Have the patient actively rotate the head towards the abducted arm or add a fifth person to do the same. In patients with learning disorders this should be performed every 3 or 4 hours, sustaining the movement in an alternating fashion in a constant rhythm for 15 to 20 minutes at a time.

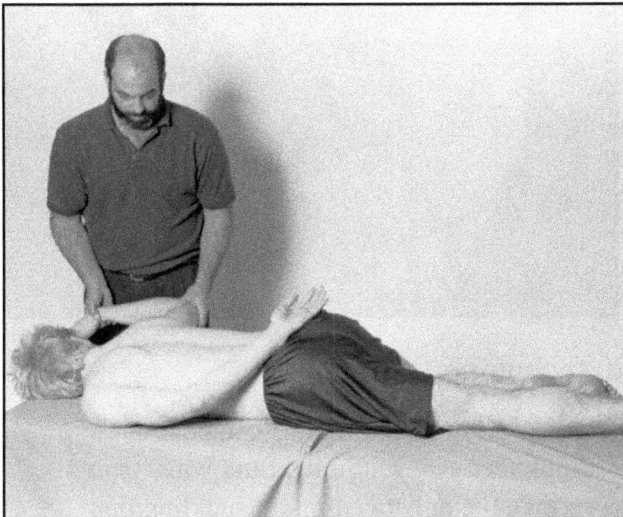 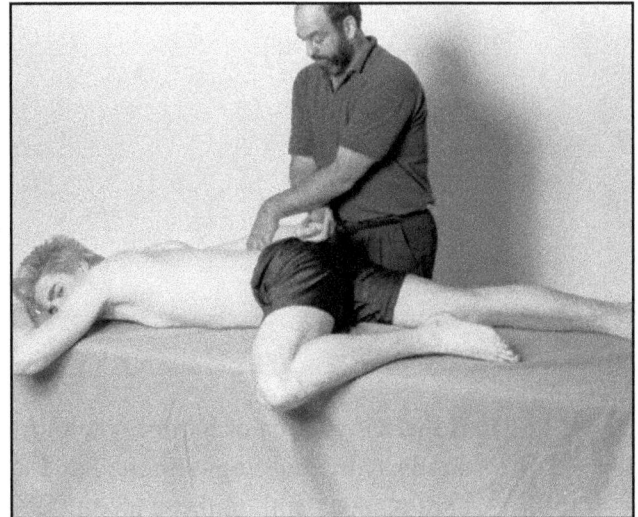

A   Homolateral Re-Patterning   B
Alternate Between A and B

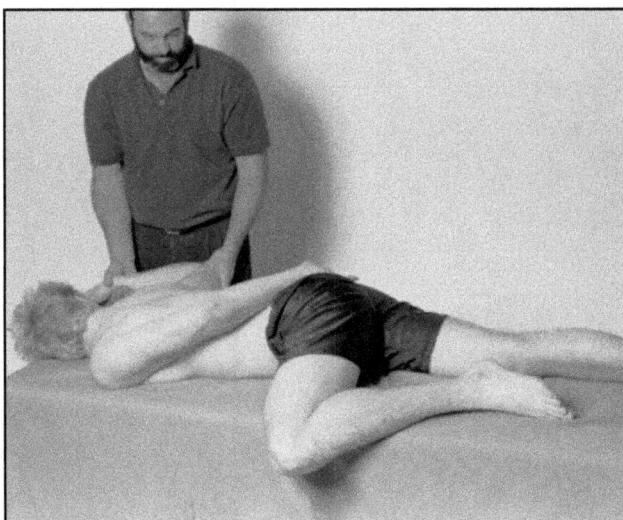 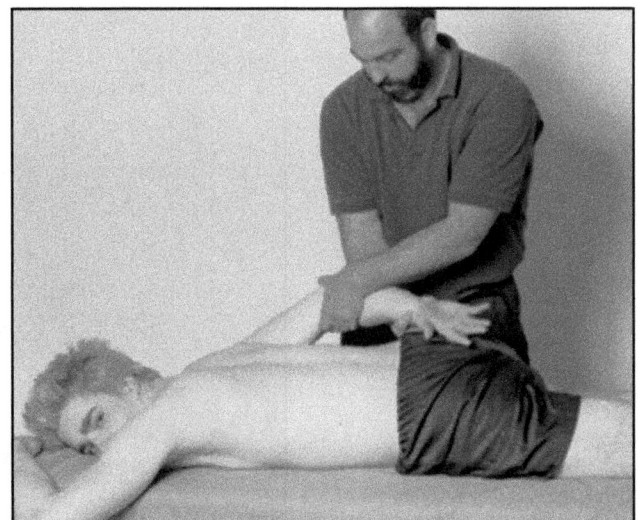

A   Cross Re-Patterning   B
Alternate Between A and B

Overlapping or Compressed Sutures:
Articular and Membranous Approaches

The operator can quickly scan the major sutures of the head, noting any prominences or areas of rigidity. These would include the coronal suture, the sagittal suture, the lamboidal suture, and the temporoparietal suture. Four quadrant diagnosis using the vault hold should also be performed to assess associated disturbances in CRI.

Treatment can be carried out by:
1) Sending a fluid wave from the cruciate suture in the middle of the hard palate to the area of rigidity or maximal overlapping where the operator has contact with a v-spread;

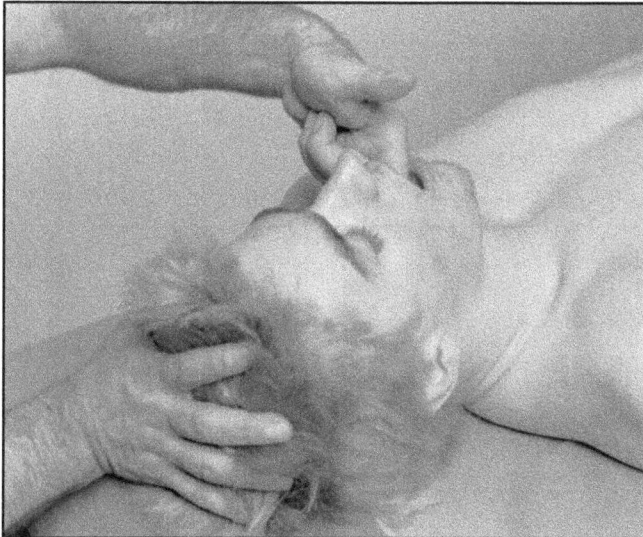
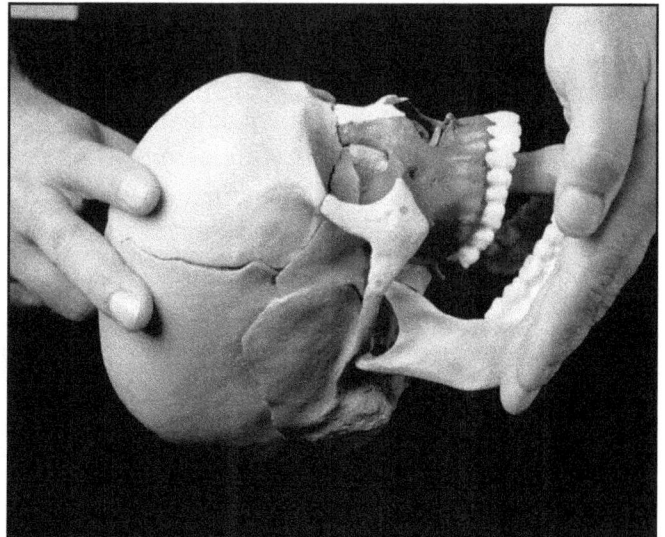

V- Spread Technique

2) If there is an area of hardness within the osseous bony structure, this can be treated similarly by molding with the hand while simultaneously sending a fluid wave from the hard palate. Both of these techniques incorporate the enhanced infant suckling that results from inserting the finger into the location of the hard palate.

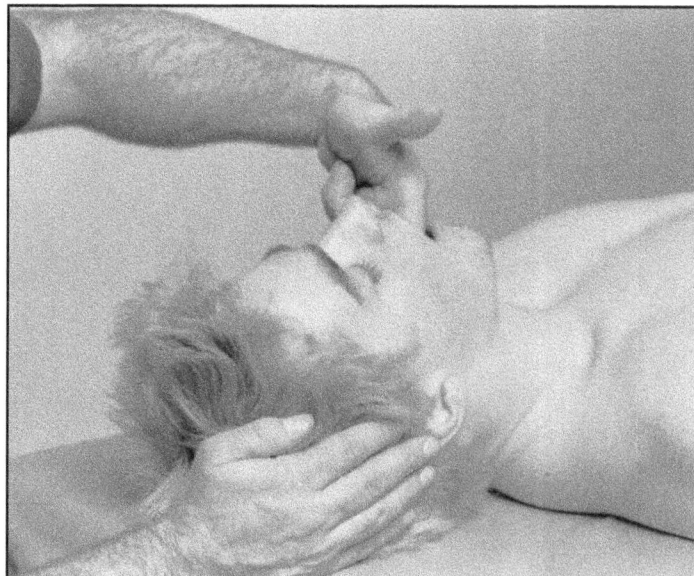

Hand Molding Technique

3) An alternative approach using the four quadrant technique (pterion and asterion) can be applied using compression and shearing forces in the directions of ease around any restricted suture (see pgs. 168-169). Remember that most overlapping sutures occur in association with disturbances in a more central location, either articular (i.e., SBS compressions), or membranous (i.e., Sutherland fulcrum or dural tube restrictions.)

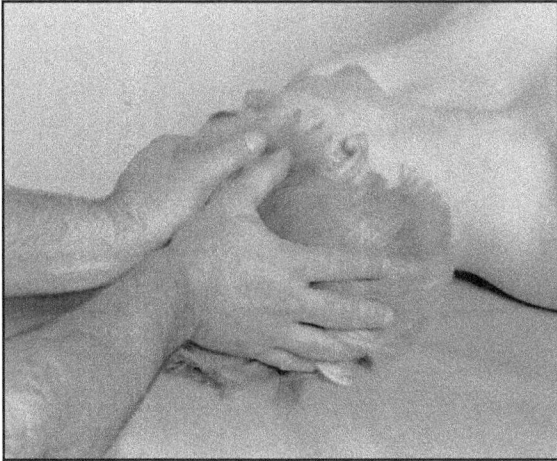
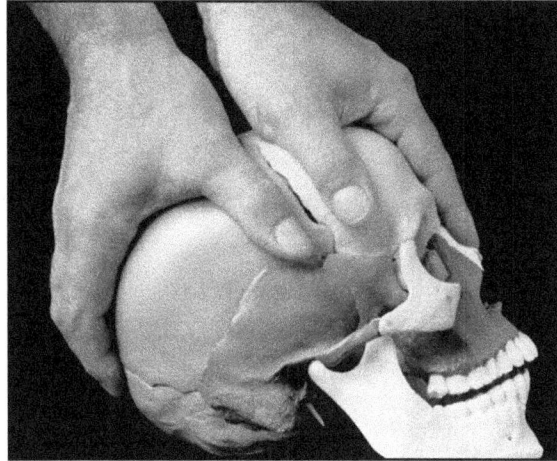

Pterion Treatment

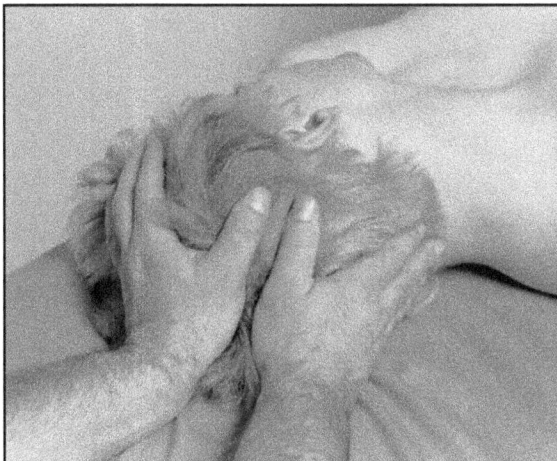
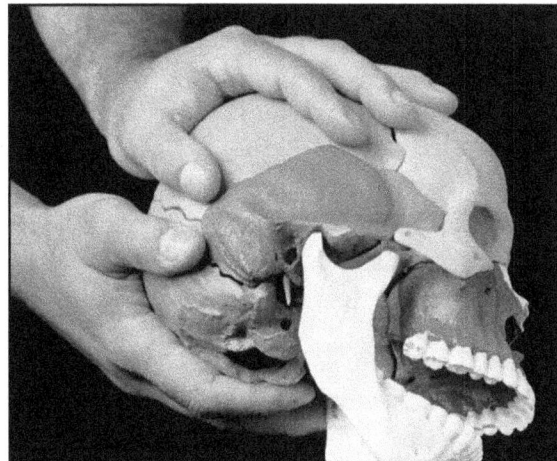

Asterion Treatment

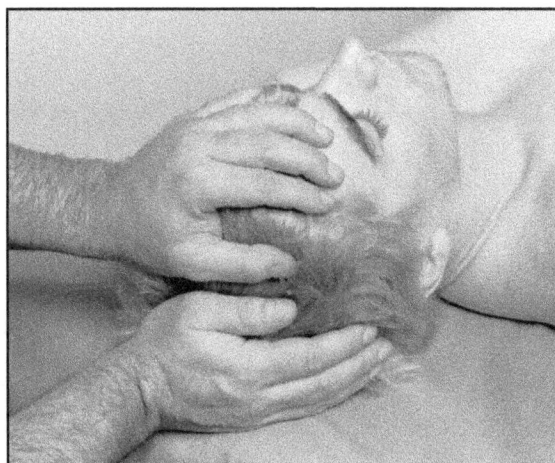

Other Sutures (i.e. Coronal) Treatment

Osteopathic View of Health and Illness

I. Promoting the developing infant's own homeostatic mechanisms is preferable to treating symptoms. Carefully observing signs and symptoms within the infant and avoiding the impulse to immediately take the baby to the doctor or make some other type of medical diagnosis will usually allow a natural resolution of the problem.

    A. Careful notation of the physical and emotional circumstances surrounding the problem will often reveal the underlying cause or reason for the behavior

    B. Observation of the child's behavior with respect to:

        1. Timing and type of crying or other verbal and non-verbal communication.

        2. Closeness to meal time, nap time, diaper time.

        3. Dynamics between mother and father or others in proximity to the infant.

II. Natural medicine works extremely well with children.

    A. Breast milk.

    B. Change in diet.

    C. Homeopathy.

    D. Acupuncture and herbs.

    E. Touch/massage.

III. Osteopathic evaluation should be initiated as soon as possible after birth, and subsequently as needed for emerging problems. Treatment principles focus on addressing homeostatic mechanisms and functions (i.e. The autonomic relations of the sympathetic and parasympathetic nervous systems, and respiratory and circulatory mechanisms of the venous, arterial and lymphatic systems) rather than the diseased organ or tissue.

    A. Treat parent to bring them into closer relation to their tidal body and to help them deal with their own disturbed midline function, shock and psychoemotional traumas.

    B. The association of difficult labor with many infant and childhood illnesses and problems is a primary consideration. Regardless of any problems or illnesses that develop, and hopefully before they develop, osteopathic intervention should be provided until the disturbances in the mechanism are normalized.

    C. Midline function of the body should be restored through assessment and treatment of sacrosternal and occipitosternal axis disturbances.

IV. Traditional diagnostic categories often obstruct inherent healing capacity through psychoemotional and belief structures of the parents.

    A.   Acutally, childhood illnesses often stimulate growth and development.

        1.   Immune function.

        2.   Respiratory function.

        3.   Metabolic function.

        4.   Behavioral function.

Related Health Topics

I.   Nighttime parenting.

    A. As soon as possible, feeding should be decreased at night in order to encourage a distinction between daytime and nighttime activity. Nighttime feedings do encourage nighttime awakenings.

    B. Under extreme circumstances, such as colic, nighttime feedings can be helpful. Frequently, colic is associated with cranial base dysfunction, food sensitivities or immaturity of the gastrointestinal system.

    C. Sleep disturbances are often related to upper airway congestion, which may also be related to teething. Teething may also be accompanied by fever, loose watery stools and irritability.

II.   Upper respiratory congestion and ear infections have relationships to the autonomic nervous system, as well as respiratory/circulatory mechanics, that can be treated osteopathically. Eustachian tube and temporal bone relations may also have important influences on fluid and membranous balance.

III. Asthma is a complex syndrome which can involve structural abnormalities of the upper thoracic spine and vagus nerve function, as well as the gastroesophogeal junction and sacrum; however, additional influences are common from nutritional and environmental irritants, as well as stress. Remember, illness is often a behavioral expression of fear, neglect, or other psychological stress. See Pediatric Ecology.

IV.   Learning and emotional disabilities.

    A. Issues of failure and inadequacy underlie behavioral problems in the development of such illnesses during infancy and childhood. Parental responses may reinforce these behaviors and often reflect unresolved parental feelings of failure and inadequacy.

    B. One in 5 children have developmental problems related to learning or emotional disabilities.

        1. Birth trauma highly associated.

        2. Only 10% of newborns have free cranial mechanisms.

        3. Neurologic development occurs in geometric forms/pathways during third trimester to 2 years of age.

        4. Severe SBS strain patterns are commonly associated.

    C. Observe child's structure and motor behaviors.

        1. Arching neck and back.

        2. Persistent facial and head asymmetry.

        3. Early fontenelle closure.

        4. Asymmetrical ocular movements.

5. Irritability, poor gastrointestinal function.

6. Breathing pattern.

7. Wakefulness, sedation, listlessness.

8. Muscle tone, reflexes and posture.

    a. Pull up to sitting from supine with traction on arms.

9. Creeping coordination.

V.   Cerebral Palsy

    A.   Diagnosis made after the age of 3 based on:

        1. Disturbed reflex equilibrium

        2. Poor postural strength and associated asymmetry

        3. Altered musculoskeletal reflexes

        4. Spasticity.

    B. Osteopathicly the problem is often associated with condylar compression and fascial tension in the cranial cervical and cervical thoracic region.

    C. Baby throws head back into spasms, rolls onto side to arch back.

    D. Congestion in the fourth ventricle due to condylar compression leads to stasis of fluid in the respiratory centers of the brain stem.

    E. Masking is a technique that stimulates the inhalation reflex by reducing oxygen, increases external rotation of the temporal bones and helps to reverse hypoxia.

VI.   Downs Syndrome

    A. Associated with deceleration of Neurologic development.

    B. Trisomy 21 may not be the only factor since some trisomy 21s have no mongoloidisim.

    C. Consistent lesion between the pre and post sphenoid with an associated defect in pituitary function (hypopituitarism, x-ray exam documents a vertically directed, straight, sphenobasilar synchrondosis).

    D. Hypotonic and hyperplastic muscular activity is often associated with delayed ocular development, strabismus and altered sphenoidal relations.

    E.   Structural abnormalities include:

        1. Depressed nasion.

        2. Palate high in the center with a flat form on the periphery.

        3. Dentition is abnormal, but health of teeth is good.

        4. There is a large anterior fontanel with delayed closure.

VII. Visual Disturbances

    A.   Far-sightedness, or hyperopia, is associated with flexion of the sphenoid or a superior vertical strain. The orbit becomes short and widened.

    B.   Near-sightedness, or myopia, is related to sphenoid in extension or an inferior vertical strain where the orbit is longer and narrower.

    C.   Strabismus.

        1.   Visual axis are divergent (not aligned).

        2.   The most common causes of strabismus are structural and neurologic defects of the eye muscles, their attachments or their enervation.

        3.   Divergence can be a paralytic phenomenon or the action of the muscular component is restricted or impaired by mechanical or neurologic factors, or non paralytic where the ocular muscles and innervations are normal.

            a.   Both cases deserve attention to the anatomic relations between the sphenoid and orbital structures.

            b.   Neurologic features of eye movement and possible entrapment sites include:

                1) <u>abducens nerve</u>, the clivus of the sphenoid, the cavernous sinus and the supraorbital fissure.

                2) <u>trochlear nerve</u>, the free border of the tentorium, cavernous sinus and supraorbital fissure.

                3) <u>oculomotor nerve</u>, superior cerebellar artery, cavernous sinus and supraorbital fissure.

VIII. Upper Respiratory Tract and Ear Infections

    A.   Fluid stasis is an underlying mechanism in all infectious problems.

    B.   Mobilization of respiratory circulatory mechanics as well as fluid potency have profound influences on host healing and regulatory responses.

    C.   Additionally, specific areas of involvement have autonomic nervous reflex changes that can be treated osteopathically, particularly in the thoracic spine and rib cage.

    D.   Particular attention should be paid to the developing eustacian tube which has a horizontal orientation through much of the childhood years.

        1.   This leads to difficulty in drainage of fluids from the inner ear.

        2.   Osteopathic evaluation and treatment of the temporal bone mechanics plays an important role in assisting with fluid drainage from this area.

        3.   Additionally, the temporal bones have an association with optimal respiratory mechanics, which can have a beneficial influence on infections of both the upper and lower respiratory tract.

Pediatric Ecology

Health Promotion is different from Disease Prevention and Crisis Management

Osteopathic philosophy has always stressed the importance of enhancing those mechanisms within a system that are designed to optimize functional performance and efficiency. As individuals we must meet the challenges of system interplay at many different levels. The individual exists within the larger context of his or her genetic makeup, which exists in the larger context of the family, as well as the environmental systems in which we live. Additionally, this interface occurs over time, during which there are many phases of growth, development and maturity. The manner in which each of these systems functions plays a significant role in the current and future life of each individual.

Pediatric ecology is the study of how these systems interface within the life and lifetime of an individual. Each system is referred to as a vector with unique characteristics that contribute to the opportunities and challenges occurring in an individual's life.

The three vectors we will discuss are:

1. The self vector, essentially the soul of the individual, that is comprised of the tidal body having its origins in the embryonic stage of development. This vector embodies the awareness of the self, its true nature and its purpose, as well as the will and intention to express that nature and purpose, and the ability to evolve through a balanced interplay of physical, emotional, intellectual, intuitive and spiritual life functions.

2. The genetic vector, which begins at about the sixth week of gestation, bringing to bear metabolic, structural and psychoemotional characteristics that will interplay with the self and all its aspects. Genetic characteristics include predisposition to illness, immunologic function, factors of growth, development and longevity, as well as autonomic balance and response to stress.

3. The environmental vector, embodies aspects of both family systems and the culture at large, which dictates various types of values and lifestyles, as well as socioeconomic factors, which influence social class, nutrition, health care access, education, etc.

Within each vector, there are strengths and weaknesses, and the doctor-patient interaction can be directed to maximize strengths and minimize vulnerabilities as they are identified in all three vectors. In the osteopathic approach, we still stress the primary importance of enhancing the inherent mechanisms within each vector that are designed to maximize its total function. However, most important is the inherent potency of the self and the tidal body to manifest the greatest health and vitality in all three vectors.

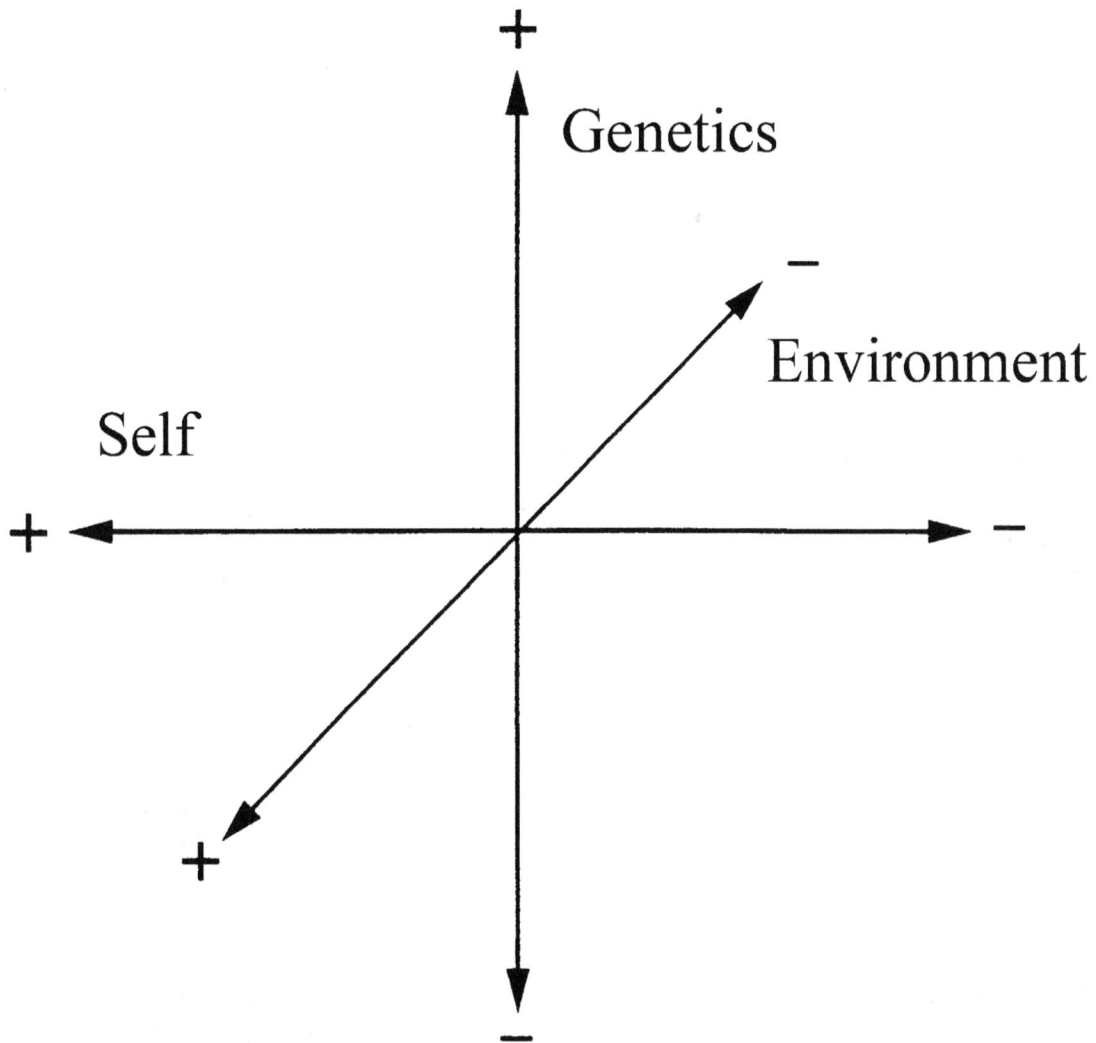

Fig. 28: Pediatric Ecology

Developmental Interfaces in Pediatric Ecology

1. The individual's <u>inherent capacity for health</u> and wellness occurs as a result of the interface between the self and the genetic vector.

2. <u>Attachment and bonding</u> and the effect of touch on infant development occurs in the relationship between parents and infant in the environmental vector.

3. <u>Growth and development</u> from infancy to childhood interfaces the family and larger environment with the individual and their genetics. Here, the choices that the parents make for introducing new experiences to the developing child play a significant role.

4. <u>Biobehavioral shifts</u> occur during childhood, due to both natural and traumatic 'life changing' events. These stimulate physical, emotional, intellectual, and spiritual life changes in the individual (self). Such changes may significantly influence the relationships between the individual and family as well as the larger environment.

5. In <u>Adolescence</u>, the individual develops more independence and life direction, but also more risk for exposure to physical and emotional insult. Family, friends, mentors, education and lifestyle habits all have important influences on the adolescent striving to achieve a sense of identity and belonging.

6. <u>Adulthood</u> focuses aspects of maturity that may or may not have completely occurred, which influence coping strategies for dealing with life's responsibilities and stresses, as well as its joys and successes. Life choices are somewhat determined at this point with respect to preferences and lifestyle habits, but can be influenced by education and personal motivation to be healthier and to avoid illness. Physical, psychological, and/or spiritual crises often occur in the third or fourth decade of life (e.g.. chronic pain)

7. <u>Parenthood</u> involves a significant shift in self-awareness, self-expression and psychospiritual focus, usually requiring advice, support, compassion and coping with constant change. Realize that most parents are experiencing a second childhood themselves as they re-evaluate their family upbringing, relationships and values. Often this is associated with "mid-life crisis" or other breakdown in the individual's self-concept.

Family Systems Assessment from the Osteopathic Perspective

This can be a difficult and frustrating aspect of doctor-patient relations, but equally rewarding. The study of family systems can be a revelation in itself for our own family origins. Osteopathic philosophy suggests a unique approach to family system assessment and treatment. Similar to treatment using manual medicine techniques, we can facilitate the release of blockages within the structure and function of the family system itself and its following components:

1. <u>Safety and trust</u>; *the whole is greater than the sum of its parts, consider the unity of the whole system and its complex dynamics when studying the individual parts.* Physical or verbal betrayal of safety and/or trust sets a tone of fear and unbridled emotion that is one of the most damaging influences on the unity of a family system. Children's feelings of inadequacy, shame and guilt are reinforced by behaviors that violate personal safety and dignity. These betrayals are usually cloaked behind a thin veil of denial and projection of responsibility onto others or extenuating circumstances.

2. <u>Self acceptance/forgiveness</u>; understand that attention-getting behaviors, power struggles and rebellion are often reactions to feeling inadequate, worthless or unimportant within the family system. They are difficult feelings to accept and forgive. The ability to discuss openly and without criticism feelings of fear, anger, loss, shame, etc., facilitates the establishment of safety and trust necessary to create a more positive family unity. Discussing personal boundaries and discipline related to crossing those boundaries is essential, as is accepting the validity of our own and others' feelings. This level of self-acceptance and forgiveness of past and current indiscretions is necessary for self-respect. As the health care provider, we can take the time to help children and parents to understand their feelings and feel the acceptance and respect from you, who are an authority figure in their life. Open communication has an infectious quality to *stimulate the positive self-regulating and healing mechanisms* inherent in family systems.

3. <u>Needs assessment/support</u>; *structure and function are reciprocally related.* As members of the family feel more safety and trust, accepting and expressing their feelings without blame or guilt, they can own their own experience in the family and begin to communicate more clearly their needs to each other, without fear of rejection. Additionally, discipline becomes an easier task of offering other family members choices of various behaviors which might satisfy their needs. Individuals can then make their own choices as to which behaviors most effectively satisfy their needs without causing problems for others. Parents and children have different needs, and one is not necessarily more important than the other. We can help the child to understand and verbalize their needs more clearly through our therapeutic interactions.

4. <u>Family empowerment/creativity</u>. The osteopathic principle that applies here is the *rule of the artery is supreme.* The bloodline of every family is the natural expression of love and intimacy. Heart-felt love nurtures a sense of belonging and has a profound influence on the unity of the family system. From this comes a natural ease in family relations that leads to a sense of vitality and creativity. Family activities which might nurture this kind of emotion include participating in music or singing, art, sports, camping, group cooking, etc. Bringing ourselves and our patients into contact with the tidal body facilitates this kind of psychoemotional process.

213

5. <u>Active listening</u>. An exercise to practice with your patients as well as your own family and loved ones is the following:

(1) Listen to what needs are being expressed when strong emotions are being exchanged.

(2) Repeat back what you understand has happened or what was said.

(3) Pose as a question a need you perceive not being fulfilled, then wait for a response.

(4) Remove criticisms, judgments and coercive tendencies, as well as any expectations of a particular outcome.

(5) Nurture a respectful, yet playful interaction that accepts the needs and differences of individuals. Everyone has their own way of perceiving and processing information and situations. Everyone has their own schedule and way of learning. Helping an individual to recognize their unique strengths and weaknesses can help them deal more effectively with these differences. Repeat what you understand their response to mean and help them clarify it themselves.

(6) Always give others a chance to respond to observations or requests made. Let others choose for themselves so they can learn responsibility for their own actions and be better able to fulfill their needs. Discuss various choices or options and the consequences and potential successes of each.

(7) Everyone must realize their own purpose and life design, which usually is not the same as the expectations of parents or other family members.

(8) Help individuals make agreements that support their choices and make note of any goals or promises for future follow-up. Take seriously these commitments, for the ability to keep one's word is the only thing that has any real power.

Our deepest fear is not that we are inadequate. Our deepest fear is that we are powerful beyond measure. It is our light, not our darkness, that frightens us. We ask ourselves, who am I to be brilliant, gorgeous, talented and fabulous? Actually, who are you not to be? You are a child of God. Your playing small doesn't serve the world. There's nothing enlightened about shrinking so that other people won't feel insecure around you. We were born to manifest the glory of God within us. It's not just in some of us; it's in everyone. And as we let our own light shine, we unconsciously give other people permission to do the same. As we are liberated from our own fear, our presence automatically liberates others.

Nelson Mandela, president, Republic of South Africa
from his 1994 inaugural speech

Level IV Course Schedule- Day 1

8:00 a.m.	*(0900)*	Course Introduction and Objectives

8:30 a.m.   *(0930)*   Lecture: Embryology

- Osteopathic Embryology
- Embryonic Intelligence; its design and function

9:45 a.m.   *(1045)*   Break

10:00 a.m.   *(1100)*   *Table Session* - Breath of Life

10:30 a.m.   *(1130)*   Lecture: Maternal and Fetal Relationships; Fetal Stimulation

11:30 a.m.   *(1230)*   Table Demonstration - Treatment of Mother before Delivery

- Fetal Release
- Thoracolumbar and Lumbosacral Release
- Seated Hip Release

11:45 a.m.   *(1245)*   Lunch

1:00 p.m.   *(1400)*   Lecture:

- Birth Mechanics
- Infant Anatomy
- Principles of Newborn Treatment

2:45 p.m.   *(1545)*   Break

3:00 p.m.   *(1600)*   Table Demonstration

- Newborn Examination and Treatment

4:00 p.m.   *(1700)*   Table Demonstration and Treatment Session of Mother after Delivery

- Seated Sacral Release
- Thoracolumbar and Lumbosacral Release
- Seated Hip Release

5:00 p.m.   *(1800)*   Adjourn

Level IV Course Schedule- Day 2

8:00 a.m.	(*0900*)	Discussion
8:15 a.m.	(*0915*)	Lecture:

       • Perinatal Health Promotion

       • Brain Function and Neurologic Organization

9:15 a.m.	(*1015*)	*Table Session*- Overlapping Sutures; Articular and Membranous Approaches
9:45 a.m.	(*1045*)	Break
10:00 a.m.	(*1100*)	Lecture:

       • Infant Stimulation

       • Movement Patterning

11:00 a.m.	(*1200*)	*Table Session* - Re-patterning

       • Homolateral and Cross Pattern Movements; Four Operator Teams

11:45 a.m.	(*1245*)	Lunch
1:00 p.m.	(*1400*)	Lecture - Osteopathic View of Health and Illness

       • Selected Health Topics

2:45 p.m.	(*1545*)	Break
3:00 p.m.	(*1600*)	Lecture - Osteopathic Pediatric Ecology

       • Developmental Interfaces

       • Family Systems

5:00 p.m.	(*1800*)	Adjourn

Level IV Course Schedule- Day 3

8:00 a.m.   (*0900*)   Discussion

8:15 a.m.   (*0915*)   Pediatric Screening Examination and Record Keeping

8:45 a.m.   (*0945*)   Case Study No. 1 - Instructor Demonstration

9:45 a.m.   (*1045*)   Break

10:00 a.m.   (*1100*)   Case Studies Nos. 2, 3 and 4 - Assessment by Class Participants

10:45 a.m.   (*1145*)   Case Evaluation and Treatment by Instructor and Class Participants Together

11:45 a.m.   (*1245*)   Lunch

1:00 p.m.   (*1300*)   Case Studies Nos. 5, 6 and 7 - Assessment by Class Participants

1:45 p.m.   (*1445*)   Case Evaluation and Treatment by Instructor and Class Participants Together

2:45 p.m.   (*1545*)   Discussion

3:00 p.m.   (*1600*)   Adjourn

OSTEOPATHIC CLINICAL PROBLEM SOLVING

The osteopathic approach to patient care considers the patient as an integrated whole with dynamic interplay between structure and function. Problem solving begins with a detailed history and physical examination to consider all the possible etiologies related to the patient's present health status. From an osteopathic perspective, old illnesses and injuries leave their imprint on body structure and function, often making the patient more vulnerable to developing future problems. Even routine childbirth is considered to be a potential 'traumatic' event in the patient's history.

In the osteopathic approach to problem solving, patient complaints are evaluated independently, problem by problem, as well as in light of their relation to the patient's overall structure and function. This requires focused local inspection as well as examination of more distal structures for relevant clinical associations. Distal structures may have associations which can be primary (causal) or contributory to the area of the patient's chief complaint. Such associations can be mechanically linked (e.g. tendonitis), neurologically linked (e.g. radiculopathy), or viscerally linked (e.g. angina).

For example, a shoulder problem may be due to local injury to the capsule or to myotendinous insertions, or to more distal problems in the rib cage, thoracic outlet, cervical spine, gall-bladder, or opposite hip extensors. A good history and physical examination should serve to screen out these and other potential problems and help localize the clinical nature of the patient's chief complaint.

Management of problems associated with the patient's chief complaint may require emergent intervention or specialty referral for appropriate medical treatment as with an acute cholelithiasis or a stress fracture. In these situations, osteopathic manipulative treatment may also be helpful as adjunctive care. In many cases, osteopathic diagnosis and treatment alone will be effective in addressing the various mechanical, neurologic and visceral aspects and interrelationships associated with the patient's chief complaint.

OSTEOPATHIC PROBLEM SOLVING MATRIX

An osteopathic screening examination with the goal of determining where the patient's problem areas are, should include: 1) gait analysis and 2) regional tests to evaluate structural landmarks, tissue resistance, and mobility. In addition to standard neurologic and orthopedic assessments, specific osteopathic tests should be carried out to evaluate possible nerve entrapment and myofascial/dural tension signs. Various approaches to locating areas of primary restrictions in the body and visceral structures can also be incorporated including palpating peripheral reflections of the cranial rhythmic impulse (CRI) or 'listening' techniques. Additionally, viscerosomatic or Chapman's reflexes may be present, also signifying the presence of visceral influences within the patient's musculoskeletal system.

Osteopathic scanning and segmental examinations further localize problems to specific areas and define their structural and functional characteristics so that specific therapeutic measures can be applied. Management of the whole patient requires consideration of the inter-relationships of the various problems identified, as well as further work-up of any potential health risks.

Table 13: EXAMINATION OF THE ADULT PATIENT

SCREENING TESTS: To locate problems, regionally

1. Gait Analysis:

Forefoot pronation
Ankle eversion
Knee rotation and extension
Hip extension
Pelvic weight shift/mobility

Lumbar side bending
Thoracic cage mobility
Shoulder position
Arm swing
Head position

2. Static Landmarks

Scoliosis
Kyphosis
Lordosis

Head
Shoulder
Scapula
Iliac crest
Trochanter
Feet

3. Tissue Resistance to Pressure

4. Dynamic Testing

Standing
Pelvis
    Stork Test
Lumbar
    Rotation
    Side bending
    Flexion
Lower extremity
    Hip shift
    One leg stand
    Knee extension
Sitting
Upper extremity
    Forearm
    Pronation
Thoracic cage
    Side bending
    Rotation
    Flexion/extension
Cervical spine
    Side bending
    Rotation
    Flexion/extension

Supine
Pelvis
    Traction test
    Pelvic rock
Thoracolumbar spine
    Sit-up test
Head and cervical spine
    Head lift
    Jaw abduction
    Vault hold
Upper extremity
    Shoulder abduction
Lower Extremity
    Side bending
Costal cage
    Respiratory motion
    Sternal compliance
Prone
Pelvis
    Sacral rock
    Hip extension
Thoracic spine
    Push-up
Side-lying
Lower extremity
    Hip abduction

SCANNING TESTS: To localize segmentally, exact areas of dysfunction

1. Global "Listening"

2. Following Reflections of Peripheral CRI to Most Proximal Area of Assymetric Function

3. Tissue Texture Abnormalities

Moisture
Hardness

Temperature
Color

SEGMENTAL TESTING: To characterize dysfunction structurally and functionally

Ankle/foot
Knee
Hip/groin
Pelvis
Sacrum

Lumbar spine
Thoracic spine
Rib cage
Cervical spine
Head

Sternoclavicular
Acromioclavicular
Glenohumeral
Elbow
Wrist/hand

220

Bibliography of Research Related to Cranial Osteopathy and Fetal and Infant Development

The research and writings presented on the following pages have been referenced by category for ease of use. The research categories and subcategories are arranged as follows:

History of Cranial Osteopathy
The Motile Brain and Central Nervous System
  The Histochemistry of the Contractile Elements of the Brain, Astroglia, and Oligondendroglia
  Observations and Measurements of CNS, Brain and Spinal Cord Motility
  The Microscopic Anatomy of the Neural and Non-neural Brain Cells and Tracts
Reciprocal Tension Membrane: The Dura Mater of the Brain and Spinal Cord
Cerebrospinal Fluid Hydraulics
  Pressure Fluctuations and Tidal Movements of Cerebrospinal Fluid
  Flow Dynamics and Pathways of Cerebrospinal Fluid
  Cerebrospinal Fluid Physiology
The Osseous-Articular Mechanism
  Osteokinematics and Arthrokinematics of the Skull Bones and Joints
  Suture Structure and Function
  Embryology, Growth, Development, and Aging of the Skull Bones and Sutures
Involvement of the Sacrum in the Craniosacral System
Clinical Research in Cranial Osteopathy
  Trauma Management in Cranial Osteopathy
  Cranial Osteopathy Applications to Pediatrics
  Cranial Osteopathy Palpatory Skills
  New Techniques to Examine and Treat the Craniosacral System
  The Clinical Effects of Cranial Somatic Dysfunction
Pulsatile Phenomena Not Related to Arterial Pulses or Cardiac Rhythms
  Instrumental Detection and Measurement of the CRI and Other Pulses
  Clinical Correlations with Impulses
Pulmocardiovascular Research Related to Cranial Osteopathy
Striated Muscle Anatomy and Function Related to Cranial Osteopathy
Bound Volumes Related to Cranial Osteopathy
Fetal and Infant Stimulation and Development
  General Development
  Brain Development
  Lateralization in Infants
  Cognitive Development
  Infant Intelligence
  Language Development
  Prenatal Stimulation
  Visual Stimulation
  Auditory Stimulation
  Vestibular Stimulation
  Motor Development and Stimulation
  Tactile Stimulation
  Gustatory Stimulation
Sleep-Wake Cycles in Infants and Children
Oxytocin, Behavior, and Development

A large portion of this bibliography was compiled from the Cranial Academy's "Bibliography of Research Related to Osteopathy in the Cranial Field". We would like to express our appreciation to the Cranial Academy and especially Hollis King, DO, PhD, FAAO, for allowing us to reprint this important compilation of reference material. Questions or inquiries about membership may be directed to: The Cranial Academy, 8202 Clearvista Parkway, Suite 9-D, Indianapolis, Indiana 46256

History of Cranial Osteopathy

Becker RF. Cranial therapy revisited. *Osteopath Ann* 1977;5:14-40 and 71

Blum CL. Biodynamics of the cranium: a survey. *J Craniomandib Pract* 1985164-171

Ferre JC, Barbin JY. The osteopathic cranial concept: fact or fiction? *Surg Radiol Anat* 1991;13:165-170.

Handy CL. A history of cranial osteopathy. *J Am Osteopathic Assoc* 1948;47:269-72.

Kappler RE. Osteopathy in the cranial field: Its history, scientific basis, and current status. *The Osteopathic Physician* 1979; Feb:13-18.

Retzlaff EW, Mitchell FL Jr, Eds. *The Cranium and Its Sutures*. Berlin, Heidelberg, New York. Springer-Verlag. 1987.

Wales AL. The work of William Garner Sutherland, DO DSc (Hon.) *J Am Osteo Assoc* 1972;71:788-793.

The Motile Brain and Central Nervous System

Johnson PC. *Peripheral circulation*. New York: Wiley Medical (Chap. 12 - Brain), 1978.

Lumsden CE, Pomerat CM. Normal oligodendrocytes in tissue culture. *Exp Cell Res* 1951;2:103-114

Vern BA, Schuette WH, Leheta B, et al. Low-frequency oscillations of cortical oxidative metabolism in waking and sleep. *J Cereb Clood Flow Metab* 1988;8:215-226

The Histochemistry of the Contractile Elements of the Brain, Astroglia, and Oligodendroglia

Abd-El-Bassett EM, Federoff S. Actin and actin-binding proteins in differentiating astroglia in tissue culture. *J Neurosci Res* 1991;30:1-17.

Abd-El-Bassett EM, Federoff S. Contractile units in stress fibers of fetal human astroglia in tissue culture. *J Chem Neuroanat* 1994;7:113-122.

Berridge MJ, Rapp PE. A comparative survey of the function, mechanism and control of cellular oscillators. *J Exp Biol* 1979;81:217-279.

Dani JW, Chernjavsky A, Smith SJ. Neuronal activity triggers calcium waves in hippocampal astrocyte networks. *Neuron* 1992;8:429-440.

Duffy S, MacVicar BA. Potassium-dependent calcium influx in acutely isolated hippocampal astrocytes. *Neuroscience* 1994;61(1):51-61.

Finkbeiner S. Calcium waves in astrocytes - filling in the gaps. *Neuron* 1992;8:1101-1108.

Groschel-Stewart U, Unsicker K, Leonhardt H. Immunohislochemical demonstration of contractile proteins in astrocytes, marginal glial and ependyman cells in rat diencephalon, *Cell Tissue Res* 1977;180:133-137.

Grundke-Iqbal I, Tung YC, Wisniewski HM. Alzheimer paired helical filaments: Immunochemical identification of polypeptides, *Act Neuropathol* 1984;62:259-267.

Jian X, Hidaka H. Schmidt JT. Kinase requirements for retinal growth cone motility. *J Neurobiol* 1994;25(10):1310-1328.

222

Jou MJ, Peng Ti, Sheu SS. Histamine induces oscillations of mitochondrial free Ca^{2+} concentration in single cultured rat brain astrocytes. *J Physiology* 1996497(2);299-308.

Jurzak M, Muller AR, Gerstberger R. Characterization of vasopressin receptors in cultured cells derived from the region of rat brain circumventricular organs. *Neuroscience* 1995;65(4):1145-1159.

Levasseur JE, et al. Detailed description of cranial window technique for acute and chronic experiments. *Stroke* 1975;6:308-317.

Mobley PL, Hedberg K, Bonin L, Chen B, Griffith OH. Decreased phosphorylation of four 20-kDa proteins precedes staurospohne-induced disruption of the actin/myosin cytoskeleton in rat astrocytes. *Exp Cell Res* 1994;214:55-66.

Porter JT, McCarthy KD. Adenosine receptors modulate [Ca2l] in hippocampal astrocytes In Situ. *J Neurochem* 1995;65:1515-1523.

Scordilis SP, Anderson JL, Pollack R, Adelstein RS. Characterization of rnyosin-phospharylating system in normal murine astrocyles and derivative SV40 wild-type and 4-mutant transformants. *J Cell Biol* 1977;74:940-949.

Sontheimer H. Voltage-dependent ion channels in glial cells. *GLIA* l994;11:156-172.

Van den Pol AN, Finkbeiner SM, Cornell-Bell AH. Calcium excitability and oscillations in suprachiasmatic nucleus neurons and glia *in vitro. J Neurosci* 1992;12(7):2648-2664.

Wang Z, Tymianski M, Jones OT, Nedergaard M. Impact of cytoplasmic calcium buffering on the spatial and temporal characteristics of intercellular calcium signals in astrocytes. *J Neurosci* 1997;1 7(19):7359-7371.

Zohar M, Salomon Y. Mechanism of action of melanocortin peptides: Possible role in astrocyle regulation. *J Molecular Neurosci* 1993;4(l):55-62.

Observations and Measurements of CNS, Brain and Spinal Cord Motility

Alperin N, Vikingstad EM, Gomez-Anson B, Levin DN. Hemodynamically independent analysis of cerebrospinal fluid and brain motion observed with dynamic phase contrast MRI. *Magn Reson Med* 1996;35:741-754.

Britt RH, Rossi GT. Quantitative analysis of methods for reducing physiological brain pulsation. *J Neurosci Methods* 1982;6:219-229.

Enzmann DR, Pelc NJ. Brain motion: Measurement with phase-contrast MR imaging. *Radiology* 1992;1 85:653-   660.

Feinberg DA. Modern concepts of brain motion and cerebrospinal fluid flow. *Radiology* 1992;185:630-632.

Feinberg DA, Mark AS. Human brain motion and cerebrospinal fluid circulation demonstrated with MR velocity   imaging. *Radiology* 1987;163:793-799.

Greitz D, Wirestam R, Franck A, Nordell B, Thomsen C, Stahlberg F. Pulsatile brain movement and associated hydrodynamics studied by magnetic resonance phase imaging. *Neuroradiology* 1992;34:370-380.

Kaufman B, David GJ. A method of intracranial volume calculation. *Invest Radiol* 1972;7:533-538.

Maier SE, Hardy CJ, Jolesz FA. Brain and cerebrospinal fluid motion: Real-time quantification with M-mode MR imaging. *Radiology* 1994;193:477-483.

Podlas H, Lewer-Allen K, Bunt EA. Computed tomography studies of human brain movements. *South African J of Surgery* 1984;22(l):57-63.

Pomerat CM. Rhythmic contracting of Schwann cells. *Science* 1959;130:1759.

Poncelet BP, Wedeen VJ, Weisskoff RM, Cohen MS. Brain parenchyma motion: Measurement with cine echo-planar MR imaging. *Radiology* 1992;185:645-651.

Schooley TL. The force behand the craniosacral mechanism. *Journal of the Osteopathic Cranial Assoc.* (With discussion by Paul E. Kimberly). 1048:3-7.

Zanakis MF, Marmora M, Morgan M, Lewandoski MA. Application of the CV4 technique during objective measurement of the CRI [abstract]. *J Am Osteopath Assoc* 1996;96(9):552.

The Microscopic Anatomy of the Neural and Non-neural Brain Cells and Tracts

Baorto DM, Melledo W, Shelanski ML. Astrocyte process growth induction by action breakdown. *J Cell Biol* 1992;1 17(2):357-367.

Gabrion J, Peraidi S, Faivre-Bauman A, Klotz C, Ghandour MS, Paulin D, Assenmacher I, Tixier-Vidal A. Characterization of ependyrnal cells in hypothalamic and choroidal primary cultures. *Neuroscience* 1988;24(3):993-1007.

LaVail JH, Winston KR, Tish A. A method based on retrograde intraaxonal transport of protein for identification of cell bodies of origin of axons terminating within the CNS. *Brain Res* 1973;58:470-477.

Padmanabhan J, Shelanski ML. Process formation in astrocytes: Modulation of cytoskeletal proteins. *Neurochem Res* l998;23(3):377-384.

Maynard EA, Schultz RL, Pease DC. Electron microscopy of the vacular bed of rat cerebral cortex. *Am J Anat* 1957;100:409-433.

Maynard EA, Schultz RL, Pease DC. Electron microscopy of neuron and neuroglia of the cerebral cortex and corpus callosum. *Am J Anat* 1957;100-409-433.

Smith SJ. Do astrocytes process neural information? In Yu, ACH, Hertz L, Norenberg MD, Sykova E, Waxman SG. (Eds) *Prog Brain Res*, Vol 94. Elsevier Science Publishers; 1992.

Reciprocal Tension Membrane: The Dura Mater of the Brain and Spinal Cord

Asboe-Hansen G. *Connective tissue in health and disease.* Ejnar Munkagaarad, Copenhagen; 1954.

Gross J. Structural and chemical studies on connective tissue. In Bunim JJ, Ed. *Research and education in rheumatic diseases - Transaction of the 1st National Conference at the National Institute of Health.* Bethesda, Maryland. November 10, 1953.pp23-38.

Gross J, Schmitt FO. The structure of human skin collagen as studied with the electron microscope. *J Exp Med* 1948;88:555-568.

Hack GD, Koritzer RT, Robinson WL, Greenman PE. Anatomic relation between the rectus capitus posterior minor muscle and the dura mater. *Spine* 1995; 20(23)L 2484-2488.

Kerr CV. The role of fascia in osteopathy. *J Am Osteop Assoc* May 1936.

Kostopoulos DC, Keramidas G. Changes in elongation of falx cerebri during craniosacral therapy techniques applied on the skull of an embalmed cadaver. *J Cranialmandibular Practice* 1992;10:9-12.

Upledger JE, Vredovoogd JD. *Color Slide Set of theIntracranial Membrane System* Unity Center for Health, Education and Research; 1983

Cerebrospinal Fluid Hydraulics

Pressure Fluctuations and Tidal Movements of Cerebrospinal Fluid

Adolf RJ, Fukusumi H, Fowler NO. Origin of cerebrospinal fluid pulsations. *Am J Physiol* 1967;212:840-846.

Bering EA. Choroid plexus and arterial pulsation of cerebrospinal fluid: demonstration on the choroid plexuses as a cerebrospinal fluid pump. *AMA Arch Neurol Psych* 1955;73165-172.

Bering EA. Demonstration of the choroid plexuses as the generator of the force for flow of fluid and ventricular enlargement. *J Neruosurg* 1962;19:405-413.

Bering EA. Choroid plexus and arterial pulsation of cerebrospinal fluid: demonstration on the choroid plexuses as a cerebrospinal fluid pump. *AMA Arch Neurol Psych* 1955;73165-172.

Bering EA. Demonstration of the choroid plexuses as the generator of the force for flow of fluid and ventricular enlargement. *J Neruosurg* 1962;19:405-413.

Cardoso ER, Rowan JO, Galbraith S. Analysis of the cerebrospinal fluid pulse wave in intracranial pressure. *J Neurosurg* 1983;59:817-821.

Chu D, Levin DN, Alperin N. Assessment of the biomechanical state of intracranial tissues by dynamic MRI of cerebrospinal fluid pulsations: A phantom study. *Magn Reson Imaging* 1998;16(9);1043-1048.

Foltz EL, Aine C. Diagnosis of hydrocephalus by CSF pulse wave analysis: a clinical study. *Surg Neurol* 1981;15:283-293.

Michael DK. The cerebrospinal fluid: values for compliance and resistance to absorption. *J Am Osteopath Assoc* 1975;74:146-158.

Pelc NJ. Flow quantification and analysis methods. MRI Clinics of North America. 1995;3 (3):413-424.

Sibayan RQ, Begeman PC, King AI, Gurdjian ES, Thomas LM. Experimental hydrocephalus: ventricular cerebrospinal fluid pressure and waveform studies. *Arch Neurol* 1970;23:165-172.

Flow Dynamics and Pathways of Cerebrospinal Fluid

Antoni N. Pressure curves from the cerebrospinal fluid in animals. *Acta Medicus Scandinavia* 1946;170:439-462, Supplement.

Blackfan KD, Dandy WE. An experimental and clinical study of internal hydrocephalus. *J Am Med Assoc* 1913;61:2216

Bowsher D. *Cerebrospinal fluid dynamics in health and disease*. Charles C. Thomas, Springfield;1960.

Bradbury MWB, Cserr HF, Westrop RJ. Drainage of cerebral interstitial fluid into deep cervical lymph of the rabbit. *Am J Physiol* 1981;240(9):F329-F336.

Brierley JB. The penetration of particulate matter from the cerebrospinal fluids into the spinal ganglia, peripheral nerves, and the perivascular spaces of the central nervous system. *J Neurol Neurosurg Psychiatry* 1950;13:203-215.

Brierley JB, Field EJ. The connexions of the spinal sub-arachnoid space with the lymphatic system. *J Anat* (London) 1948;82:153-166.

Cushing H. The third circulation and its channels. *Lancet* 1925;2:251-857.

Drinker CK, Yoffey JM. *Lymphatics, lymph and lymphoid tissue*. Harvard University Press, Cambridge; 1941.

Du Bolay GH. Pulsatile movements in the CSF pathways. *Br J Radiol* 1966;39:255-262.

Du Bolay GH, O'Connell J, Currie J, Bostick T, Verity P. Further investigations on pulsatile movements in the cerebrospinal fluid pathways. *Acta Radiologica Diagnostica* 1972;13:496-523.

Elman R. Spinal arachnoid granulations with especial reference to the cerebrospinal fluid. *Johns Hopkins Hospital Bulletin*. 1923;34:99-104.

Enzmann DR, Pelc NJ. Cerebrospinal fluid flow measured by phase-contrast cine MR. *Am J Neuroradiology*1993;14:1301-1307.

Enzmann DR, Pelc NJ. Normal flow patterns of intracranial and spinal cerebrospinal fluid defined with phase-contrast cine MR imaging. *Radiology* 1991;178:467-474.

Erlingheuser RF. Circulation of the cerebrospinal fluid through the connective tissue system. *AAO Yearbook* 1959:77-87.

Faber WM. The nasal mucosa and the subarachnoid space. *Am J Anat* 62:121-148.

Feinberg DA. Modern concepts of brain motion and cerebrospinal fluid flow. *Radiology* 1992;185:630-632.

Feinberg DA, Mark AS. Human brain motion and cerebrospinal fluid circulation demonstrated with MR velocity imaging. *Radiology* 1987;163:793-799.

Fowler FD, Gammill JC, Martin J. Distribution of radioactive colloidal gold in cats. *J Neuropathol Exp Neurol* 1954;13:435-447.

Goldensohn E, Whitehead RW, Parry TM, Spencer JN, Grover FF, Draper WB. Studies on diffusion respiration and high concentration of carbon dioxide on cerebronspinal fluid pressure of anesthetized dogs. *Am J Phys* 1951;165:334-340.

Greitz D. Cerebrospinal fluid circulation and associated intracranial dynamics: A radiologic investigation using MR imaging and radionuclide cistrernography. *Acta Radiol* (Suppl) 1993;386:1-23.

Greitz D, Wirestam R, Franck A, Nordell B, Thomsen C, Stahlberg F. Pulsatile brain movement and associated hydrodynamics studied by magnetic resonance phase imaging. *Neuroradiology* 1992;34:370-380.

Gross J, Schmitt FO. The structure of human skin collagen as studied with the electron microscope. *J Exp Med* 1948;88:555-568.

Hassin GB. The cerebrospinal fluid pathways. *J Neuropathol Exp Neurol* 1947;6:172-176. Katzenelbogen S. *Cerebrospinal fluid and its relation to the blood*. The Johns Hopkins Press, Baltimore; 1935.

Kennedy JJ. Tubular structure of collagen fibrils. *Science* 1955;121:673-674.

Maier SE, Hardy CJ, Jolesz FA. Brain and cerebrospinal fluid motion: Real-time quantification with M-mode MR imaging. *Radiology* 1994;193:477-483.

O' Connell JEA. The vascular factor in intracranial pressure and the maintenance of the cerebrospinal fluid circulation. *Brain* 1943;66:204-228.

Pollay M, Davson H. The passage of certain substances out of the cerebrospinal fluid. *Brain* 1963;86:137-150.

Schmitt FO, Hall CE, Jakus MA. Electron microscope investigations of the structure of collagen. *J Cell Comp Physiol* 1943;20:11-33.

Simmons WJ. The abosorption of labeled erythrocytes from the subarachonoid space in rabbits. *Australian J Experimental Biology and Med Sci* 1953;31-77-83.

Somberg HM. The relation of the spinal sub-arachnoid and the perineural spaces. *J Neuropathol Exp Neurol* 1947;6:166-176.

Sweet WH, Locksley H. Formation, flow and resorption of cerebronspinal fluid in man. *Pro Soc Exp Biol and Med* 1953;84:397-402.

Weed LH. The cerebrospinal fluid. *Physiol Rev* 1922; 2:171-203.

Wyckoff RWG. The fine structure of connective tissues. In: Ragan C (ed) Josiah Macy, Jr. Foundation Conferences on Connective Tissues, no 3, pp 38-91; 1952.

Cerebrospinal Fluid Physiology

Davson H. *Physiology of the ocular and cerebrospinal fluids*. Little, Brown and Co., Boston; 1956.

Halliburton WD. Presidential address: The possible functions of the cerebrospinal fluid. *Proc R Soc Med*. London. 10:(Section of Neurology) 1-12. November, 1916.)

The Osseous-Articular Mechanism

Currey JD. The adaptation of bones to stress. *J Theor Biol* 1968;20:1-106.

Moss ML. Experimental alteration of sutural area morphology. *Anat Rec* 1957;127:569-589.

Moss ML. The pathogenesis of premature cranial synostosis in man. *Acta Anat* 1959;37:51-370.

Retzlaff EW, Roppel R, Becker RF, Mitchell FL Jr, Upledger J. Craniosacral mechanisms. *J Am Osteopath Assoc* 1976;76:123.

Osteokinematics or Arthrokinematics of the Skull Bones and Joints

Adams T, Heisey RS, Smith MC, Briner BJ. Parietal bone mobility in the anesthetized cat. *J Am Osteopath Assoc* 1992;92(5):599-622.

Baker EG. Alteration in width of maxillary arch and its relation to sutural movement of cranial bones. *J Am Osteopath Assoc* 1971;70:559-564.

Chan Han Sun, Liu Y King. The asymmetric response of a fluid filled spherical shell - a mathematical simulation of a glancing blow to the head. *J Biomech* 1974;7:43-59.

Heifitz MD, Weiss M. Detection of skull expansion with increased intracranial pressure. *J Neurosurg* 1981;55:811-812.

Heisey SR, Adams T. Role of cranial bone mobility in cranial compliance. *Neurosurgery* 1993;33(5):869-876.

Herring SW, Teng S, Huang X, Mucci RJ, Freeman J. Patterns of bone strain in the zygomatic arch. *Anatomical Rec* 1996;246-446-457.

Lewandoski MA, Drasby E, Morgan M, Zanakis MF. Kinematic system demonstrates cranial bone movement about the cranial sutures [abstract]. *J Am Osteopath Assoc* 1996;96(9):551.

Michael DK. A preliminary study of cranial bone movement in the squirrel monkey. *J Am Osteopath Assoc* 1975;74:866-869.

Michael DK, Retzlaff EW. A preliminary study of cranial bone movement in the squirrel monkey. *J Am Osteopath Assoc* 1975;74:866-880.

Retzlaff EW, Michael DK, Roppel RM. Cranial bone mobility. *J Am Osteopath Assoc* 1975;74:869-873.

Retzlaff EW, Michael DK, Roppel RM. Cranial bone mobility. *J Am Osteopath Assoc* 1975;74:138-146.

Rogers JS, Witt PL. The controversy of cranial bone motion. *JOSPT* 1997;26(2):95-102.

St Pierre N, Roppel R, Retzlaff E. The detection of relative movements of cranial bones. [abstract]. *J Am Osteopath Assoc* 1976;76:289.

Zanakis MF, Cebelenski RM, Dowling D, Lewandoski MA, Lauder CT, Kircher BA, Hallas BH. The cranial kinetogram: Objective quantification of cranial mobility in man [abstract]. *J Am Osteopath Assoc* 1994;94(9):761.

Zanakis MF, Zhao H, Schatzer M, Zaza W, Morgan R, Dyer D, Abboud A. Studies of the cranial rhythmic in man using a tilt table [abstract]. *J Am Osteopath Assoc* 1996;96(9):552.

Zanakis MF, Zaza W, Zhao H, Morgan R, Schatzer M. Objective measurement of the cranial rhythmic impulse in children [abstract]. *J Am Osteopath Assoc* 1996;96(9):552.

Zanakis MF, Morgan M, Storch I, Bele M, Carpentieri A, Germano J. Detailed study of cranial bone motion in man [abstract]. *J Am Osteopath Assoc* 1996;96(9):552.)

Zanakis MF, Marmora M, Banihashem M, Lewandoski MA, Kircher KT, Dowling D. Effect of observer participation on the dynamics of cranial mobility in man [abstract]. *J Am Osteopath Assoc* 1995;95(9).

Suture Structure and Function

Ashley-Montagu MF. Aging of the skull. *Am J Phys Anthropol* 1938;23:355-375.

Bolk L. On the premature obliteration of sutures in the human skull. *Am J Anat* 1915;17:495-523.

Bradley JP, Levine JP, Bleweti C, Krummel T, McCarthy JG, Longaker MT. Studies in cranial suture biology: *In vitro* cranial suture fusion. *Cleft Palate Craniofac J* 1996;3(2):150-156.
Buckland-Wright JC. The shock-absorbing effect of cranial sutures in certain mammals. *J Dent Res* (s) 1972;51:1241.

Burstone CJ, Shafer WG. Sutural expansion by controlled mechanical stress in the rat. *J Dent Res* 1959;38:534-540.

Cohen MM. Sutural biology and the correlates of craniosynostosis. *Am J Med Genet* 1993;47:581-616.

Cooper RR, Misol S. Tendon and ligament insertion. *J Bone Joint Surg* 1970;52-A:1-20.

Diamant J, et al. Collagen: ultra structure and its relation to mechanical properties as a function of aging. *Proc R Soc* London 1972;180:293-315.

Dolan KJ. Cranial suture closure in two species of South American monkeys. *Am J Phys Anthrop* 1971;35:109-118.

Giblin N, Alley A. Studies in skull growth. Coronal suture fixation. *Anat Rec* 1944;88:143-153.

Herring SE. Sutures - a tool in functional cranial analysis. *Acta Anat* 1972;83:222-247.

Hubbard RB. Flexure of layered cranial bone. *J Biomech* 1971;4-251-263.

Hubbard RB, Melvin JW, Barodawala IT. Flexure of cranial sutures. *J Biomech* 1971;4:491-496.

Hurrell DJ. The nerve supply of bone. *J Anat* 1937;72:54-61.

Isotupa K, Koski K, Makinen L. Changing architecture of growing cranial bones at sutures as revealed by vital staining with Alizarin Red S in the rabbit. *Am J Phys Anthropol* 1965;23:19-22.

Jaslow CR. Mechanical properties of cranial sutures. *J Biomech* 1990;23(4):313-321.

Jones L, Retzlaff E, Mitchell FL Jr, Upledger J, Walsh J. Significance of nerve fibers interconnecting cranial suture vasculature, the superior sagittal sinus, and the third ventricle. *J Am Osteopath Assoc* 1982;82:113.

Jones SJ. Secretory territories and rate of matrix production of osteoblasts. *Calc Tiss Res* 1974;14:309-315.

Khouw FE, Goldhaber P. Changes in vasculature of the periodontium associated with tooth movement in the rhesus monkey and dog. *Arch Oral Biol* 1970;15:1125-1132.

Kokich VG. Age changes in the human frontozygomatic suture from 20 to 95 years. *Am J Orthodont* 1976;69:411-430.

Kokich VG, Shapiro PA, Moffett BC, Retzlaff EW. Craniofacial sutures. *Aging in nonhuman primates*. New York: Van Nostrand Reinhold, pp 356-368, 1979.

Koskinen L, Isotupa K, Koski K. A note on craniofacial sutural growth. *Am J Phys Anthropol* 1976;45:511-516.

Latham RA. The sliding of cranial bones at sutural surfaces during growth. *J Anat* 1968;103:593.

Latham RA, Burston WR. The postnatal patterns of growth at the sutures of the human skull. *Dent Practit* 1966;17:61-67.

Lin KY, Nolen AA, Gampper TJ, Jane JA, Opperman LA, Ogle RC. Elevated levels of transforming growth factors Beta 2 and Beta 3 in lambdoid sutures from children with persistent plagiocephaly. *Cleft Palate Craniofac J* 1997;34(4):331-337.

Madeline LA, Elster AD. Suture closure in the human chondrocranium: CT assessment. *Radiology* 1995;196:747-56

Magoun H. New knowledge of the skull. *J. Amer. Osteopath Assoc* 1973;73, 250/11-252/14.

Markens LS, Oudhof HAJ. Morphological changes in the coronal suture after replantation. *Acta Anat* 1980;107:289-296.

McDowell EM, Trump BF. Histological fixatives suitable for diagnostic light and electron microscopy. *Arch Pathol Lab Med* 1976;100:405-414.

Moss ML. Fusion of the frontal suture in the rat. *Am J Anat* 1958;102:141-165.

Moss ML. Inhibition and stimulation of sutural fusion in the rat calvaria. *Anat Rec* 1960;136:457-467.

Opperman LA, Passarelli RW, Morgan EP, Reintjes M, Ogle RC. Cranial sutures require tissue interactions with dura mater to resist osseous obliteration in vitro. *J Bone Miner Res* 1995;10:1978-1987.

Opperman LA, Sweeney TM, Redmon J, Persing JA, Ogle RC. Tissue interactions with underlying dura mater inhibit osseous obliteration of developing cranial sutures. *Developmental Dynamics* 1993;1 98:312-322.

Oudhof HAJ. Sutural growth. *Acta Anatom* 1982;112:58-68.

Persson M. *Odontologisk Revy.* CWK Gleerup (Lund) 1973;24:1-146.

Popevec JP, Biggert TP, Retzlaff EW. Histological techniques for cranial bone studies. *J Am Osteopath Assoc* 1976;75:606-607.

Pritchard JJ. Repair of fractures of the parietal bone in rats. *J Anat* 1946;80:55-60.

Quigley MB. Perforating (Sharpey's) fibers of the periodontal ligament and bone. *Ala J Med Sci* 1970;7:336-342.

Retzlaff EW, Jones L, Mitchell FL Jr, Upledger J. Possible autonomic innervation of cranial sutures of primates and other mammals [abstract]. *Brain Research* 1973;58:470-477.

Retzlaff EW, Jones L, Mitchell FL Jr, Upledger J, Walsh J. Possible autonomic innervation of cranial sutures of primates and other mammals. *Anat Rec* 1982;202:156A.)

Retzlaff EW, Michael D, Roppel RM, Mitchell FL Jr. The structures of cranial bone sutures. *J Am Osteopath Assoc* 1976;75:106-107,607-608.

Retzlaff EW, Mitchell FL Jr, Eds. *The Cranium and Its Sutures*. Berlin, Heidelberg, N.Y. Springer-Verlag. 1987.

Retzlaff EW, Mitchell FL Jr, Upledger J. Nerve fibers present within the parietal cranial bones of primates. *J Am Osteopath Assoc* 1981;80:753-754.

Retzlaff EW, Upledger J, Mitchell FL Jr, et al. Aging of cranial sutures in humans. *Anat Rec* 1979;193:663.

Retzlaff EW, Mitchell FL Jr, Upledger J, Biggert T. Aging of cranial sutures in *Macaca nemestrina*. *Anat Rec* 1978;190:52.

Retzlaff EW, Mitchell FL Jr, Upledger J, Biggert T. Nerve fibers and endings in cranial sutures. *J Am Osteopath Assoc* 1978;77:100-101.

Retzlaff EW, Mitchell FL Jr, Upledger J, Biggert T. Sutural collagenous bundles and their innervation in *Saimiri sciureus*. *Anat Rec* 1977;187:692.

Retzlaff EW, Mitchell FL Jr, Upledger J, Vredevoogd J, Walsh J. Neurovascular mechanisms in cranial sutures [abstract]. *J Am Osteopath Assoc* 1980;80-218-219.

Retzlaff EW, Mitchell FL Jr, Upledger J, Vredevoogd J, Walsh J. Nerve fibers present within the parietal cranial bones of primates [abstract]. *J Am Osteopath Assoc* 1981;80(11):753-754.

Retzlaff EW, Mitchell FL Jr, Upledger J, Vredevoogd J, Walsh J. Light and scanning microscopy of nerve fibers within the parietal bones of primates. *Anat Rec* 1981;199:21.)

Retzlaff EW, Mitchell FL Jr, Walsh J, Wendecker A. The role of the cranial ligaments in primates. *Anat Rec* 1985;211:159-160.

Retzlaff EW, Upledger J, Mitchell FL Jr, Walsh J, Vredevoogd J. Age related changes in human cranial sutures. 23rd Annual Am Osteopath Assoc, res conv, p 14; 1979.

Retzlaff EW, Upledger J, Mitchell FL Jr, Walsh J. Aging of cranial sutures in humans. [abstract]. *Anat Rec* 1979;193:663.

Retzlaff EW, Upledger JE, Vredevoogd JD. Cranial suture morphology. Second World Congress on Pain, Int Assoc Study Pain 1:68 1978.

Retzlaff EW, Walsh J, Mitchell FL Jr, Vredevoogd J. Histological detail of cranial sutures as seen in plastic embedded specimens [abstract]. *Anat Rec* 1984;198-145A.

Retzlaff EW, Walsh J, Mitchell FL Jr, Vredevoogd J. Histological detail of cranial sutures as seen in plastic embedded specimens. *Anat Rec* 1984;208:145A.

Retzlaff EW, Walsh J, Mitchell FL Jr, Vredevoogd J. Structure of cranial sutures in plastic embedded tissues. *J Am Osteopath Assoc* 1984;84:212.

Robinson RA, Watson ML. Electron microscopy of bone. Transactions of the fifth conference. New York: Josiah Macy, Jr., Foundation, p 72; 1953.

Sevier AC, Munger BL. A silver method for paraffin sections of neural tissue. *J Neuropath Exp Neurol* 1965;24:130-135.

Smith HG, McKeown M. Experimental alteration of the coronal sutural area: a histological and quantitative microscopic assessment. *J Anat* 1974;118:543-559.

Sperino G. *Anatomia Umana*, (transl.), 1981;vol 1, pp 202-203.

Todd WT, Lyon DW Jr. Endocranial suture closure - Its progress and age relationship: Part I. Adult males of white stock. *Am J Phys Anthropol* 1924;7(3):325-384.

Todd WT, Lyon DW Jr. Cranial suture closure - Its progress and age relationship: Part II. - Ectocranial closure in adult males of white stock. *Am J Phys Anthropol* 1925;8(1):23-45.

Todd WT, Lyon DW Jr. Cranial suture closure - Its progress and age relationship: Part III. - Endocranial closure in adult males of negro stock. *Am J Phys Anthropol* 1925;8(1):47-71.

Todd WT, Lyon DW Jr. Suture closure - Its progress and age relationship: Part IV. - Ectocranial closure in males of negro stock. *Am J Phys Anthropol* 1925;8(2):149-168.

Verhuist J, Onghena P. Cranial suture closing in *Homo sapiens:* evidence for circaseptennian periodicity. *Ann of Hum Biol* 1997;24(2):141-156.

Vis JH. Histological investigation into the attachment of tendons and ligaments to the mammalian skeleton. *Proc Acad Sci Amst* (Series C) 1957;60:147-157.

Embryology, Growth, Development, and Aging of the Skull Bones and Sutures

Brodie AG. On the growth pattern of the human head from the third month to the eighth year of life. *Am J Anat* 1941;68:209-262.

Clark LC Jr. Discussion (page 668) of: Evidence for the participation of serotonin in mental processes, by DW Wooley and EN Shaw. *Ann N Y Acad Sci* 1957;66:649-667.

Cleall JF, et al. Growth of the craniofacial complex in the rat. *Am J Orthod* 1974;60:368-381.

Cohen MM Jr, Walker GF, Phillips C. A morphometric analysis of the craniofacial configuration in achondroplasia. *J Craniofacial Genet Dev Biol* (Suppl I), 1985;pp 139-155.

Dovesmith EE. The growing skull and the injured child. *AAO Yearbook* 1967;34-39.

Duterloo HS, Enlow DH. A comparative study of cranial growth in Homo and Macaca. *Am J Anat* 1970;7:357-368.

Giblin N, Alley A. Studies in skull growth. Coronal suture fixation. *Anat Rec* 1944;88:143-153.

Hecht JT, et al. Computerized tomography of the foramen magnum: achondroplastic values compared to normal standards. *Am J Med Genet* 1985;20:55-360.

Horton WA, Rotter JJ, Rimoin DL, Scott Cl Jr, Hall JG. Standard growth curves for achondroplasia. *J Pediatr* 1978;93 (Suppl 3):435-438.

Hoyte DAN. Experimental investigations of skull morphology and growth. *Int Rev Gen Exper Zool* 1966;2:345-407.

Kokich VG. Age changes in the human frontozygomatic suture from 20 to 95 years. *Am J Orthodont* 1976;69:411-430.

Kokich VG, Shapiro PA, Moffett BC, Retzlaff EW. Craniofacial sutures. *Aging in nonhuman primates*. New York: Van Nostrand Reinhold, pp 356-368, 1979.

Koski K. Cranial growth centers: facts of fallacies? *Am J Orthodont Oral Surg* 1968;54:566-583.

Koskinen L, Isotupa K, Koski K. A note on craniofacial sutural growth. *Am J Phys Anthropol* 1976;45:511-516.

Latham RA. The sliding of cranial bones at sutural surfaces during growth. *J Anat* 1968;103:593.

Madeline LA, Elster AD. Suture closure in the human chondrocranium: CT assessment. *Radiology* 1995;196:747-56

Moss ML, Baer MI. Differential growth of the rat skull. *Growth* 1956;20:107-120.

Moss ML, Young RW. A functional approach to craniology. *Am J Phys Anthropol* 1960;18:281-292.

Opperman LA, Passarelli RW, Morgan EP, Reintjes M, Ogle RC. Cranial sutures require tissue interactions with dura mater to resist osseous obliteration in vitro. *J Bone Miner Res* 1995;10:1978-1987.

Opperman LA, Sweeney TM, Redmon J, Persing JA, Ogle RC. Tissue interactions with underlying dura mater inhibit osseous obliteration of developing cranial sutures. *Developmental Dynamics* 1993;1 98:312-322.

Oudhof HAJ. Sutural growth. *Acta Anatom* 1982;112:58-68.

Persson M. *Closure of facial sutures: a preliminary report*. Transactions of the European Orthodontic Society; 1976.

Persson M. *Odontologisk Revy*. CWK Gleerup (Lund) 1973;24:1-146.

Persson M, Thilander B. Palatal suture closure in man from 15 to 35 years of age. *Am J Orthod* 1977;72:42-52.

Pritchard JJ, Scott JH, Girgis FG. The structure and development of cranial and facial sutures. *J Anat* 1956;90:73-86.

Retzlaff EW, Mitchell FL Jr, Eds. *The Cranium and Its Sutures*. Berlin, Heidelberg, New York. Springer-Verlag. 1987

Retzlaff EW, Upledger J, Mitchell FL Jr, et al. Aging of cranial sutures in humans. *Anat Rec* 1979;193:663.

Retzlaff EW, Mitchell FL Jr, Upledger J, Biggert T. Aging of cranial sutures in *Macaca nemestrina*. *Anat Rec* 1978;190:52.

Retzlaff EW, Upledger J, Mitchell FL Jr, Walsh J, Vredevoogd J. Age related changes in human cranial sutures. 23rd Annual Am Osteopath Assoc, res conv, p 14; 1979.

Revelo B, Fishman LS. Maturational evaluation of ossification of the midpalatal suture. *Am J Orthod Dentofac Orthop* 1994;105:288-92.

Scott JH. Growth at facial sutures. *Am J Orthod* 1956;42:381-387.

Simmons DR, Peyton WT. Premature closure of the cranial sutures. *J Pediatr* 1947;31:528-547.

Singer R. Estimation of age from cranial suture closure - a report on its unreliability. *J Forens Med* 1953;1:1 52-59.

Slavkin HC. Developmental craniofacial biology. Philadelphia: Lea and Febiger, pp 1-464; 1979.

Todorov AB, Scott CI Jr, Warren AE, Leper JD. Developmental screening tests in achondroplastic children. *Am J Med Genet* 1981;9:19- 23.

Young RW. The influence of cranial contents on postnatal growth of the skull in the rat. *Am J Anat* 1959;105:383-415.

Involvement of the Sacrum in the Craniosacral System

Levy LM, DiChiro G, McCullough DC, et al. Fixed spinal cord: Diagnosis with MR imaging. *Radiology* 1988;169:773-778.

Mitchell FL Jr. Roentgenographic measurement of sacroiliac respiratory movement. *J Am Osteopath Assoc* 1970;69:81-82.

Mitchell FL Jr. Voluntary and involuntary respiration and the craniosacral mechanism. *Osteopath Ann* 1977;5:52-59. Reprinted in *Collected osteopathic papers*, M Tilley (ed), New York: Insight Publishing; 1979.

Mitchell FL Jr, Pruzzo NA. Investigation of voluntary and primary respiratory mechanisms. *J Am Osteopath Assoc* 1970;70:149-153.

Pruzzo NA. Lateral double-exposure technique and associated principles in examination of the lumbar spine. *The DO* 1970;10:20-24.

Pruzzo NA. Lateral lumbar spine double-exposure technique and associated principles. *J Am Osteopath Assoc* 1970;69:84-86.

Weisl H. The articular surfaces of the sacro-iliac joint and their relation to the movements of the sacrum. *Acta Anat* 1954;22:1-14.

Weisl H. The movements of the sacro-iliac joint. *Acta Anat* 1955;23:80-91.

Zanakis MF, Dimeo J, Madonna S, Morgan M, Drasby E. Objective measurement of the CRI with manipulation and palpation of the sacrum [abstract]. *J Am Osteopath Assoc* 1996;96(9):551.

Clinical Research in Cranial Osteopathy

Bertelsen TI. *The premature synostosis of the cranial sutures*. Copenhagen: Ejnar Munksgaard; 1958.

Trauma Management Using Cranial Osteopathy

Anderson JM, Kaokan MS, Felsenthal G. Brain injury obscured by chronic pain: a preliminary quantitative probe of beat to beat cardiovascular control. *Science* 1981;213:220

Arbuckle BE. *The selected writings of Beryl E. Arbuckle, DO, FACOP*. National Osteopathic Institute and Cerebral Palsy Foundation; 1977.

Arbuckle BE. Subclinical signs of trauma. *J Am Osteopath Assoc* 1958;58:160-166.

Becker RE. Craniosacral trauma in the adult. *Osteopath Ann* 1976;213-225.

Binder L. Presisting sypmtoms after mild head injury: a review of post concussive syndrome, *J. Clin Exp Neuropsychol* 1986;8:4

Esselman PC, Uomoto JM. Traumatic brain injury and chronic pain: differential types and rates by head injury severity. *Arch Phys Med Rehabil* 1991;72:774

Frymann VM. The trauma of birth. *Osteopath Ann* 1976;4:22-31.

Horn LJ. Post-concussive headache. *Physical medicine and rehabilitation: State of the art reviews*. 1992;6:69-78

Lippincott HA. Case of birth injury or cranial trauma. *AAO Yearbook* 1948:158.

Magoun HI Sr. Trauma: a neglected cause of cephalgia. *J Am Osteopath Assoc* 1975;74:88-98.

Miyasaka-Hiraga J, Tanne K, Nakamura S. Finite element analysis for stresses in the craniofacial sutures produced by maxillary protraction forces applied at the upper canines. *Br J of Orthod* 1994;21(4):343-248.

Zasler ND. Neuromedical diagnosis and management of post-concussive disorders. *Physical medicine and rehabilitation: state of the art reviews* 1992;6:33-67

Cranial Osteopathy Applications to Pediatrics

Arbuckle BE. The cranial aspect of emergencies of the newborn. *J Am Osteopath Assoc* 1948;47:507-511.

Arbuckle BE. Scoliosis capitis. *J Am Osteopath Assoc* 1971;70:559-564.

Austin JJM, Gooding CA. Roentgenographic measurement of skull size in children. *Radiology* 1971;99:641-646.

Degenhardt BF, Kuchera ML. The prevalence of cranial dysfunction in children with a history of otits media from kindergarten to third grade. *J Am Osteopath Assoc* 1994;94:754

Dobbing J, Sands J. Vulnerability of developing brain. IX. The effect of nutritional growth retardation on the timing of the brain growth-spurt. *Biol Neonate* 1971;19:63-378.

Dovesmith EE. The growing skull and the injured child. *AAO Yearbook* 1967;34-39.

Easa D, Tran A, Bingham W. Noninvasive intracranial pressure measurement in the newborn: an alternate method. *Am J Dis Child* 1983;137:332-335.

Frymann VM, Carney RE, Springall P. Effect of osteopathic medical management on neurological development in children. *J Am Osteopath Assoc* 1966;65:1059-1075

Frymann VM. Learning difficulties of children viewed in the light of the osteopathic concept. *J Am Osteopath Assoc* 1976;6-61.

Frymann VM. Relation of disturbances of craniosacral mechanisms to symptomatology of the newborn: study of 1250 infants. *J Am Osteopath Assoc* 1966;65:1059-1075.

Frymann VM. The trauma of birth. *Osteopath Ann* 1976;4:22-31.

Lippincott RC. Interesting cases of infantile paralysis. *AAO Yearbook* 1947:109.

Magoun HI Sr. Idiopathic adolescent spinal scoliosis: a reasonable etiology. *The DO* 1973;13:6-13.

Mitchell FL Jr, Brooks HD, Bunnel WB. You can help children with scoliosis. *Patient Care* 1981;April 30.

Peters JE, Romine JS, Dykman RA. A special neurological examination of children with learning disabilities. *Dev Med Child Neurol* 1975;1563-78.

Rosenberg JG, Weller GM. Minor physical anomalies and academic performance in young schoolchildren. *Dev Med Child Neurol* 1973;15:131-135.

Upledger JE. The relationship between craniosacral examination findings and the problems of special education students. Am Osteopath Assoc Res Conf. 1978.

Upledger JE. The relationship of craniosacral examination findings in grade school children with developmental problems. *JAOA* 1978;77:760-776.

Upledger JE, Vredevoogd JD, Retzlaff EW, Raynesford AK, Howard TF. Autistic children: preliminary physiological, structural and craniosacral evaluations. 23rd Ann Am Osteopath Assoc Res Conv, p 34. 1979.

Walsh P, Logan WJ. Continuous and intermittent measurement of intracranial pressure by Ladd monitor. *J Pediatrics* 1983;102(3):439-442.

Woods RH. Structural normalization in infants and children with particular reference to disturbances of the central nervous system. *J Am Osteopath Assoc* 1973;72:81-86.

Cranial Osteopathy Palpatory Skills

Armitage P. Diagnostic touch: its principles and applications. Society of Osteopaths, Cranial Group. *Newsletter* II 1981;7-12.

Becker RE. Diagnostic touch: its principles and application, part IV. *AAO Yearbook* 1965;165-177.

Drengler KE, King HH. Inter-examiner reliability of palpatory diagnosis of the cranium [abstract] *J Am Osteopath Assoc* 1998;98(7):387.

Frymann VM. Palpation: part I, II, III, & IV, its study in the workshop. *AAO Yearbook* 1963;16-31.

Greenman PE. Roentgen findings in the craniosacral mechanism. *J Am Osteopath Assoc* 1970;70:1-12.

Kaltenbom FM. *Manual therapy for the extremity joints specialized techniques: tests and joint-mobilization.* Oslo: Olaf Norlis Bokhandel, pp 1-142; 1976.

Lay EM. Teaching cranial therapy to undergraduates. *Osteopath Ann* 1976;4:62-72.

Mitchell FL Jr. The training and measurement of sensory literacy in relation to osteopathic structural and palpatory diagnosis. *J Am Osteopath Assoc* 1976;75:874-884.

Mitchell FL Jr, Roppel RM, St Pierre N. Accuracy and perceptual decisional delay in motion perception. *J Am Osteopath Assoc* 1978;78:149.

Mitchell FL Jr, Roppel RM, St. Pierre N. Accuracy and perceptual decisional delay in motion perception [abstract]. *J Am Osteopath Assoc* 1978;77:475.

Page-Echols W, Page-Echols W, Retzlaff E, Mitchell FL Jr. Respiratory kinematics of ribs and sacrum: natural history and physical diagnosis interrater reliability. *J Am Osteopath Assoc* 1982;82:112.

Roppel RM, St Pierre N, Mitchell FL Jr. Measurement of accuracy in bimanual perception of motion. *J Am Osteopath Assoc* 1978;77:475.

Salter MVV, Hicks JL. ATP causes release of intracellular Ca^{2+} via the phospholipase Cbeta/IP_3 pathway in astrocytes from the dorsal spinal cord. *J Neurosci* 1995;15(4):2961-2971.

Upledger JE. The reproducibility of craniosacral examination findings: A statistical analysis. *J Am Osteopath Assoc* 1977;76:890-899.

Upledger JE, et al. The reproducibility of craniosacral examination findings: a statistical analysis. *J Am Osteopath Assoc* 1977;76:67-76.

Upledger JE, Karni S. Bioelectric and strain measurements during cranial manipulation. *J Am Osteopath Assoc* 1978;77:476.

Upledger JE, Karni S. Mechano-electric patterns during craniosacral osteopathic diagnosis and treatment. *J Am Osteo-path Assoc* 1979;78:782-791.

Wirth-Pattullo V, Hayes KVV. Interrater reliability of cranialsacral rate measurements and their relationship with subjects' and examiners' heart and respiratory rate measurements, *Phys Ther* 1994;74(10):908-916.

Woods JM, Woods RH. A physical finding related to psychiatric disorders. *J Am Osteopath Assoc* 1961;60:988-993.

New Techniques to Examine and Treat the Craniosacral System

Bilkey WJ. Cranial suture manipulation in the treatment of torticollis. *J Manual Med* 1992;(6):212-214.

Blood SD. The craniosacral mechanism and the temporomandibular joint. *J Am Osteopath Assoc* 1986;86:512-519.

Blum CL. Cranial therapeutic approach to cranial nerve entrapment Part I: Cranial nerves III, IV, and VI. *ACA J Chiropract* 1988;22(7);63-67.

Blum CL. Cranial therapeutic approach to cranial nerve entrapment Part II: Cranial never VII. *ACA J Chiropract* 1990;27(7):108.

Blum CL, Curl DD. The relationship between sacro-occipital technique and sphenobasilar balance. Part one: The key continuities. *Chiropractic Technique* 1988; 10(3);95-99.

Blum CL, Curl DD. The relationship between sacro-occipital technique and sphenobasilar balance. Part two: Sphenobasilar strain stacking. *Chiropractic Technique* 1988; 10(3);101-109.

Brock M, Dietz H. Eds. *Intracranial pressure.* Springer-Verlag, New York; 1972.

Dufour G. The dysgnathogenic distress syndrome. *J Prosthet Dent* 1983;3:403-414.

Gehin A. *Atlas of manipulative technique of cranium and face.* Portland, OR: Eastland Press; 1985.

Gelb HL. Effective management of the craniomandibular syndrome. Chap. 11 pp 288-369. *Clinical management of head, neck and TMJ pain and dysfunction.* Philadelphia, PA: Saunders; 1977.

Greenman PE (ed). Concepts and mechanisms of neuromuscular functions. An international conference. Berlin, Heidelberg, New York, Tokyo: Springer Verlag; 1984.

Greenman PE, Mein EA, Andary M. Craniosacral manipulation. Physical Medicine and Rehabilitation Clinics of North America. 1996;7(4):877-896.

Hoover HV. Craniosacral therapy and the general practitioner. *AAO Yearbook,* 1969;pp 112-115.

Hussar CJ, Retzlaff EW, Mitchell FL Jr, Kalbfell JJ, Briner BJ. Combined osteopathic and dental treatment of cephalgia. *J Am Osteopath Assoc* 1985;85:605-606.

Lavitan S. The whiplash syndrome in the light of the craniosacral mechanisms. *J Clin Chiropract* 1977;2:28.

Lay EM. The osteopathic management of temporomandibular joint dysfunction. In: Harold Gelb (ed) *Clinical management of head, neck and TMJ pain and dysfunction.* Philadelphia: Saunders; 1977.

Lay EM. The osteopathic management of trigeminal neuralgia. *J Am Osteopath Assoc* 1975;74:55-71.

Lippincott HA. Basic principles of osteopathic technique. *AAO Yearbook* 1961:45.

Lippincott HA. Corrective technique for the sacrum. *AAO Yearbook* 1958:57.

Lippincott HA. Depressed sacrum *AAO Yearbook* 1965:206.

Lippincott HA. The osteopathic technique of Wm G Sutherland, DO. *AAO Yearbook* 1949;1. 1964; reprinted in *AAO Yearbook*, p138.

Lippincott HA. Respiratory technique developed by William G. Sutherland. *AAO Yearbook* 1948:31.

Lippincott RC. Cranial osteopathy. *AAO Yearbook* 1947; p103.

Lippincott RC. "Old timer's" osteopathy. *AAO Yearbook* 1943-44:24.

Miller HC. Head pain. *J Am Osteopath Assoc* 1972;72:135-143.

Mitchell FL Jr. Office management of acute torticollis. *Osteopath Ann 1974*;2:22-27.

Mitchell FL Jr, Mitchell PKG. *The muscle energy manual, Volume One: Concepts and mechanisms, the musculoskeletal screen, cervical region evaluation and treatment* (1995); *Volume Two: Evaluation and treatment of the thoracic spine, lumbar spine, and rib cage* (1998); *Volume Three* (est.1999 pub). East Lansing: MET Press.

Retzlaff EW, et al. The piriformis muscle syndrome. *J Am Osteopath Assoc* 1974;73:1-8.

Retzlaff EW, Furda A, Maynard M, Mitchell FL Jr. Differential biochemical diagnosis of back pain. *J Am Osteopath Assoc* 1984;84:217.

Retzlaff EW, Mitchell FL Jr, Eds. *The Cranium and Its Sutures*. Berlin, Heidelberg, New York. Springer-Verlag. 1987.

Royder JO. Structural influences in temporomandibular joint pain and dysfunction. *Clinical Management of Head, Neck and TMJ Pain and Dysfunction: A Multidisciplinary Approach to Diagnosis and Treatment*, edited by Harold Gelb, DDS, Philadelphia, W.B. Saunders Co., 1985.

Speransky AD. *A basis for the theory of medicine*. International Publishers, New York; 1043.

Spiering N. Manipulative procedures ftilized during obstetrical delivery. *J Am Osteopath Assoc* 1980;80:219.

Sutherland WG. Philosophy of osteopathy; and; its application by the cranial concept. Transcript of lecture by WG Sutherland. Second annual convention of the Osteopathic Cranial Association, July 18, 1948. Boston, Mass; 1948. Sperino G. *Anatomia Umana*, (transl.), 1981;vol 1, pp 202-203.

Travell J. The myofascial genesis of pain. *Postgrad Med* 1952;11:425-434.

Upledger JE. The goal of therapy. *The DO* 1978;18:112-117.

Upledger JE. Integration of acupuncture and manipulation. *Osteopath Med* 1977;2:19.

Upledger JE, Retzlaff EW, Vredevoogd JD. Diagnosis and treatment of temporoparietal suture head pain. *Osteopath Med* 1978;3:19-26.

The Clinical Effects of Cranial Somatic Dysfunction

Blum CL. The effect of movement, stress and mechanoelectric activity within the cranial matrix. *Int J Orthodontics* 1987;25(1-2);1-8.

Blum CL. Spinal/cranial manipulative therapy and tinnitus: A case history. *Chiropractic Technique* 1988;10(4):163-167.

Greenman PE, McPartland JM. Cranial findings and iatrogenesis from craniosacral manipulation in patients with traumatic brain syndrome. *J Am Osteopath Assoc* 1995;95:182-191

Magoun HI Sr. The cranial concept in general practice. *Osteopath Ann* 1976;4:32-42.

Magoun HI Sr. Dental equilibration and osteopathy. *J Am Osteopath Assoc* 1975;74:981-990.

Magoun HI Sr. The dental search for a common denominator in craniocervical pain and dysfunction. *J Am Osteopath Assoc* 1979;78:1-6.

Magoun HI Sr. Entrapment neuropathy in the cranium. *J Am Osteopath Assoc* 1968;67:643-652.

Magoun HI Sr. Entrapment neuropathy of the central nervous system, Part II. cranial nerves I-IV, VI-VIII, XII. *J Am Osteopath Assoc* 1968;67:779-787.

Magoun HI Sr. Entrapment neuropathy of the central nervous system, Part III. cranial nerves V, IX, X, XI. *J Am Osteopath Assoc* 1968;67:889-899.

Magoun HI Sr. Osteopathic approach to dental enigmas. *J Am Osteopath Assoc* 1962;62:110-118.

Magoun HI Sr. A pertinent approach to pituitary pathology. *The DO* 1971;11:133-141.

Magoun HI Sr. The temporal bone: trouble maker in the head. *J Am Osteopath Assoc* 1974;73:825-835.

Magoun HI Sr. Whiplash injury: a greater lesion complex. *J Am Osteopath Assoc* 1964;63:524-535.

Mathews MO. Personal monograph entitled *The ecology of pain*. 1979;32 pages.

Mitchell FL Jr. Toward a definition of somatic dysfunction. *Osteopath Ann* 1980;7:12-25. Also reprinted in *J Soc Osteopaths*, Maidstone, Kent, UK; 1980.

Morey LW Jr. Uses Of cranial manipulative therapy. *Osteopath Med* 1978;3:43-52.

Rein G. Biological effects of quantum fields and their role in the natural healing process. The Center for Frontier Sciences 1998;7(l):16-23.

Retzlaff EW. Reflex mechanisms and their clinical significance. *Osteopath Ann* 1974;2:40-43.

Retzlaff EW. Structural and functional concepts of craniosacral mechanisms. In: Philip E. Greenman (ed) *Concepts and mechanisms of neuromuscular functions*. Springer-Verlag, Berlin Heidelberg New York, pp 111-128. 1980.

Retzlaff EW, Mitchell FL Jr, Hussar C, Walsh J. The role of the Vth cranial nerve in the TMJ syndrome. *Anat Rec* 1983;205:161A.

Retzlaff EW, Mitchell FL Jr, Hussar C, Walsh J. The role of the proprioprioceptive component of the fifth nerve in the temporomandibular joint syndrome. 1983.

Retzlaff EW, Mitchell FL Jr, Upledger J. Efficacy of cranial sacral manipulation: the physiological mechanism of the cranial sutures. *J Soc Osteopath* 1982-83;12:8-12.

Upledger JE, Retzlaff EW. Cranial suture pain. Second World Congress on Pain. *Int Assoc Study Pain*, vol 1, p 120. 1978.

Upledger JE, Vredevoogd JD. Management of autogenic headache. *Osteopath Ann* 1979;7:21 30.

White WK, White JE, Baldt G. The relation of the craniofacial bones to specific somatic dysfunctions: a clinical study of the effects of manipulation. *J Am Osteopath Assoc* 1985(85):603-604.

Pulsatile Phenomena Not Related to Arterial Pulses or Cardiac Rhythms

Instrumental Detection and Measurement of the CRI and Other Pulses

Cope M, Dunlap SH. Calibration of a device for the measurment of the Cranial Rhythmic Impulse. J. Am. Osteopath Assoc 1983;83(1):60/132

Frymann VM. A study of the rhythmic motions of the living cranium. *J Am Osteopath Assoc* 1971;70:1-18.

Hamer J, Alberti E, Hoyer S, Wiedemann K. Influence of systemic and cerebral vascular factors on the cerebrospinal fluid pulse waves. *J Neurosurg* 1977;46:36-45.

Lockwood MD, Degenhardt BF. Cycle-to-cycle variability attributed to the primary respiratory mechanism. *J Am Osteopath Assoc* 1998;3:137-141.

Moskolenko YE. The phenomenology and mechanisms of cranial bone fluctuations. Paper presented at Proceedings of 1 Russian Symposium. St. Petersburg, Russia, May 27-29, 1998.

Moskolenko YE, Kravchenko T, Chervotok A, Shalaev V. Application of bio-impedence for the study of hemo and CSF dynamics in the human head. Proceedings of the X International Conference on Electrical Bio-Impdenece. International Committee for Promotion of Research in Bio-Impedence European Uniton, Barcelona, Spain, 1988.

Moskolenko YE, Kravchenko T, Chervotok A, Sharapov K. Bioengineering support of the cranial osteopathy treatment. Med Biol Eng Comput. 1995:34 (Suppl 1, Part 2: 185-186).

Moskolenko YE, Wainshtein G, Kravchenko T, Vorobjev, Semernia V. Informational meaning of local brain electrical impedence pulse fluctuation. Proceedings of the IX International Conference on Electrical Bio-Impedence. Gersing E, Schaefed M. Eds. Goltze Drunck, Gottingen, German, 1995:87-90.

Myers R. Measurement of small rhythmic motions around the human cranium *in vivo. Australian J of Osteopathy* 1998;9(2):6-13.

Retzlaff EW, Michael DK, Roppel RM. Cranial bone mobility. *J Am Osteopath Assoc* 1975;74:869-873.

Retzlaff EW, Michael DK, Roppel RM. Cranial bone mobility. *J Am Osteopath Assoc* 1975;74:138-146

Tettambel M. Recording of the cranial rhythmic impulse. *J Am Osteopath Assoc* 1978;78:149.

Tettambel M, Cicora RA, Lay EM. Recording of the cranial rhythmic impulse [abstract]. *J Am Osteopath Assoc* 1978;78:149.

Urayama K. Origin of lumbar cerebrospinal fluid pulse wave. *Spine* 1994;19(4):441-445.

Wallace WK, Avant WS, McKinney WM, Thurstone FL. Ultrasonic techniques for measuring intracranial pulsations. *Neurology* 1966;16:380-382.

Zanakis MF, Cebelenski RM, Dowling D, Lewandoski MA, Lauder CT, Kircher BA, Hallas BH. The cranial kinetogram: Objective quantification of cranial mobility in man [abstract]. *J Am Osteopath Assoc* 1994;94(9):761.

Zanakis MF, Dimeo J, Madonna S, Morgan M, Drasby E. Objective measurement of the CRI with manipulation and palpation of the sacrum [abstract]. *J Am Osteopath Assoc* 1996;96(9):551.

Zanakis MF, Marmora M, Morgan M, Lewandoski MA. Application of the CV4 technique during objective measurement of the CRI [abstract]. *J Am Osteopath Assoc* 1996;96(9):552.

Clinical Correlations with Impulses

Karni Z, Upledger JE, Mizrahi J, Heller L, Becker E, Najenson T. Examination of the cranial rhythm in long-standing coma and chronic neurologic cases. In Upledger JE, Vredevoogd JD. *Craniosacral Therapy.* Eastland Press, Seattle. 1983;275-281.

Norton JM. A tissue pressure model for palpatory perception of the cranial rhythmic impulse. *J Am Osteopath Assoc* 1991;91(10):975-994.

Pulmocardiovascular Research Related to Cranial Osteopathy

Akselrod S, Gordon D, Ubel FA, et al. Powers spectrum analysis of heart rate fluctuation: a quantitative probe of beat to beat cardiovascular control. *Science* 1981;213:220

Diehl RR, Diehl B, Sitzer M, et al. Spontaneous oscillations in cerebral blood flow velocity in normal humans and in patients with carotid artery disease. *Neurosci Lett* 1991;127:54

Grossman P. Respiration, stress, and cardiovascular function. *Psychophysiology* 1983;20:284

Kleiger RE, Miller JP, Bigger JT, et al. Decreased heart rate variability and its association with increased mortality after acute myocardial infarction. *Am J Cardiol* 1987;59:256

McCraty R, Atkinson M, Tiller WA. New electrophysiological correlates associated with intentional heart focus. *Subtle Energies* 1995;4:251-268

Ori Z, Monir G, Weiss J, et al. Heart rate variability: *Ambulatory Electrocardiograph* 1992;10:499-537

Pomeranz B, Macaulay JB, Caudill MA. Assessment of autonomic functions in humans by heart rate spectral analysis. *Am J Physiol* 1985;248:H151-H158

Stroufe LA. Effects of depth and rate of breathing on heart rate and heart rate variability. *Psychophysiology* 1971;8:648

Yeragani VK, Pohl R, Berger R, et al. Decreased HRV in panic disorder patients: a study of power-spectral analysis of heart rate. *Psychiatry Res* 1993;46:89-93

Striated Muscle Anatomy and Function Related to Cranial Osteopathy

Hack GD, Koritzer RT, Robinson WL, Greenman PE. Anatomic relation between the rectus capitus posterior minor muscle and the dura mater. *Spine* 1995; 20(23)L 2484-2488.

Hoyt WH, Hadley, et al. Osteopathic manipulation in the treatment of muscle contraction headache. *J Am Osteopath Assoc* 1979;78:322-325.

Hoyte DAN, Enlow DH. Wolff's law and the problem of muscle attachment on resorptive surfaces of bone. *Am J Phys Anthropol* 1966;24:205-214.

Mitchell FL Jr, Mitchell PKG. *The muscle energy manual, Volume One: Concepts and mechanisms, the musculoskeletal screen, cervical region evaluation and treatment* (1995); *Volume Two: Evaluation and treatment of the thoracic spine, lumbar spine, and rib cage* (1998); *Volume Three* (est.1999 pub). East Lansing: MET Press.

Ramfjord SP. Bruxism, a clinical and electromyographic study. *J Amer Dent Assoc* 1961;62:21-44.

Washburn SL. The relation of the temporal muscle to the form of the skull. *Anat Rec* 1947; 99:239-248.

Bound Volumes Related to Cranial Osteopathy

Bertelsen TI. *The premature synostosis of the cranial sutures*. Copenhagen: Ejnar Munksgaard; 1958.

Bowsher D. *Cerebrospinal fluid dynamics in health and disease*. Charles C. Thomas, Springfield;1960.

Drinker CK, Yoffey JM. *Lymphatics, lymph and lymphoid tissue.* Harvard University Press, Cambridge; 1941.

Feely RA. *Clinical Cranial Osteopathy*. Indianapolis, IN: The Cranial Academy; 1988.

Gray's anatomy, edited by Williams PL, Warwick R. Philadelphia, PA: Sanders; 1980.

Hruby RJ. *Craniosacral osteopathic technique: A manual*. Second Ed. 4061 Shoals Drive, Okemos, MI 48864. Institute of Osteopathic Studies; 1996.

Kimberley PE. *An outline of osteopathy in the cranial field*. 1980 Kirksville, Missouri, 1998 The Cranial Academy, Indianapolis, Indiana (rev ed).

Liem T. *Kraniosackrale osteopathie: Ein prakti;sches lehrbuch*. Hipprokrates; 1998.

Lippincott RC, Lippincott HA. *A manual of cranial technique*. Academy of Applied Osteopathy; 1948.

Magoun HI Sr. *Glossary of terms relating to osteopathy in the cranial field*. Sutherland Cranial Teaching Foundation; 1971.

Magoun HI Sr. *Osteopathy in the Cranial Field*;(1951, 1st edn; 1976, 3rd edn). Kirksville, MO: Journal Printing Company; 1976.

Moskolenko YE. Ed. *Biiophysical aspects of cerebral circulation*. Pergamon Press, Oxford; 1980.

Retzlaff EW. Structural and functional concepts of craniosacral mechanisms. In: Philip E. Greenman (ed) *Concepts and mechanisms of neuromuscular functions*. Springer-Verlag, Berlin Heidelberg New York, pp 111-128. 1980.

Retzlaff EW, Mitchell FL Jr, Eds. *The Cranium and Its Sutures*. Berlin, Heidelberg, New York. Springer-Verlag. 1987

Salinas C. *Craniofacial anomalies: new perspectives*. Liss, New York, pp 1-172. 1982.

Still AT. *Philosophy of osteopathy*. Journal Printing Company. Kirksville, MO; 1899.

Sutherland AS, Wales AL. *Contributions of thought: collected writings of William Garner Sutherland, DO, DSc(Hon.)* Sutherland Cranial Teaching Foundation; 1967.

Sutherland WG. *The Cranial Bowl*. Published by the author. Mankato, Minnesota; 1939. (Available through The Cranial Academy).

Sutherland WG. *Teachings in the Science of Osteopathy*. Edited by Anne L. Wales, DO, Sutherland Cranial Teaching Foundation; 1990.

Truhlar RE (ed). Doctor AT Still in the living: his concepts and principles of health and disease. Privately published by Robert E Truhlar, 31437 Shaker Boulevard, Chagrin Falls, Ohio. 1950.

Tucker EE, Wilson PT. *The theory of osteopathy*. Journal Printing Company, Kirksville, MO; 1936.

Upledger JE. *Craniaosacral therapy II: Beyond the dura*. Eastland Press, Seattle; 1987.

Upledger JE, Vredevoogd JD. *Craniosacral therapy*. Eastland Press, Chicago; 1983.

Wales AL, Sutherland AS. Eds. *Contributions of thought: The collected writings of William Garner Sutherland, DO*. The Sutherland Cranial Teaching Foundation. Rudra Press, Portland, Oregon; 1998.

Fetal and Infant Stimulation and Development

General Development

Berntson GG, Cacioppo JT, Quigley KS. Autonomic determinism: the modes of autonomic control, the doctrine of autonomic space, and the laws of autonomic constraint. *Psychological Review* 1991;98:459-487

Cohen LB, Salapatak P. Infant perception: from sensation to cognition — Vol I: *Basic Visual Processes*, and Vol. II: *Perception of Space, speech, and sound*, (Academic Press, London, 1975): 1-771.

Connolly KJ, Prechtl HR. Maturation and Development: Biological and Psychological Perspectives. Clinics in Developmental Medicine 77/78, *Developmental Psychobiology* 1982 15(3): 275-277.

Cornell EH, Gottfried AW. Intervention with premature infants, *Child Development* 1976;47:32-39

Emde RN. Changing Models of infancy and the Nature of Early Development: Remodeling the Foundation, *J. of the Am. Psychoanalytic Assoc.*, 1981 Vol. 29, No. 1

Friedman S, Sigman M. *Preterm birth and psychological development*, Academic Press, NY, NY 1981.

Greenberg D, O'Donnell W. Infancy and the optimal level of stimulation. *Child Development* 1972;43:639-645..

Hofer NA. The Roots of Human Behavior: An Introduction to the Psychobiology of Early Development., *Developmental Psychobiology* 1982 15(1):89-91.

Humphrey T. Function of the nervous sytem during prenatal life. *Physiology of the Perinatal Period*. U Stave ed. Appleton-Century-Crofts, New York;1970

Klaus MH, Fanaroff AA. Bach, Beethoven, or Rock-and How Much? T. *Journal of Pediatrics* 1976; Feb: 300

Lamb NE. Paternal Influences on Early Socio-Emotional Development, *J. Child Psychol. Psychiat.*, 1982 Vol. 23, No. 2:185-190.

Leib SA, et al. Effects of early intervention and stimulation on the preterm infant. *Ped.* 1980;Vol. 66, July :83-90.

Levine S. Stimulation in infancy. *Scientific American* 1960;Vol. 202:81-86.

Lewis AM, Baryels B, et al. State as a determinant of infants' heart rate response to stimulation *Science* 1967;155:486-488.

Lipsitt IW, Rovee-Collier CK. Advances in Infancy Research, Volume 1. Ablex Publishing, Norwood NJ. 1982

Marshall N. The Brain: A Chilling Effect. *Psychology Today*, 1982;Feb:92.

Myers BJ. Early Intervention Using Brazelton Training with Middle-Class Mothers and Fathers. *Child Development* 1982 53:462-471.

Pines M. Baby, You're Incredible. *Psychology Today* (February 1982): 48-53.

Pines M. A head start in the nursery. *Psych. Today*, Sept. 1979 :56-68

Pines M. Infant Stim. *Psychology Today* (June 1982):48-54.

Pines M. Superkids. *Psych. Today*, Jan. 1979:53-63.

Porges SW. Vagal tone: A physiological marker of stress vulnerability. *Pedatrics* 1992;90:498-504

Quinn S. Your Baby's Smarter Than You Believe," *Families* (May 1982):24-28.

Restak RN. Newborn Knowledge. *Science* 82 (January-February):58-65.

Riesen A. Stimulation as a requirement for growth and function in behavioral development. *Functions of Varied Exerience* Dorsey Press, Homewood, Ill., 1961 :57-80.

Rinn WE. The neurophysiology of facial expression: a review of the neurological and psychological mechanisms for producing facial expression. *Psychological Bulletin* 1984;95:52-57

Rutter M. The long-term effects of early experience Develop. *Med. Child Neurol.*1980:800-815.

Sawin DB, Parke, RD. Fathers' affectionate stimulation and caregiving behaviors with newborn infants. *The Family Coordinator* 1979;Vol. 28, No. 4: 509.

Segal J, Yahroes H. Bringing up mother," *Psych Today* Nov. 1978:90-96

.Senn MJ. Early childhood education:for what goals? Children 1969;16 (Jan.-Feb):8-13.

Soboloff HR. Early intervention- fact or fiction? *Develop. Med. Child Neurol.* 1981; 23:261-266.

Vuori L, et al. Food supplementation of pregnant women at risk of malnutrition and their newborns' responsiveness to stimulation. *Develop. Med. Child Neurol.* 1980;22:61-71

Yarrow LJ. Rubenstein JL, et al. Dimensions of early stimulation and their differential effects on infant development. *Merrill-Palmer Quarterly* 1972;18:205-218.

Brain Development

Arbib MA. Visuomotor coordination: from neural nets to schema theory. *Cognition and Brain Theory* 1981;4:23-39.

Brandt I. Brain growth, fetal malnutrition, and clinical consequences. *J. of Perinatal Medicine* 1981;1:3-26

Brown S. Sex differences in the brain. *Childbirth Educator* 1982; Spring:27-30.

Carter S, Greenough W. Sending the right sex messages. *Psychology Today* Sept. 1979: 112

Connolly KJ, Precht HR eds. *Maturation and development: biological and psychological perspectives. clinics in developmental medicine*, Spastics International Medical Pulbications, Suffolk, England;1981, p. 1-315.

Coursin DB Nutrition and brain development in infants. *Merrill-Palmer Quarterly*, 1972; 18(2):177-202.

Dobbing J. Human brain development and its vulnerability. *Biologic and Clinical Aspects of Brain Development*, Mead Johnson Symposium on Perinatal and Developmental Medicine No. 6 (December 8-11,1974).

Dobbing J, Sands J. The quantitative growth and development of the human brain. *Arch Dis Child* 1973;48:757-767.

Dobbing J, Sands J. Timing of neuroblast multiplication in developing human brain. *Nature*1970;226:.639-640.

Fisch RO, Bilek MK, Horrobin JM, Chang PN. Children with superior intelligence at 7 years of age: a prospective study of the influence of perinatal medical, and socioeconomic factors. *American U. Diseases of Children* 1976;130(5): 481-487.

Goleman D. Special abilities of the sexes: do they begin in the brain? *Psych. Today*, Nov. 1978, :48-54.

Hakim AM, Moss G, Scuderi D. The p entose phosphate pathway in brain during development," *Biol. Neonate* 1980 ;37:15-21.

Hunt N. Male/female brains. *Self* (March 1982):57-58.

Hobbs SH. *Malnutrition, environment and behavior: new perspectives*, Cornell Univ Press, Ithaca, New York 1979.

MacLean PD. *The triune brain in evolution*. Plenum press, New York; 1990

Marshall MW. Heredity and nutrition. *The Science Teacher* 1970;37:26

Marshall NK. A chilling effect. *Psychology Today* (February 1982): 92.

Martinez JA. New publications in language, mind, and brain. *Devel. Med. Child Neurol.* 1981;23:97-100.

Marx JL. The two sides of the brain. *Science* 1983;220:488-490

Narawong D, Hecox K. Sensory evoked potentials in neonates. Perinatology-Neonatology 1982; 6(3):33-42

Purpura DP. Dendritic differentiation in human cerebral cortex: normal and aberrant developmental patterns. *Advances in Neurology* 1975;12:91-134.

Reinis S, Goldman JM. *The development of the brain. biological and functional perspectives* C.C. Thomas, Springfield, Ill; 1980.

Robinson R. Equal recovery in child and adult brain? *Dev. Med. Child Neurol.* 1981; 23:379-383.

Rodier PM. Chronology of neuron development: animal studies and their clinical implications. *Develop. Med. Child Neurol.* 1980:525-545.

Sidman RK, Rakic P. Neuronal migration, with special reference to developing human brain: a review. *Brain Research* 1975;62:1-35

Sternberg RJ, Davidso, JE. The mind of the puzzler. *Psychology Today* (June 1982):37-44.

Tanaka H., et al. Experimental studies on male alcoholism on fetal development. *Brain Dev.* (1982): 1-6.

Wigglesworth JS. Brain development and the structural basis of perinatal brain damage. *Perinatal Brain Insult*, Mead-Johnson Symposium on Perinatal and Developmental Medicine, No. 17, Marco Island, Dec. 7-11, 1980.

Reinis S, Goldman JM. *The development of the brain, biological and functional perspectives*. Springfield, ILL.: C. C. Thomas (1980).

Wyden B. Growth:45 crucial months. *Life* (December 17, 1971): 63-64.

Wynn M, Wynn A The importance of maternal nutrition in the weeks before and after conception. *Birth* 1982;9:1

Zamenhof S, Van Marthens E. Distribution of nutrients between fetal brain and body during rat development. *Biol. Neonate* 1982; 41: 63-73

Lateralization in Infants

Buchsbaum N. Tuning in on hemispheric dialogue. *Psych. Today*, Jan. 1979. p.100.

Dawson G. Cerebral lateralization in individuals diagnosed as autistic in early childhood. *Brain and Language* 1982;15:353-368.

Dean RS. Personality and lateral preference patterns in children. *Clinical Neuropsychology*, Vol. III, No. 4.

Fox N, Lewis M. Motor asymmetries in preterm infants: effects of prematurity and illness. *Developmental Psychobiology* 1982;15(1):19-23.

Lewkowicz ., Turkewitz, G. Influence of hemispheric specialization in sensory processing on reaching in infants: age and gender related effects. *Developmental Psychology*, 1982;18(2):301-308.

Ross ED, Homan RW, Buck R. Differectial hemispheric lateralization of primary and social emotions. *Neuropsychiatry, Neuropsychology, and Behav. Neurology* 1994;7:1-19

Taylor HG, Heilman KM. Monaural recall and the right-ear advantage. *Brain and Language* 1982;15:334-339.

Cognitive Development

Cline V. How to raise your child's I.Q. *Families*, Feb. 1982:23-28.

Cline V. *How to make your child a winner*, (N.Y.:Walker and Co., 1980).

Clinton M. Baby is smarter than you think. *Families*, May 1982.

Eastman C. How to smarten up your baby *Self*, March 1982, p. 61.

Graves P. The functioning fetus. *The course of life: psychoanalytic contributions toward understanding personality development. vol. 1: infancy and early childhood* S. Greenspan & G. Pollock, eds, National Institute of Mental Health, 1980, p. 236

Greenough W, Volkman F. Rearing complexities affect branching of dendrites in rats. *Science* 1972;176:1445-1447.

Gutalius M, Kirsch A, et al. Promising results from a cognitive stimulation program in infancy. Clinical Pediatrics 1972; 12:585-893

Horowitz F, et al. The effectiveness of environmental intervention programs. *Review of Child Developmental Research* 1973;3:331-402

Jensen A. How much can we boost IQ and scholastic achievement? *Harvard Educ. Review* 168;39:1-14.

Kagan J. Do infants think? *ScientificAmerican* 1972;226:74-82.

Marquis P. Cognitive stimulation. *American Journal Diseases of Children* 1976;130:410-415.

Meyer C. Homework in the crib. *McCalls* 1972;99:55

Pines M., A child's mind is shaped before age 2. *Life* Dec. 17, 1971, p. 68-88.

Restak R. Newborn knowledge. *Science* 1982;82:59-65.

Rosenzweig M, Bennett E, et al. Brain changes in response to experience. *Sci American* 1972;226:22-29.

Scott J. Critical periods in behavioral development. *Science* 1962;138:949-958.

Steinberg RJ. Who's intelligent? *Psychology Today*, April 1982, 30-40.

Infant Intelligence

Berbaum ML, MarkusGB, Zajonc RB. A closer look at Galbraith's 'Closer Look'. *Developmental Psychology* 1982;18(2):174-180.

Cline VB. How to raise your child's I.Q. *Families* (February 1982): 23-28.

Flavell JH. On cognitive development. *Child Development* 1982 53: 1-10.

Galbraith RC. Sibling spacing and intellectual development: a closer look at the confluence model. *Developmental Psychology*, 1982;18(2):151-173.

Kopp CB, Vaughn BE. Sustained attention during exploratory manipulation as a predictor of cognitive competence in preterm infants. *Child Development* 1982:53: 174-182.

Pines M. The I.Q.'s connected to the heartbeat," *Science* 1982:82:70-71.

Restak R. Islands of genius. *Science* 1982:82:62-67.

Ruddy MG, Bornstein MH. Cognitive correlates of infant attention and maternal stimulation over the first year of life, *Child Development* 1982;53:183-188.

Rice B. Brave new world of intelligence testing. *Psych. Today*, Sept. 1979, p. 27-41

Sternberg RJ. Stalking the IQ quark. *Psych. Today*, Sept. 1979 p. 42-54

Sternberg RJ. Who's intelligent? *Psychology Today* (April 1982): 30-40.

Sullivan, MW. Reactivation: priming forgotten memories in human infants. *Child Development* 1982;53:516-523.

Zigler E, Abelson WD, Trickett PK, Seitz V. Is an intervention program necessary in order to improve economically disadvantaged children's IQ scores? *Child Development* 1982:53 340-348.

Language Development

Ambrose JA. The development of the smiling response in early infancy. in B.M. Foss (Ed.) *Determinants of Infant Behavior, Vol. 1* N.Y. Wiley and Sons, 961.

Bishop DVM. Plasticity and specificity of language localization in the developing brain. *Develop. Med. Child Neurol.* 1981;23:251-255.

Cadden V. The miracle of the smiling face. *Working Mother* (April 1982)

Eimas PD, et al. Speech perception in infants *Science* 1971;171:303-306.

Haugan G, McIntire R. Comparisons of vocal imitation, tactile stimulation, and food as reinforcers for infants' vocalizations. *Developmental Psychology* 1972;6:201-209..

Gardner H., Do babies sing a universal song? *Psychology Today* (December 1981): 70-76.

Leventhal, SA, Lipsitt LP. Adaptation, pitch discrimination, and sound localization in the neonate. Child Development 1954;33:759-767.

Lewis MM. *Language, thought and personality in infancy*,:C. Harrapt, London 1963.

Ling D, Ling A. Communication development in the first three years of life. *J. of Speech and Hearing Research* 1974;17:146-159

Martin GB, Clark RD. Distress crying in neonates: species and peer specificity Developmental Psychology 1982;18(1):3-9.

Morse PA. The discrimination of speech and nonspeech stimuli in early infancy. *J. Experimental Child Psychology* 1972;14:477-492.

Olson DR. *The social foundations of lanauage and thought: essays in honor of Jerome S. Bruner.* Norton, New York; 1980

Oviatt SL. Inferring what words mean: infants' comprehension of common object names. *Child Development* 1982;53:274-277.

Petersen GA, Sherrod KB. Relationship of maternal language to language development and language delay of children. *American Journal of Mental Deficiency* 1982;86(4):391-398.

Roe KV, McClure A, Roe A. Vocal interaction at 3 months and cognitive skills at 12 years. Developmental Psychology 1982;18(1):15-16.

Rosenthal MK. Vocal dialogues in the neonatal period. Developmental Psychology, 1982;18(1):17-21.

Trehub S. Infants' sensitivity to vowel and tonal contrasts *Developmental Psychology* 1973;9:91-96.

Prenatal Stimulation

Bradley RM, Mistretta CM. Fetal sensory receptors.*Psychological Review* 1975;55(3):352-382.

Cook RO, Konishi T, Salt AN, Hamm CW, Lebetkin EH., Koo JT. Brainstem-evoked rtsponses of guinea pigs exposed to high noise levels in utero. *Developmental Psychobiology* 1982;15:95-104.

Lumley J. The image of the fetus in the first trimester. *Birth and the Family Journal* 1980;7(1):5-14.

Oehler S. Sensory processing abilities of the premature infant *J. Calif. Perinatal Assoc.* 1983;3(1):55-63.

Okamoto Y, Kirikae T. Electroencephalographic studies of brains of fetus and premature children. *J.Jap. Ob-Gyn Soc* 1951;3:461

Verny T. *The secret life of the unborn child.* Simon & Schuster, N.Y. 1981

Salk L. The heartbeat rhythm as a prenatal stimulus: experiments, observations, and thoughts. *Amer. Orthopsych. Assoc. Meeting*, N.Y., March 1965.

Visual Stimulation

Apostolakis E, Cha C. Visual preferences of preterm and term neonates. *J. California Perinatal Assoc*, 1982;11(3):61-64.

Bloom K. Eye contact as a setting event for infant learning. J. Experimental Child Psychology 1974;17:250-263.

Bower T. The visual world of the infant. *Scientific American* 1966;215:80-92.

Bushnell IWR. Discrimination of faces by young infants. *J. of Experimental Child Psychology* 1982;33:298-308.

Butterworth G, Jarrett N, Hicks L. Spatiotemporal identity in infancy: perceptual competence or conceptual deficit? *Developmental Psychology* 1982;18(3):435-449.

Cadden V. The miracle of the smiling face. *Working Mother*, April 1982: 68-114.

Cohen L. The effect of stimulus complexity on infant visual attention & habituation. *Child Development* 1975;46:611-617.

Dubowitz LMS, Dubowitz V, Morante A., Verghote M. Visual function in the preeterm and fullterm newborn infant. *Develop. Med. Child Neurol.* 1980: 465-475.

Fagan J. Infant color perception *Science* 1974;183:973-975.

Fantz RL. Pattern vision in young infants. *Psychological Record* 1958;8:43-49.

Fantz RL. Maturation of pattern vision in infants during the first six months. *J. Comparative and Physiological Psychology* 1962;55: 907-917.

Hainline L, Lemerise E. Infants' scanning of geometric forms varying in size. *Journal of Experimental Child Psychology* 1982;33:235-256.

Haith MM. The response of the human newborn to visual movement. *J Exp Child Psychiat* 1966;3: 235243.

Hellman H. Guiding light. *Psychology Today* April   1982: 22-26.

Hershenson J. Visual Discrimination in the Human Newborn. J. Comp & Physiological Psychology 1964;58: 270-276.

Hofsten C. Eye-hand coordination in the newborn. *Developmental Psychology* 1982;18(3):450-461.

Hunter PJL. Babies Eyes. *New Health Visit Community Nurse* 1977;13:14-17.

Korner A, Grobstein, R. Visual alertness as related to soothing in neonates: implications for maternal stimulation and early deprivation. Child Development 1966;42:867-876.

Krantz DH, Human color vision, *Contemporary Psychology* 1982;17(2): 88-91.

Leehey S, Moskoxita A. Orientational anistropy in infant vision *Science* 1975;190: 900-902.

Lewis M. Infants' responses to facial stimuli during the first year of life. *Devel Psycholog* 1969;1(2)

Maurer D, Maurer C. Newborn babies see better than you think. *Psychology Today* (Oct. 1976): 85-88.

Melhuish EC. Visual attention to mother's and stranger's faces and facial contrast in 1-month-old infants. *Developmental Psychology*, 1982;18(2):229-231.

Mellor DH, Fielder AR. Dissociated visual development: electradiagnostic studies in infants who are 'slow to see'. *Develop.Med. Child Neurol.* 1980;22:327-335.

Miranda SB. Visual abilities and pattern preferences of premature infants and fullterm neonates. *J. Experimental Child Psychology* 1970;10:189-203.

Mitchell DE. *Neuralbiology of vision*, New York, Plenum Press 1979.

Molfese-Hones VL. Individual differences in neonatal preference for planometric and stereometric patterns. *Child Development* 1972;43:1289-1296.

Rubenstein J. Maternal attentiveness and subsequent exploratory behavior in the human infant. *Child Development* 1967;38:1089-1099.

Ruff HA. Effect of object movement on infant's detection of object structure. *Developmental Psychology* 1982;18(3):462-472.

Ruff H, Birch H. Infant visual fixation: the effec.t of concentricity and curvilinearity and number of directions,. *J. Experinental Child Psychology* 1974;18:460-473.

Sherick I, et al. Some comments on the significance and development of midline behaviour during infancy. *Child Psych. Human Dev.* 1976;6:170-183.

Shodell M The curative light *Science* 82 (April):47-51.

Slater AM, Findlay J. Binocular fixation in the newborn baby. *J. Experimental Child Psychiatry* 1975;20:248-273.

Thomas H. Visual fixation responses to infants to stimuli of varying complexity. *Child Devel.* 1965:35: 629-638.

Auditory Stimulation

Akaan-Penttilia E. Middle ear mucosa in newborn infants. *Acia Otolaryrngol* 1982;83:251-259.

Bernard J, Sontag LW. Fetal reactivity to tonal stimulation: a preliminary report. *J. Genet. Psych.* 1947;70:205.

Bundy RS, Colombo J, Singer J. Pitch perception inyoung infants. *Developmental Psychology* 1982;18(1):10-14.

Canter R. Too loud for her, too soft for him. *Psychology Today*, April 1980, 19-20.

Cook RO, Konishi T, Salt AN, Hamm CW, Lebetkin EH, Koo J. Brainstem-evoked responses of guinea pigs exposed to high noise levels in utero. Developmental Psychobiology 1982;15(2):95-104.

DeCasper AJ, Sigafoos AD. The intrauterine heartbeat as a potent reinforcer for newborns. *Infant Behav. Dev.* 1983;6:19-25.

Dunkle T. The sound of silence *Science* 1982;82, 30-33.

Dwornicka C, et al. Attempt at determining fetal reaction to acoustic stimulation. *Acta Otolaryng.* (Stockholm)1964;57:571.

Forbes HS, Forbes NB. Fetal sense reactions: hearing. *J. Comp. Psychology* 1927;7:353

Francis M. What music can do for your baby. *American Baby* August 1973.

Gardner H. Do babies sing a universal song? *Psychology Today*, Dec. 1981, 70-76.

Gardner H. The music of the hemispheres. *Psychology Today* June 1982:91-92.

Gelman, SR, Woods S, Spellacy WM, Abrams RM. Fetal movements in response to sound stimulation. *A. J. Ob, Gyn.* 1982;143(4):484-485.

Graham FK, Clifton RK, Hatton HM. Habituation of heart rate response to repeated auditory stimulation during the first five days of life. *Child Development* 1968;39(1):35-52.

Johanson B, Wedenberg E, Westin B. Measurement of tone response by the human fetus: a preliminary report. *Acta Otolaryng* (Stockholm) 1964;57:188

Katz V. Relationship between auditory stimulation and the developmental behaviour of the premature infant. *Nursing Research Conference* 1971;7:103-117

Lathom WB. Survey of current functions of a music therapist. *Journal of Music Therapy* 1982;19(1):2-27.

Morse PA, Eilers ER, GavinWJ. The perception of the sound of silence in early infancy. *Child Development* 1982;53:189-195.

Murooka H, Koie Y, Suda N. Analyse des Sons Entra Uterus et Leurs Effect Tranquillisants sur Le Nouveau-Ne. *J. Gynec. Obstet. Biol. Reprod.* 1976;5:367-376.

Murooka H. *Lullaby from the Womb* Capitol Records.

Murphy KP, Smyth CN. Response of fetus to auditory stimulation. *Lancet* 1962;1:972.

Palmquist H. The effect of heartbeat sound stimulation on the weight Development of newborn infants. *Child Dev* 1975;46:292-295.

Pieper A., Sinnesempfindungen des Kindes vor Seiner Geburt *MSCHR. Kinderheilk* 1924;29:236

Riese M. Hypersensitivity to auditory stimulation during administration of the neonatal neurobehavioral assessment scale. *Developmental Medicine and Child Neurology* 1980;22:404-405.

Salk L. The role of the heartbeat in the relations between mother and infant. *Scientific American* 1973;220: 24-29.

Salk L. The effects of the normal heartbeat sound on the behavior of the newborn infant; implications for mental health. *World Mental Health* 1960;4:168-175.

Salk L. The importance of the heartbeat rhythm to human nature: theoretical, clinical, and experimental observations. *Proceedings of the Third World Congress of Psychiatry*, Univ. Toronto Press, Totonto; 1961.

Salk L. Mother's heartbeat as an imprinting stimulus. *Transaction of the New York Academy of Sciences* Ser. 2, Vol. 24 (1962):753-763.

Salk L. The heartbeat rhythm as a prenatal stimulus: experiments, observations, and thoughts. *American Orthopsychiatry Association Meeting*, New York, March 1965.

Smyth CN, Bench RJ. Fetal response to audiogenic stimulation as an indication of neurological function. *Digest 7th International Conf. Med. Biol. Engineer* 1967, p. 137.

Sontag LW, Wallace RF. The movement response of the human fetus to sound stimuli. *Child Dev.* 1935;6:253-258.

Specter GA, Cowen EL. A pilot study in stimulation of culturally deprived infants. *Child Psychiatry and Human Development* 1971;1:168-177.

Voldrich L. Ulehlova L. Correlation of the development of acoustic trauma to the intensity and time of acoustic overstimulation. *Hearing Research* 1982;6:1-6.

Wedenberg E. Prenatal Tests of Hearing. *Acta Otolarnyngology Suppl.* 1965;27: 205-211

Weiland JH. Heartbeat rhythm and maternal behavior. *J. of the American Academy of Child Psychiatry* 1964;3:161-164.

Wennberg RP, Ahlfors CE, Bickers R, McMurtry CA, Shetter JL. Abnormal auditory brainstem response in a newborn infant with hyperbilirubinemia: improvement with exchange transfusion. *The Journal of Pediatrics* (April 1982).

Vestibular Stimulation

Ayres AJ, et al. Hyperresponsivity to touch and vestlbular stimulation as a predictor of and response to sensory integration procedures by autistic children. *AJOT* 1980;34:375-381.

Bairstow PJ, Laszlo JI. Kinaesthetic sensitivity to passive movements and its relationship to motor development and motor control. *Develop. Med. Child Neurol* 1981;23:506-616.

Caffey J. The whiplash shaken infant syndrome: manual shaking by the extremities with whiplash-induced intracranial and ontraocular bleedings, linked with Residual permanent brain damage and mental retardation. *Pediatrics*, 1974;54(4):396-403

Couper JL. Dance therapy effects on motor performance of children with learning disabilities. *Phys. Ther.* 1981;61:23-26.

Espenschade AS, Eckert HM, Merrill CE. Motor development. *Am. Jo. of Mental Deficiency*, 1981;86(2)

Friedman DG, et al. Effects of kinesthetic stimulation on weight gain and on smiling in premature infants. *annual meeting of American Orthopsychiatric Association*, San Francisco, April 15, 1969.

Gellhorn E. Motion and emotion: the role of proprioception in the physiology and pathology of emotions. *Psychological Review* 1964;71:457-472

Kantner RM, Kantner B, Clark DL. Vestibular stimulation effect on language development in mentally retarded children. *The American Journal of Occupational Therapy*, 1982;36(1):36-41

Kavanagh CA, Banco L. The infant walker. *Am. J. Dis. Child.* 1982;136(3):205-206.

Kramer LJ, Pierpont ME. Rocking waterbeds and auditory stimulation to enhance growth of preterm infants. *J. Ped.* 1976;88:297-299.Hohlstein RR. The development of prehension in normal infants. *The American Journal of Occupational Therapy*, 1982;36(3):170-176.

Laszlo J I, Bairstow PJ. The measurement of kinaesthetic sensitivity in children and adults. *Develop. Med. Child Neurol* 1980;22:454-464.

Magrun W, et al. Effects of vestubular stimulation on spontaneous use of verbal language in developmentally delayed children. *AJOT* 1981;35:101-104.

Parber DE. The vestibular apparatus. *Scientific American* 1980;243:118-121.

Porter L. The role of activity in growth and development. *Phillipine J. of Nursing* 1971;40:91-94.

Rausch CB. Effects of tactile and kinesthetic stimulation on premature infants. *JOGN Nursing* 1981;10(1):34-40.

Sellick KJ, Over R. Effects of vestibular stimulation on motor development of cerebral-palsied children. *Develop. Med. Child Neurol* 1980;22:476-483.

Weeks ZR. Effects of vestibular system on human development overview of functions and effects of stimulation. *AJOT* 1979;33:376-381.

Weeks ZR. Effects of vestibular system on mentally retarded, emotionally disturbed and learning disabled individuals, part 2. *AJOT*, 1979;33:450-457.

Motor Development and Stimulation

Ainsworth M. *Infancy in Uganda: infant care and the growth of love* Johns Hopkins Press, Baltimore;1967.

Dubowitz V. Postnatal maturation of peripheral nerves in preterm and fullterm infants, Journal of Pediatrics 1971;79:915.

Sertel H, et al. Peripheral nerve maturation in English, West Indian, and Turkish newborn infants. *Developmental Medicine and Child Neurology* 1976;18:493-497.

Super CM. Environmental effects on motor development: the case of 'African infant precocity'. *Developmental Medicine and Child Neurology* 1976;18:561-567

Zelaso PR. Walking in the newborn. *Science* 1972;76:314.

Tactile Stimulation

Bernstein L. The effects of variations in handling upon learning and retention. *J. Comparative and Physiological Psychology* 1957;50:162-167.

Burke D, GRandevia SC, McKeon B, Skuse NP. Interactions between cutaneous an muscle afferent projections to cerebral cortex in man. *Electroencephalography and Clinical Neurophysiology* 1982;53:349-360

Hasselmeyer EG. The premature neonate's responses to handling. *American Nurses' Association* 1964;11:15-24.

Lipsitt LP, Levy N. Electrotactual thresholds in the neonate. *Child Development* 1959;30:547-554.

Older J. Touching and birthing *Aust. NZ J. Obstet Gynecol.* 1983;23(3):161-164.

Powell LF. The effect of extra stimulation and maternal involvement on the development of low birth weight infants and on maternal behavior. *Child Development* 1974;106-113

Rausch CB. Effects of tactile and kinesthetic stimulation on premature infants. *JOGN* 1981;10(1):34-40.

Rice R. Caressing and Cuddling helps a baby grow. *Psychology Today* January 1976:101

Rose SA, Schmidt,K, et al. Cardiac and behavioral responsivity to tactile stimulation in premature and full-term infants. *Developmental Psychology* 1976;12:311-320.

Scarr-Salapatek S, Williams M. A stimulation program for low-birthweight infants. *American Journal of Public Health* 1972;62:662-667.

Smeiglio V. (Ed.) *Newborns and parents: parent infant contact and newborn sensory stimulation.* Lawrence Elbaum Press; 1981

Solkoff N, et al. Effects of handling on the subsequent development of premature infants. *Developmental Psychology* 1969;1:760-765.

Solkoff N, Matuszak D. Tactile stimulation and behavioral development among low-birthweight infants. *Child Psychiatry and Human Development* 1975;6:33-36.

Turkewitz G. A sensory basis for the lateral difference in the newborn's response to somesthetic stimulation. *J. Experimental Child Psychology* 1974;18:304-312.Lamb M. Second thoughts on first touch. *Psychology Today*, April 1982:9-11.

Wilson JM The value of touch in psychotherapy. *Amer. J. Orthopshychiat.* 1982;52(1):65-72

Gustatory Stimulation

Aloe L, Calissano P, Levi-Montalcina R. Effects of oral administration of nerve growth factor and of its antiserum on sympathetic ganglia of neonatal mice. *Developmental Brain Research* 1982;4: 31-34.

Brown JW. Prenatal development of the human nucleus abiguus during the embryonic and early fetal periods. *American J. of Anatomy* 1990;189:267-283

Crook C. Functional aspects of the chemical senses in the newborn period. *Develop. Med. Child Neurol.* 1981;23:247-259.

Hopkins DA. The dorsal motor nucleus of the vagus nerve and the nucleus ambiguus: structure and connections. *Cardiogenic reflexes: Report of an international symposium*, PN Williams ed. Oxford Univ. Press, Oxford; 1987

Nysenbaum AN, Smart JL. Sucking behavior and milk intake of neonates in relation to milk fat content. *Early Human Development* 1982;6:205-213.

Turner J, Schwab ME, Thoenen H. Nerve growth factor stimulates neurite outgrowth from goldfish retinal explants: the influence of a prior lesion. *Developmental Brain Research* 1982; 4:59-66.

Uvnas-Moberg K. Gastrointestinal hormones in mother and infant. *Acta Pediatrica Scand.* 1989;351:88-93

Sleep-Wake Cycles in Infants and Children

Anders TF. Neurophysiological studies of sleep in infants and children. *J. Child Psychol. Psychiat.* 1982;23(1):75-83.

Becker PT, Thoman EV. Intense rapid eye movements during active sleep: an iIndex of neurobehavioral instability. *Developmental Psychobiology* 1982;15(3):203-210.

Carse EA, Wilkinson AR, Whyte PL, Henderson-Smart DJ, Johnson P. Oxygen and carbon dioxide tensions, breathing and heart rate in normal infants during the first six months of life. *J. of Dev. Physiology* Apr. 1981:85-100.

Crowell DH, et al. Daytime sleep stage organization in three-month-old infants. *Electroencephalography and Clinical Neurophysiology* 1982;53:36-47.

Drewett RF. Returning to the suckled breast: A further test of Hall's hypothesis. *Early Human Development* 1982;6:161-163.

Ellingson RJ, Peters JF, Nelson B. Respiratory pauses and apnea during daytime sleep in normal infants during the first year of life: longitudinal observations. *Electroencephalography and Clinical Neurophysiology* 1982;53:48-59.

Fagioli I, Salzarulo P. Sleep states development in the first year of life assessed through 24 hr recordings. *Early Human Development* 1982;6:215-228.

Hakamada S, et al. Body movements during sleep in full-term newborn infants. *Brain & Devel.* 1982;4(1):51-55.

Hofer MA, Shair H. Control of sleep- wake states in the infant rat by features of the mother-infant relationship *Developmental Psychobiology* 1982;15(3):229-243

Mukhtar AI, Cowan FN, Stothers JK. Cranial blood flow and blood pressure changes during sleep in the human neonate. *Early Human Development* 1982;6:59-64.

Nijhuis JG, et al. Are there behavioural states in the human fetus? *Early Human Dev.* 1982;6:177-195.

Radvanyi-Bouvet MF, Monset-Couchard M, Morel-Kahn F, Vicente G, Dreyfus-Brisac D. Expiratory patterns during sleep in normal full-term and premature Neonates. *Biol. Neonate* 1982;41:74-84.

Wu H, et al. Factors affecting sleep spindle activity during infancy. *Develop. Med. Child Neurol* 1980;22:344-351.

Oxytocin, Behavior and Development

Carter CS. Oxytocin and sexual behaviour. *Neurosci. Biobehav. Rev* 1992;16:131-144

Carter CS, Williams JR, Witt DM, Insel TR. Oxytocin and social bonding. *Ann. N Y Acad. Sci.* 1992:652:201-211

Keverne EB, Kendrick KM. Oxytocin facilitaion of maternal behaviour. *Ann. N Y Acad. Sci.* 1992:83-101

Uvnas-Moberg K, Bruzelius G, Alster P, Lundeberg T. The antiociceptive effect of non-noxious sensory stimulation is partly mediated through oxytogenic mechanisms. *Acta. Physiol. Scand.* 1993;149:199-204

Uvnas-Moberg K. Oxytocin and Behaviour. *Ann Med.* 1993;26:315-317

Uvnas-Mober K. Role of efferent and afferent vagal nerve activity during reproduction: integrating function of oxytocin on metabolism and behaviour. *Psychoneuroendocrinology* 1994;19:687-695

SFIMMS SERIES IN NEUROMUSCULOSKELETAL MEDICINE

AUTHORS: Harry Friedman D.O., Wolfgang Gilliar D.O., Jerel Glassman D.O.

Osteopathic approaches to patient care offer the practitioner a variety of problem-solving and treatment options. Palpatory skill development establishes a basis for diagnostic assessment of neuromusculoskeletal function and its integrative role in maintaining health and overcoming disease. Osteopathic treatment and problem-solving skills apply a holistic approach that considers the therapeutic response of the whole patient. A variety of diagnostic and treatment methods have been developed to maximize outcomes.

This series of Osteopathic manipulative medicine texts presents a comprehensive course of instruction, including theory, palpation, diagnosis, and treatment. The thoughtful student will appreciate the detail and clarity of topic presentation and the sequence of skills development. Quality close-up photographic visuals accurately depict the table sessions using human and anatomic models.

COUNTERSTRAIN APPROACHES IN OSTEOPATHIC MANIPULATIVE MEDICINE

* Basic and intermediate level instructional manual
* Theoretical principles of indirect technique and spontaneous release by positioning
* Diagnostic application of tender point palpation for each body region
* Multiple therapeutic procedures presented for each tender point

MYOFASCIAL AND FASCIAL-LIGAMENTOUS APPROACHES IN OSTEOPATHIC MANIPULATIVE MEDICINE

* Basic and advanced level instructional manual
* Detailed connective tissue anatomy and physiology
* Theoretical principles of myofascial and fascial-ligamentous release
* Diagnostic and treatment approaches for each body region, including a myofascial screening exam
* Release enhancing maneuvers and multiple operator techniques
* Includes approaches of Dr.'s Ward, Chila, Becker, Barral and Sutherland

OSTEOPATHIC MANIPULATIVE MEDICINE APPROACHES TO THE PRIMARY RESPIRATORY MECHANISM

* Basic, intermediate, and advanced level instructional manual
* Anatomic relations and physiologic principles underlying the cranial concept
* Palpation exercises designed to facilitate diagnostic touch throughout the body
* Diagnostic and treatment approaches focus on fluid, membranous (dural), muscular, articular and bony aspects of the cranial mechanism, including a cranial screening exam
* Includes multiple operator techniques and approaches to infants and children

FUNCTIONAL METHODS IN OSTEOPATHIC MANIPULATIVE MEDICINE

* Presents Functional Methods approach developed by William L Johnston DO FAAO
* 2 basic level courses to cover all body regions
* Presents a unique palpation based understanding of the functional relationships between all body regions
* Diagnostic principles based on passive motion testing
* Treatment elegantly applies palpation based findings to restore proper relationships between body regions

email: admin@sfimms.com
www.sfimms.com